CANCER IN TRANSPLANTATION - PREVENTION AND TREATMENT

Transplantation and Clinical Immunology
Symposia Fondation Marcel Mérieux

VOLUME 27

Cancer in Transplantation: Prevention and Treatment

Proceedings of the 27th Conference on Transplantation and Clinical Immunology, 22—24 May 1995

organized by
Fondation Marcel Mérieux and Université Claude Bernard-Lyon I

Edited by

J.L. Touraine
J. Traeger
H. Bétuel
J.M. Dubernard
J.P. Revillard
C. Dupuy

KLUWER ACADEMIC PUBLISHERS

DORDRECHT / BOSTON / LONDON

A C.I.P. Catalogue record for this book is available from the Library of Congress.

ISBN-13: 978-94-010-6563-4 e-ISBN-13: 978-94-009-0175-9
DOI: 10.1007/978-94-009-0175-9

Published by Kluwer Academic Publishers,
P.O. Box 17, 3300 AA Dordrecht, The Netherlands

Kluwer Academic Publishers incorporates
the publishing programs of
D. Reidel, Martinus Nijhoff, Dr W. Junk and MTP Press.

Sold and distributed in the U.S.A. and Canada
by Kluwer Academic Publishers,
101 Philip Drive, Norwell, MA 02061, U.S.A.

In all other countries, sold and distributed
by Kluwer Academic Publishers Group,
P.O. Box 322, 3300 AH Dordrecht, The Netherlands

Printed on acid-free paper

Table of Contents

Contributors

E. ALAMARTINE
Hopital Nord
Avenue Albert Raimond
42277 St Priest en Jarrest
France

A. BAZARBACHI
Hôtel Dieu
Serv. d'Hématologie
1, Place Parvis de Notre Dame
75004 Paris
France

H. BISMUTH
Centre Hépato-biliaire
Hôpital Paul Brousse
14, Av Paul Vaillant Couturier
94800 Villejuif
France

JY. BLAY
Centre Léon Bérard
28, Rue Laënnec
69373 Lyon 8
France

C. BRECHOT
Carcinogenèse Hépatique et
Virologie Moléculaire – INSERM U 370
CHU Necker
156, rue de Vaugirard
75730 Paris 15
France

J. BRISSINCK
East Anglian Blood Transfusion Centre
Long Road
Cambridge CB 2 2PT
UK

D. CANTAROVICH
CHRU Hôtel Dieu
Néphrologie
Place Alexis Ricordeau
BP 1005
44000 Nantes
France

P. COCHAT
Hôpital Edouard Herriot
Pavillon S – Néphrologie
5, place d'Arsonval
69437, Lyon
France

J. DANTAL
CHU Hôtel Dieu
Néphrologie
Place Alexis Ricordeau
BP 1005
44035 Nantes
France

J. DICKMAN
Children's Hospital of Pittsburgh
Dept. of Pathology
3705 Fifth Avenue
PA 15213, Pittsburgh
USA

E. DROUET
Faculté de Pharmacie de Grenoble
Domaine de la Merci
38706 La Tronche
France

J.L. Touraine et al. (eds.), Cancer in Transplantation. Prevention and Treatment, xiii–xv.

A. DURANDY
Hôpital Necker Enfants Malades
INSERM U 429
Pavillon Kirmisson
149, rue de Sèvres
75743 Paris
France

D. EMILIE
Unité INSERM 131
32, rue des Carnets
92140 Clamart
France

S. EUVRARD
Hôpital Edouard Herriot
Dermatologie
Place d'Arsonval
69437 d'Arsonval
69437 Lyon
France

U. FREI
Standort Wedding
Universitätsklinikum Rudolf Virchow
Postfach 65 02 69
13353 Berlin
Allemagne

M. F. GAGNADOUX
Hôpital Necker – Enfants Malades
Néphrologie – Pédiatrie
149, rue de Sèvres
75743 Paris CEDEX 15
France

J.L. GARNIER
Hôpital Edouard Herriot
Pavillon P
5, Place d'Arsonval
69437 Lyon
France

G. KARAM
Hôpital Hôtel Dieu
Clinique Urologique
Place Alexis Ricordeau
44035 Nantes
France

V. LAMARQUE
Laboratoires Sandoz
14, Bd Richelieu
92500 Rueil Malmaison
France

V. LEBLOND
Hôpital Pitié Salpetrière
41, Bd de l'hôpital
75103 Paris
France

N. LEFRANCOIS
Hôpital Edouard Herriot
5, Place d'Arsonval
Pavillon P
69437 Lyon
France

M. MASUCCI
Karolinska Institutet
Box 280
Microbiology and Tumor Biology
Center
S 17177 Stockholm
Sweden

P. MATHEVET
Hôpital Edouard Herriot
5, Place d'Arsonval
Gynécologie Obstétique
69437N Lyon
France

G. OPELZ
Abteilung Transplantations
Immunologie
Institut für Immunologie
Im Neuenheimer Feld 305
69120 Heidelberg
Germany

P. PATERLINI
Carcinogenèse Hépatique et
Virologie Moléculaire – INSERM U 370
CHU Necker
156, rue de Vaugirard
75730 Paris 15
France

I. PENN
Department of Surgery
University of Cincinnati Medical Center
231 Bethesda Avenue
Cincinnati OH 45267–0558
USA

M. RAPHAEL
Service d'Hématologie Biologique
Hôpital d'Avicenne
125, route de Stalingrad
93009 Bobigny
France

D. SAMUEL
Centre Hepato Biliaire
Hôpital Paul Brousse
12, Avenue Paul Vaillant Couturier
94804 Villejuif
FRANCE

A. SERGEANT
Hôpital Necker – Enfants Malades
INSERM U 412
46, Allée d'Italie
69364 Lyon 7
France

T. STEVENSON
Tenovus Research Laboratory
General Hospital
Tremona Road
Southampton SO9 4XY
UK

J. SWINNEN
Loyola University Medical Center
Section of hematology/oncology
Building 54 – 21605 First Avenue
Maywood, Illinois 60153
USA

G. TOUCHARD
Service de Néphrologie-Réanimation
CHU Poitiers
350, Avenue Jacques Coeur – BP 577
86021 Poitiers
France

J.L. TOURAINE
Hôpital Edouard Herriot
Pavillon P
5, Place d'Arsonval
69437 Lyon 3
France

N. VOORZANGER
Centre Léon Bérard
28, Rue Laënnec
69373 Lyon 8
France

A. M. WINGEN
Universitätsklinikum Essen
Hufelandstr. 55
45122 Essen 1
Germany

N. YOSHIMURA
The Second Dept. of Surgery
Kyoto Prefectural University
465 Kajii-cho Hirokoji, Kawaramachi
Kamikyo-ku
602 Kyoto City
Japan

PART ONE

Epidemiology

1. Epidemiology of cancer in transplant Patients*

ISRAEL PENN**

Observations made during the last 25–30 years have shown that organ transplant recipients are prone to develop a variety of cancers, many of which are rare in the general population. In this report we shall review the epidemiology of these malignancies, and emphasize different patterns of neoplasms seen in nonrenal allograft recipients compared with renal transplant patients, and, also, in children compared with adult recipients. This study is based on data collected by the Cincinnati Transplant Tumor Registry (CTTR) [1–4], the only worldwide repository of data on this topic, but the observations of numerous investigators is included. Up to May 1995 the CTTR has data on 8724 cancers that occurred de novo after transplantation in 8191 recipients. The patients include 6821 renal, 772 cardiac, 336 hepatic, 145 bone marrow, 54 pancreatic, 29 combined heart-lung, 29 pulmonary, 4 abdominal organ clusters, and 1 small bowel allograft recipients.

Epidemiology of posttransplant cancers

Overall the incidence of cancer is increased 3 to 4-fold in organ allograft recipients compared with age-matched controls in the general population [5, 6], but the incidence of certain neoplasms is very greatly increased [1–6]. In most studies tumors that are frequently seen in the population at large (carcinomas of the lung, breast, prostate, colon and invasive uterine cervical carcinomas) show no increase and even a decrease among transplant patients [1–5] (Table 1). Only two types of neoplasm, that are common in the general population, are also frequently encountered among transplant patients. Excluding lip cancers, the percentage of non-melanoma skin cancers in the CTTR (31%) is similar to that observed in the general population (37% of all tumors), but the incidence of squamous cell carcinomas (SCCs) is markedly increased (see below). Another neoplasm which comprises 3% of all tumors

* Supported in part by a grant from Department of Veterans Affairs.
** Professor of Surgery.

J.L. Touraine et al. (eds.), Cancer in Transplantation. Prevention and Treatment, 3–15.

Table 1. General population vs CTTR patients (% of all cancers) *(Excluding non-melanoma skin cancer and in situ cervical cancers)*

	Gen Pop[a]	Tx[b]
Carcinoma of prostate	19%	2%
Carcinoma of breast	15%	4%
Carcinomas of lung	14%	8%
Carcinoma of colon/rectum	11%	5%
Carcinomas of bladder	4%	3%
Invasive cancer of uterus (Body and cervix)	4%	2%

[a] Gen Pop = General population.
[b] Tx = Transplant recipients.

Table 2. General population vs CTTR patients (% of all cancers) *(Excluding non-melanoma skin cancer and in situ cervical cancers)*

	Gen Pop[a]	Tx[b]
Lymphomas	6%	24%
Carcinomas of lip	0.2%	7%[c]
Kaposi's sarcoma	Negligible	6%
Carcinomas of vulva/perineum	0.5%	3.5%
Carcinomas of kidney	2%	5%
Hepatobiliary cancers	1.5%	2.4%
Sarcomas (Excluding Kaposi's)	0.5%	1.7%

[a] Gen Pop = General population.
[b] Tx = Transplant recipients.
[c] 48% also had skin cancers.

in the general population is in situ carcinoma of the uterine cervix which makes up 2.5% of malignancies in the CTTR. If non-melanoma skin cancers and in situ cervical carcinomas are excluded, as they are from most cancer statistics, the CTTR findings indicate that transplant patients are prone to develop a variety of neoplasms that are uncommon in the general population (Table 2) [1–5]. These results are consistent with several epidemiologic

Table 3. Time of appearance of malignancies

Type of tumor	Range in months	Average in months	Median in months
Kaposi's sarcoma	1–225.5	21	12
Lymphomas	0.25–305.5	33	12.5
Carcinomas of kidney	1–213.5	54	40
Sarcomas (excluding KS)	2–239.5	68	43.5
Carcinomas of cervix	1.5–250	60	48
Skin cancers	1–313	75	60
Hepatobiliary carcinomas	1–289.5	82	67.5
Carcinomas of vulva/perineum	1.5–285.5	112	109
All tumors	0.25–313	61	46

studies that show 28 to 49-fold increased incidence of non-Hodgkin's lymphomas [5], 29-fold increase in lip carcinomas [7], 400 to 500-fold increase in Kaposi's sarcoma compared with controls of the same ethnic origin [8], 100-fold increased incidence of vulvar and anal carcinomas [7], 20 to 38-fold increased incidence of hepatocellular carcinomas [9], and 4.3-fold increased risk of genitourinary cancers [6] (a rather broad definition which includes carcinomas of the kidney, ureter, bladder, cervix, vulva, and vagina).

The incidence of cancer increases with the length of follow-up after transplantation. The actuarial probability of developing malignancy among patients who received cardiac transplants during childhood is 7% at 1 and 2 years, 12% at 3 years, and 15% at 4 and 5 years [10]. An Australasian study of 6596 recipients of cadaver renal transplants shows that the percent probability of developing cancer 24 years after transplantation is 66% for skin neoplasms, 27% for non-skin malignancies and 72% for any type of tumor [6]. These exceptional figures must be carefully reviewed as most of the malignancies are skin cancers (which are very common in Australia) and the number of 24 year survivors is small. Nevertheless, they stress the necessity to follow transplant patients indefinitely.

Certain patterns of tumor appearance are recognized [1–4]. In contrast with other known oncogenic stimuli in man, which often take 15 to 20 years or more before causing clinical lesions, cancers appear a relatively short time posttransplantation. The CTTR data for the various malignancies is shown in Table 3.

Most common types of malignancy

Cancers of the skin and lips

The most common tumors in the CTTR affect the skin and lips and comprise 36% of all malignancies [1–4]. They appear on sun exposed areas, particularly of the head and neck and upper limbs [1–4, 11]. They occur particularly in light-skinned individuals with blue eyes and blonde or red hair [11]. HLA antigens, which play an important role in host defense against the development of neoplasia, may contribute to the occurrence of skin cancers in some patients. A significantly increased frequency of HLA-B27, and of HLA-DR homozygosity and a significantly decreased frequency of HLA-A11 is noted in Dutch renal transplant recipients with skin cancers [12].

The incidence of skin cancers varies with the amount of sunshine exposure [1–4, 11, 13]. In regions with limited exposure, there is a four to seven fold increase [14, 15], but in areas with abundant sunlight there is an almost 21-fold increase [16] over the already high incidence found in the local population. Almost all the increment is in SCCs (see below). However, exposure to sunshine is not the only etiologic factor. A surprisingly high incidence of SCCs is recorded from areas of low sunlight in Canada, Sweden, and Great Britain and may be related to carcinomatous change in papillomavirus-induced warts, under the influence of immunosuppression, sunlight, and possibly other factors [7, 17–19]. For example, a British study of 291 renal allograft recipients showed that 59% had cutaneous warts and 22% had nonmelanoma skin cancers [19].

The incidence of skin cancers increases with the length of follow-up after transplantation as shown by an Australasian study of 6596 recipients of cadaveric renal transplants who experienced a linear increase in the incidence of skin cancer reaching 66% at 24 years posttransplantation [6]. Similarly, a Dutch study shows a 10% incidence of nonmelanoma skin cancers in renal transplant recipients at 10 years posttransplantation rising to 40% after 20 years [20].

The patterns of skin cancer in transplant patients differ in several way from those seen in the general population [1–4, 6, 11, 12]. Basal cell carcinomas (BCCs) outnumber SCCs in the general population by 5 to 1, but the opposite occurs in transplant recipients in whom SCCs outnumber BCCs by 1.8 to 1. SCC is estimated to occur at a frequency between 40 and 250 times higher than in the general population, BCC ten times higher [20] and malignant melanoma five times more commonly than expected [11]. In the general population SCCs occur mostly in persons in their 60's and 70's but the average age of transplant patients is 30 years younger [21]. In addition, the incidence of multiple skin cancers in the CTTR is remarkably high (42%) and, despite being a worldwide collection, is similar to that seen only in areas of copious sunlight [1–4, 13]. Some patients each have more than 100 skin cancers. Apparently there is a widespread skin abnormality in some patients who have areas of unstable epithelium containing multifocal premalignant and malignant lesions [10].

In the general population most lymph node metastases and deaths from skin cancer are caused by malignant melanoma. In contrast SCCs are much more aggressive in transplant patients than in the general population and account for the majority of lymph node metastases and deaths from skin cancer [1–4, 13]. In the CTTR data base 5.8% of patients with skin cancers have lymph node metastases. Of these 75% are from SCCs and only 17% from melanomas. Similarly 5.1% of patients die of skin cancer, with 60% of deaths being from SCC and only 33% from melanomas [1–4]. Patients with skin cancer are also more likely to develop other more fulminant types of malignancy than are allograft recipients without skin cancer [11].

Non-Hodgkin's lymphomas

Among posttransplant lymphomas Hodgkin's disease and plasmacytoma/myeloma are much less common than in the general population comprising less than 3% and 4% of lymphomas respectively compared with 11% and 18% respectively in the general population [1–4]. Most lymphomas in the CTTR are nonHodgkin's lymphomas (NHL) which comprise 94% of the total. As many lesions straddle the borderland between infection and neoplasia the term posttransplant lymphoproliferative disorder (PTLD) is frequently used to describe Epstein-Barr virus (EBV)-induced lymphoid proliferations [22, 23]. While EBV infection occurs in most NHLs in transplant patients some show no evidence of this virus despite a careful search for it [24]. One author suggests that PTLD encompasses four disease groups (a) uncomplicated posttransplant infectious mononucleosis (b) benign polyclonal polymorphic B-cell hyperplasia (c) early malignant transformation into polyclonal polymorphic B-cell lymphoma and (d) monoclonal polymorphic B-cell lymphoma [25]. The majority of NHL arise from B-lymphocytes but CTTR data indicate that 13% arise from T-lymphocytes, while rare cases are of null cell origin [1–4].

Fifty-three percent involve multiple organs or sites while 47% are confined to a single organ or site [1–4]. Posttransplant NHLs differ from their counterparts in the general population in several ways [1–4].

Whereas extranodal involvement occurs in from 24% to 48% of patients in the general population, it is present in 69% of NHL. Surprisingly, one of the most common extranodal sites is the central nervous system (CNS) which is involved in 22% of cases [1–4, 26]. Ten percent involve the CNS and other organs, a figure similar to the 8–12% of CNS involvement by systemic NHLs in the general population [26]. However, most lesions in transplant patients are located in the brain parenchyma whereas in the general population most involve the leptomeninges, perivascular spaces and nerve roots [26]. The other 12% are limited to the CNS in contrast with a 1–2% incidence of primary

Table 4. Involvement of the allograft by NHL

(1364 patients)	
Renal	155
Hepatic	86
Pulmonary	31
Cardiac	26
Pancreatic	9
Bone Marrow	8
Abdominal cluster organs	3
Total	318 (23%)

CNS involvement by NHL in the general population [26]. In both groups the brain parenchyma is usually involved and meningeal involvement occurs infrequently [26]. In the CTTR series, spinal cord lesions are very unusual. In this regard the lesions resemble CNS lymphomas in the general population in whom the spinal cord is affected in only 0–5% in different series [26].

A remarkable finding in the CTTR data is the frequency of either macroscopic or microscopic allograft involvement which occurs in 23% of patients with NHL (Table 4) [1–4]. In some patients the infiltrate is mistaken for rejection when allograft biopsies are studied microscopically. It is frustrating that 18% of patients with NHL die without treatment, either because the diagnosis is missed, or is made too late for effective therapy to be instituted [1–4]. Following treatment complete remissions are obtained in 40% of patients [1–4].

Kaposi's sarcoma (KS)

KS most frequently occurs in transplant patients who are Arabic, Jewish, black or of Mediterranean ancestry [1–4]. For example, it occurred in 1.6% of 820 Italian renal transplant recipients [27] and was the most common cancer in renal transplant recipients in Saudi Arabia making up 76% of all neoplasms [28].

KS affects males to females in a 3:1 ratio, far less than the 9:1 to 15:1 ratio seen with KS in the general population [1–4]. Transplant-related KS is rare in children [28]. A clinician should suspect KS whenever a transplant patient, particularly one belonging to the ethnic groups described above, presents with reddish blue macules or plaques in the skin or oropharyngeal mucosa, or has apparently infected granulomas that fail to heal [1–4]. If the diagnosis is confirmed, a thorough workup including CT scans of the chest and abdomen and upper and lower gastrointestinal endoscopy, is needed to exclude any internal visceral involvement [1–4].

Sixty percent have nonvisceral KS confined to the skin, or oropharyngolaryngeal mucosa and 40% have visceral disease, affecting mainly the gastrointestinal tract and lungs, but other organs are also affected [1–4]. In patients with nonvisceral disease the lesions are confined to the skin in 98% and the mouth or oropharynx in 2%. Patients with visceral lesions have no skin involvement in 27%, but 13% of them have oral involvement which provides an accessible site for biopsy and diagnosis [1–4]. The outlook of patients with nonvisceral disease is much more favorable than those with visceral disease, as 53% of the former group have complete remissions following treatment compared with only 27% in the latter.

Renal carcinomas

Unlike most other malignancies, which arise as complications of immunosuppressive therapy, many renal carcinomas are related to the underlying kidney disease in renal allograft recipients [1–4, 29], but no explanation is available for the small number of carcinomas that occur in hepatic or cardiac allograft recipients. Most neoplasms in renal recipients arise in their own diseased kidneys although 9% appear in the allografts from 2 to 213.5 (average 59) months after transplantation [29].

In various studies in the general population 5–10% of renal tumors are carcinomas of the pelvis [29] whereas in the CTTR series these account for 14% of tumors. The increase is almost certainly due to the high incidence of analgesic nephropathy among renal allograft recipients, which occurs in 8% of CTTR patients with carcinomas of their native kidneys [29]. This disorder is known to cause carcinomas in various regions of the urinary tract [30]. This is borne out in the CTTR series in which 68% of patients with analgesia-related renal carcinomas have similar cancers elsewhere in the urinary tract [29]. Another predisposing cause of tumors in renal transplant recipients is acquired cystic disease (ACD) of the native kidneys. It occurs in 30–95% of patients receiving long term hemodialysis [31–32], and is complicated by renal adenocarcinoma, which is increased 30–40 fold over its incidence in the general population [33]. With a successfully functioning transplant the ACD tends to regress [31], and presumably the risk of developing renal cell carcinoma also recedes. However, cases of persistence of ACD and development of renal cell carcinoma have been reported in patients with successfully functioning renal allografts [34–36]. The precise incidence of ACD-related carcinomas in renal transplant recipients is not known.

Carcinomas of the vulva and perineum

Included in this group are carcinomas of the vulva, perineum, scrotum, penis, perianal skin or anus. Females outnumber males by 2.6:1 in contrast with most other posttransplant cancers where males outnumber females by more than 2:1 [1–4]. One-third of patients have in situ lesions [37]. A worrying finding is that patients with invasive lesions are much younger (average age 42 years) than their counterparts in the general population, whose average age is usually between 50 and 70 years. Prior to the development of the neoplasm approximately one third of transplant patients had condyloma acuminata ('genital warts'), caused by human papillomavirus [37]. Female patients sometimes have multifocal lesions with neoplastic involvement not only of the vulva and perineum but also the vagina and/or uterine cervix [37].

Carcinomas of the uterus

Cervical carcinomas comprise 11% of posttransplant cancers in women in the CTTR. At least 72% of patients have in situ lesions [1–4]. As mentioned above the percentage that in situ cervical carcinomas comprise of all malignancies is no different from that in the general population. In view of the 14 to 16-fold increased incidence reported in two epidemiologic studies [38, 39] it suggests that many cases are being missed. One therefore recommends that all postadolescent female patients have regular pelvic examinations and cervical smears to detect such lesions and, also, vulvar and perineal carcinomas [1–4].

Hepatobiliary tumors

Most cases in the CTTR are hepatomas [9] and a substantial number of patients have a preceding history of hepatitis B infection [9]. Several recipients with a history of hepatitis C infection are now being reported.

Sarcomas (excluding KS)

Most involve the soft tissues or visceral organs whereas cartilage or bone involvement is uncommon [1–4]. The major types are fibrous histiocytoma (20 patients), leiomyosarcoma (15), fibrosarcoma (12), rhabdomyosarcoma (9), hemangiosarcoma (8), mesothelioma (6) and liposarcoma (5).

Other cancers

In some studies an increased incidence of other malignancies is reported. For example, the Australia and New Zealand Dialysis and Transplant Registry reports 289-fold increased incidence of endocrine cancers, 5.6-fold increase of leukemia, 2.5-fold increase in digestive organ cancers, 2-fold increase in

Table 5. Tumors in non-renal vs renal recipients

	1406 tumors (%)[a]	7318 tumors (%)[b]
Lymphomas	46	12
Skin cancers	23	39
Kaposi's sarcoma	2	4
Carcinomas of cervix	1	4
Ca of vulva/perineum	1	3
Miscellaneous	27	38

[a] In 1370 patients.
[b] In 6821 patients.

respiratory system tumors, and 4.6-fold increase of miscellaneous cancers [6].

Biological behavior of posttransplant neoplasms

Malignancies that occur in organ allograft recipients frequently demonstrate a more aggressive nature than do similar neoplasms in patients who have not undergone transplantation [40].

Tumors in renal versus nonrenal recipients

There are significant differences in tumor incidence in renal compared with nonrenal recipients (Table 5) [1–4, 41]. The striking incidence of lymphomas (46% vs 12%) in nonrenal recipients is most likely related to the intensity of the immunosuppression given to the former group. Severe rejection of a renal transplant may be managed by placing the patient on dialysis and discontinuing immunosuppressive therapy, whereas severe rejection of a cardiac, pulmonary, or hepatic allograft will result in death of the patient unless the immunosuppressive therapy is substantially increased, except in rare instances where one is fortunate enough to obtain a new organ with which to replace the failing allograft.

Many renal recipients have been followed for 10–30 years posttransplantation, whereas the follow-up in nonrenal recipients is generally much shorter. This may account for the higher incidence of late-appearing malignancies of the skin, uterine cervix, vulva and perineum in the renal recipients. The higher incidence of carcinomas of the kidney in renal recipients may reflect the influence of analgesic nephropathy and acquired cystic disease of the kidney in predisposing to renal neoplasms [29].

Table 6. Tumors in pediatric versus adult recipients

Tumor	Pediatric (%)[a]	Adult (%)[b]
Lymphoma	53	16
Skin	19	40
Sarcomas	4	1
Vulva/anus	3	3
Kaposi's sarcoma	3	4
Hepatic	3	2

[a] 430 tumors in 419 patients.
[b] 8294 tumors in 7772 patients.

Cancers in pediatric versus adult recipients

The types of neoplasms seen in pediatric organ allograft recipients (aged 18 years or less) are very different from those observed in the general childhood population and from those seen in adult organ allograft recipients (Table 6) [42].

By far the most common neoplasm observed is NHL. This is surprising as most NHLs occur in adults at a median age of 56 years and are relatively uncommon in children [42]. However children with congenital immunodeficiency disorders are prone to develop cancers, of which the most common (44%) are NHLs [43]. One reason why NHL is more common in immunodeficient pediatric patients is that children have more lymphoid tissues than adults and these become the sites of NHL when exposed to EBV infection or other stimuli [42]. Primary EBV infections are more common in children than in adults and in immunosuppressed patients are more likely to lead to NHL[42]. Even more striking is the high incidence of NHL in pediatric recipients of nonrenal organs [42], in whom they comprised 81% of all tumors.

As regards skin cancers a difference between children and adults is that melanomas make up 14% of skin cancers in the former group compared with 5% in the latter. In the general population malignant melanoma is rare during childhood yet in the CTTR series 6 of 11 melanomas occurred in patients aged 9 to 18.5 (average 12) years at the time of diagnosis of the tumor. Four of the 11 patients (36%) were bone marrow transplant recipients.

Leiomyosarcoma is very unusual in childhood. Surprisingly 4 of 15 tumors in the CTTR occurred in children and in 3 of the cases the lesion involved the allograft, although none of the donors nor any recipients of other organs from these donors had evidence of this malignancy [1–4, 42]. Three young children, two of whom developed smooth muscle tumors after liver transplantation (one of which is included in the CTTR series) and one of whom developed the tumors after combined liver and small bowel transplantation were recently reported [44]. In two patients the liver allograft was involved. Smooth muscle tumors are also seen in AIDS patients, mainly children, with liver involvement in at least 5 cases [45, 46]. Smooth muscle tumors occurring after organ transplantation contain clonal EBV, suggesting that the virus has a role in the development of these malignancies [44].

Among patients who received transplants during childhood carcinomas of the vulva and perineum occurred in 15 when they were between 20 and 39 years of age [42]. It is disturbing to see these malignancies in such young individuals particularly as they are usually seen in elderly individuals [37]. All occurred in renal allograft recipients. Fortunately 8 of the lesions were "in situ" carcinomas and were readily treatable.

For the future we must be concerned about the types of malignancy that may appear in patients who received transplants during childhood and who will have been kept on immunosuppressive therapy for several decades [42].

Acknowledgment

The author wishes to thank numerous colleagues throughout the world for generous contributions of data concerning their patients to the CTTR.

References

1. Penn I. Why do immunosuppressed patients develop cancer? In: Pimentel E, editor. CRC critical reviews in oncogenesis. Boca Raton: CRC, 1989; 1: 27–52.
2. Penn I. Depressed immunity and the development of cancer. Cancer Detect Prev 1994; 18: 241–252.
3. Penn I. The problem of cancer in organ transplant recipients: an overview. Transplant Science 1994; 4: 23–32.
4. Penn I. Malignancy. Surg Clin N Amer 1994; 74: 1247–1257.
5. Kinlen LJ. Incidence of cancer in rheumatoid arthritis and other disorders after immunosuppressive treatment. Am J Med 1985; 78: (supl1A)44–9.
6. Sheil AGR, Disney APS, Mathew TH, et al. De novo malignancy emerges as a major cause of morbidity and late failure in renal transplantation. Transplant Proc 1993; 25: 1383–4.
7. Blohme I, Brynger H. Malignant disease in renal transplant patients. Transplantation 1985; 39: 23–35.
8. Harwood AR, Osoba D, Hofstader SL, et al. Kaposi's sarcoma in recipients of renal transplants. Am J Med 1979; 67(5): 759–765.
9. Schröter GPJ, Weil R III, Penn I, et al. Hepatocellular carcinoma associated with chronic hepatitis B virus infection after kidney transplantation (Letter to the editor). Lancet 1982; 2: 381–2.
10. Bernstein D, Baum D, Berry G, et al. Neoplastic disorders after pediatric heart transplantation. Circulation 1993; 88(Pt 2): 230–7.
11. Sheil AGR. Skin cancer in renal transplant recipients. Transplant Science 1994; 4: 42–5.

12. Bouwes Bavinck JNB, Vermeer BJ, Van der Woude FJ, et al. Relation between skin cancer and HLA antigens in renal transplant recipients. New Engl J Med 1991; 325(12): 884–7.
13. Penn I. Immunosuppression and skin cancer. Clinics Plastic Surg 1980; 7: 361–8.
14. Hoxtell EO, Mandel JS, Murray SS, et al. Incidence of skin carcinoma after renal transplantation. Arch Dermatol 1977; 113: 436–8.
15. Kinlen LJ, Sheil AGR, Peto J, et al. Collaborative United Kingdom–Australasian study of cancer in patients treated with immunosuppressive drugs. Br Med J 1979; 2: 1461–6.
16. Hardie IR, Strong RW, Hartley CJ, et al. Skin cancer in Caucasian renal allograft recipients living in a subtropical climate. Surgery 1980; 87: 117–183.
17. Barr BB, Benton EC, McLaren K, et al. Human papilloma virus infection and skin cancer in renal allograft recipients. Lancet 1989; 1: 124–9.
18. Gupta AK, Cardella CJ, Haberman HF. Cutaneous malignant neoplasms in patients with renal transplants. Arch Dermatol 1986; 122: 1288–1293.
19. Glover MT, Niranjan N, Kwan JTC, et al. Non-melanoma skin cancer in renal transplant recipients: the extent of the problem and a strategy for management. Brit J Plastic Surg 1994; 47: 86–9.
20. Hartevelt MM, Bouwes-Bavinck JN, Koote AM, et al. Incidence of skin cancer after renal transplantation in the Netherlands. Transplantation 1990; 49(3): 506–9.
21. Mullen DL, Silberberg SG, Penn I, et al. Squamous cell carcinoma of the skin and lip in renal homograft recipients. Cancer 1976; 37: 729–734.
22. Nalesnik MA, Locker J, Jaffe R, et al. Experience with posttransplant lymphoproliferative disorders in solid organ transplant recipients. Clin Transplant 1992; 6: 249–252.
23. Nalesnik MA, Starzl TE. Epstein-Barr virus, infectious mononucleosis, and posttransplant lymphoproliferative disorders. Transplant Science 1994; 4: 61–79.
24. Wilkinson AH, Smith JL, Hunsicker LG, et al. Increased frequency of posttransplant lymphomas in patients treated with cyclosporine, azathioprine, and prednisone. Transplantation 1989; 47: 293–296.
25. Hanto DW. Classification of Epstein-Barr virus-associated posttransplant lymphoproliferative diseases: implications for understanding their pathogenesis and developing rational treatment strategies. Annual Rev Med 1995; 46: 381–394.
26. Penn I, Porat G. Central system lymphomas in organ allograft recipients. Transplantation 1995; 59: 240–244.
27. Montagnino G, Bencini PL, Tarantino A, el al. Clinical features and course of Kaposi's sarcoma in kidney transplant patients: report of 13 cases. Amer J Nephrol 1994; 14: 121–6.
28. Al-Sulaiman MH, Al-Khader AA. Kaposi's sarcoma in renal transplant recipients. Transplant Science 1994; 4: 46–60.
29. Penn I. Primary kidney tumors before and after renal transplantation. Transplantation 1995; 59: 480–485.
30. Catalona WJ. Urothelial tumors of the urinary tract. In: Walsh PC, Retik AB, Stamey TA, Vaughn ER Jr, editors. Campbell's urology, 6th ed. Philadelphia: Saunders Co., 1992: 1094–1158.
31. Ishikawa I. Acquired cysts and neoplasms of the kidneys in renal allograft recipients. In: Berlyne GM, editor. The kidney today. Selected topics in renal science. Basel, Karger: Contrib Nephrol, 1992: 100: 254–268.
32. Vaziri ND, Darwish R, Martin DC, el al. Acquired renal cystic disease in renal transplant recipients. Nephron 1984; 37: 203–5.
33. Clinicopathologic conference. A new chest mass in a 49-year-old man with a transplanted kidney. Amer J Med 1988; 84: 121–8.
34. Almirall J, Ricart MJ, Campistol JM, et al. Renal cell carcinoma and acquired cystic kidney disease after renal transplantation. Transplant Internat 1990; 3: 49.

35. Faber M, Kupin W. Renal cell carcinoma and acquired cystic kidney disease after renal transplantation (Letter to the editor). Lancet 1987; 1(8540): 1030–1.
36. Lien Y-H H, Kam I, Shanley PF, et al. Metastatic renal cell carcinoma associated with acquired cystic kidney disease 15 years after successful renal transplantation. Amer J Kidney Dis 1991; 18: 711–5.
37. Penn I. Cancers of the anogenital region in renal transplant recipients. Analysis of 65 cases. Cancer 1986; 58: 611–6.
38. Sillman F, Stanek A, Sedlis A, et al. The relationship between human papillomavirus and lower genital intraepithelial neoplasia in immunosuppressed women. Am J Obstet Gynecol 1984; 150: 300–8.
39. Porreco R, Penn I, Droegemueller W, et al. Gynecologic malignancies in immunosuppressed organ homograft recipients. Obstet Gynecol 1975; 45: 359–364.
40. Barrett WL, First R, Aron BS, et al. Clinical course of malignancies in renal transplant recipients. Cancer 1993; 72: 2186–9.
41. Penn I. The changing patterns of posttransplant malignancies. Transplant Proc 1991; 23: 1101–3.
42. Penn I. De novo malignancy in pediatric organ transplant recipients. J Ped Surg 1994; 29: 221–8.
43. Kersey JH, Shapiro RS, Heinitz KJ, et al. Lymphoid malignancy in naturally occurring and post bone marrow transplantation immunodeficiency diseases. In: Good RA, Lindenlaub E, eds. The nature, cellular and biochemical basis and management of immunodeficiences. Stuttgart: FK Shattaeur Verlag Symposia Medica Hoechst 1987; 21: 289–94.
44. Lee ES, Locker J, Nalesnik M, et al. The association of Epstein-Barr virus with smooth-muscle tumors occurring after organ transplantation. New Engl J Med 1995; 332: 19–25.
45. Van Hoeven KH, Factor SM, Kress Y, et al. Visceral myogenic tumors: a manifestation of HIV infection in children. Amer J Surg Path 1993; 17: 1176–81.
46. Mueller BU, Butler KM, Higham MC, et al. Smooth muscle tumors in children with human immunodeficiency virus infection. Pediatrics 1993; 91: 1020–1.

2. Multicenter analysis of posttransplant malignancies

GERHARD OPELZ, VOLKER SCHWARZ, HELEN GRAYSON,
ROBIN HENDERSON, RAIMUND SCHNOBEL,
THOMAS WUJCIAK & ANDREA RUHENSTROTH

Introduction

It is well known that transplant patients are at an increased risk of developing malignant tumors. The most striking increase, in comparison to the general population, is observed concerning the occurrence of non-Hodgkin lymphoma (NHL) [1]. We have recently quantified this risk to be approximately 20 times the background rate in the general population for kidney transplant recipients and 120 times background for heart transplant recipients [2]. In the present paper we present results of a refined analysis of risk factors associated with the occurrence of NHL. Moreover, we present results of a preliminary analysis concerning the occurrence of tumors other than NHL in recipients of different types of organ transplants.

The analysis was based on transplants reported to the Collaborative Transplant Study [3]. To eliminate the problem of "underreporting", all participating centers were asked to provide written confirmation that the posttransplant information on malignant tumors was accurate and complete. Only data from those centers who provided this verification were included in the analysis. Positive verification was received from 282 kidney transplant centers, 105 heart transplant centers and 40 liver transplant centers. The analysis was restricted to recipients of first transplants who received organs from cadaver donors. The incidence of tumors is presented as incidence per 100.000 patients.

Results

Table 1 lists the incidence of non-Hodgkin lymphoma (NHL) observed during the first posttransplant year in recipients of different types of organ transplants.

J.L. Touraine et al. (eds.), Cancer in Transplantation. Prevention and Treatment, 17–23.

Table 1. Incidence of non-Hodgkin lymphoma during the first posttransplant year

	Type of organ transplant					
	Kidney (n = 67785)	Heart (n = 10987)	Heart-lung (n = 626)	Lung (n = 895)	Liver (n = 3113)	Pancreas + kidney (n = 1720)
Observed Incidence per 100.000 patients	242	1259	5223	3063	937	347

Table 2. Incidence of non-Hodgkin lymphoma

Type of transplant	Posttransplant year					
	1	2	3	4	5	6
Kidney (n = 67785)	242	66	57	81	78	58
Heart (n = 10987)	1259	507	462	527	588	538

Incidence = incidence per 100.000 patients.

It is apparent that the frequencies of NHL vary widely, ranging from 242 per 100.000 in kidney transplant recipients to 5223 per 100.000 in heart-lung transplant recipients. NHL incidence rates in non-transplant populations of patients with similar disease background are not available for comparison. It should be noted, however, that the background rate of NHL in the general population is typically reported to be in the order of 10 cases per 100.000 [4]. We have shown earlier that, whereas the NHL incidence shows an age-dependent increase in the general population, the incidence is age-independent during the first posttransplant year in kidney and heart transplant recipients [2].

The incidence of NHL decreases substantially after the first posttransplant year, although the rates remain substantially higher than background. Table 2 shows yearly incidence rates for kidney and heart transplant recipients. The NHL incidence during subsequent years is less than one-half of the first-year rate and remains relatively constant from year to year. However, even during the sixth year after transplantation, the incidence of NHL is nearly 10 times higher in heart recipients than in kidney recipients. Year-by-year analysis of liver, lung and pancreas transplants showed a similar decrease in NHL incidence from the first to the second posttransplant year, although there was greater year-to-year variation, probably because the numbers of patients available for analysis were relatively small.

Table 3. Incidence on non-Hodgkin lymphoma during the first posttransplant year

	Type of organ transplant			
	Kidney	Heart	Liver	Pancreas + kidney
Europe	158 (n = 41062)	594 (n = 3486)	517 (n = 1271)	257 (n = 934)
North-America	335 (n = 21167)	1321 (n = 7016)	1270 (n = 1341)	527 (n = 668)

Incidence = incidence per 100.000 patients

Table 4. Incidence of non-Hodgkin lymphoma first posttransplant year

		Heart transplants
Europe	With Antibody prophylaxis (n = 2655)	640
	Without Antibody prophylaxis (n = 540)	370
North America	With Antibody prophylaxis (n = 3574)	1679
	Without Antibody prophylaxis (n = 1971)	863

Incidence = incidence per 100.000 patients

We reported previously that the incidence of NHL was significantly higher among kidney and heart recipients transplanted in North-America than among patients transplanted in Europe, and we provided circumstantial evidence that a “more aggressive” use of immunosuppressive drugs in North-America may be responsible for this difference [2]. Table 3 provides updated results as well as an extension of this observation to liver and pancreas transplants.

Interestingly, during the period following the first posttransplant year, the NHL incidence rates observed in Europe and North-America were very similar. Thus, if “more aggressive immunosuppression” indeed was the cause for the higher NHL incidence observed during the first posttransplant year in North-American patients, it would be of interest to examine the immunosuppressive treatment strategies during the patients’ early posttransplant course. An interesting variable in this context is the application of mono- or polyclonal antibody treatment for rejection prophylaxis during the first weeks after transplantation. As shown in Table 4, prophylactic antibody treatment was

Table 5. Incidence of non-Hodgkin in lymphoma per 100.000 patients cadaver kidney transplants, first posttransplant year

	Immunosuppressive regimen	CSA + STE + AZA	CSA + STE	STE + AZA
Europe	With Antibody prophylaxis	402	254	270
	Without Antibody prophylaxis	111	94	51
North America	With Antibody prophylaxis	621	379	205
	Without Antibody prophylaxis	239	195	64

CSA = Cyclosporine.
STE = Steroids.
AZA = Azathioprine.

associated with an increased NHL incidence in heart transplant recipients, both in Europe and North-America. However, in each of the 2 patient subgroups (with or without antibody prophylaxis), North-American patients had a much higher NHL incidence than European patients.

The results obtained in kidney transplant recipients were entirely consistent with those obtained in heart transplant patients. Antibody prophylaxis was associated with a higher rate of NHL occurrence both in Europe and North-America, however, the NHL incidence was higher in North-America than in Europe in each patient subset.

Whereas most heart transplant recipients received triple-drug immunosuppression including cyclosporine, azathioprine and steroids, kidney transplant recipients received different types of combination drug regimens. The 3 most commonly used immunosuppressive regimens were analyzed separately and NHL incidence rates are given in Table 5. Both in Europe and North-America, the NHL incidence was higher with the triple-drug regimen cyclosporine, azathioprine and steroids than with the combination cyclosporine and steroids without azathioprine. In each treatment subgroup, the NHL incidence was higher in patients who received prophylactic antibody treatment. Patients on steroids and azathioprine had a lower NHL incidence, with the exception of patients transplanted in Europe who received antibody prophylaxis.

It was not possible in this analysis to identify whether antibody prophylaxis with monoclonal antibodies was associated with a higher NHL incidence than prophylaxis with polyclonal antibodies, or whether products of certain

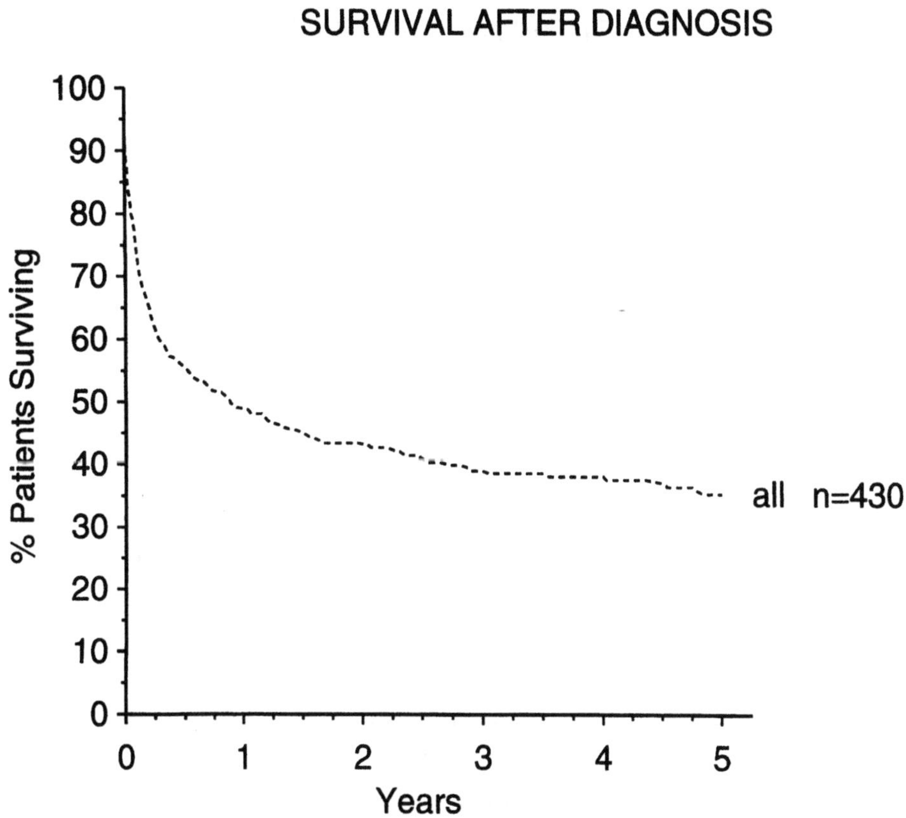

Fig. 1. Survival rate of cadaver kidney transplant recipients following the diagnosis of non-Hodgkin lymphoma. Actuarial method. The number of patients studied is indicated.

manufacturers were associated with particularly high or low NHL incidence rates.

That NHL is associated with a high risk of death is shown in Figure 1 for kidney transplant recipients and in Figure 2 for heart transplant recipients. In both groups of recipients, the patient survival rate after 3 years following the diagnosis of NHL was lower than 40%.

We have only recently embarked on an analysis of tumors other than non-Hodgkin lymphomas. Thus far, only cumulative crude incidence rates have been calculated which were not age standardized. A comparison with background incidence rates in the general population is therefore not possible. However, even at this early stage of the analysis, striking differences among the tumor incidence rates in recipients of kidney, heart or liver transplants are apparent (Table 6). These results will have to be examined in detail, considering variables such as recipients age, time of tumor occurrence, immunosuppressive treatment regimen, etc. However, from these preliminary results it

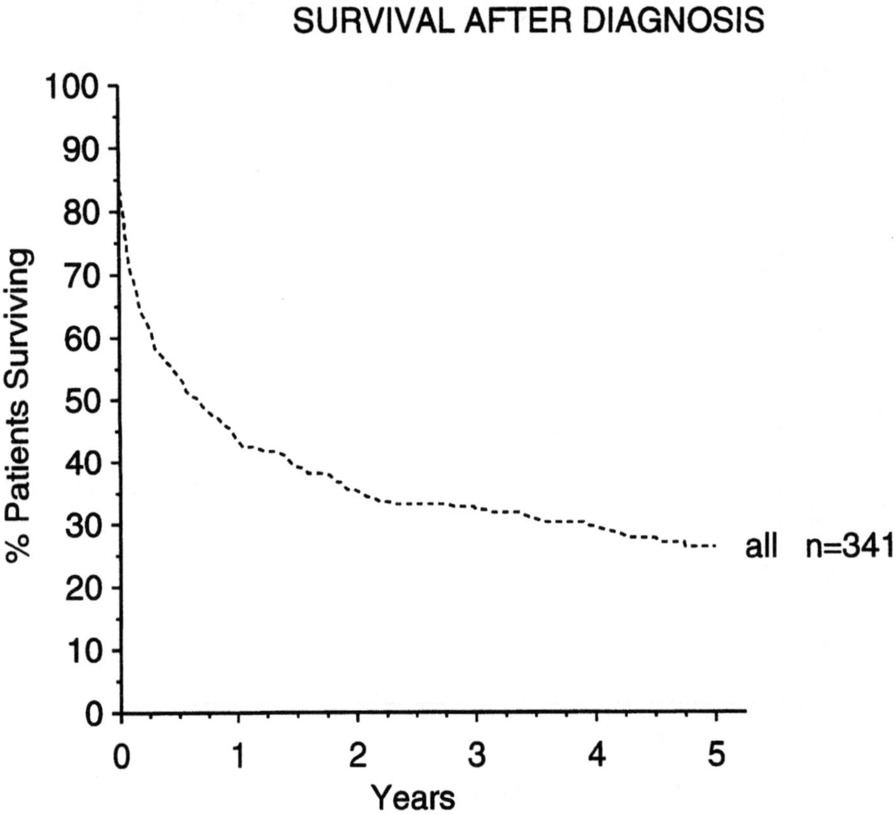

Fig. 2. Survival rate of heart transplant recipients following the diagnosis of non-Hodgkin lymphoma.

Table 6. Incidence of posttransplant De-Novo malignancies. Cumulative rates per 100.000 patients, transplant years 1985–1993

Type of tumor	Cadaver kidney transplants (n = 59476)	Heart transplants (n = 10987)	Liver transplants (n = 3113)
Melanoma	67	191	91
Kaposi sarcoma	221	146	91
Colon cancer	84	209	121
Lung cancer	226	764	121
Gallbladder/billiary tract	13	27	243
Liver cancer	47	46	548
Bladder cancer	99	82	0
Kidney cancer	225	173	0

would seem unlikely that the differences in tumor incidence shown in Table 6 would be attributable entirely to the "strength" of immunosuppressive treatment.

Acknowledgment

We thank the transplant centers participating in the Collaborative Transplant Study for providing information on posttransplant malignancies. This study was supported by a grant from Mildred Scheel Stiftung, Deutsche Krebshilfe, Bonn, Germany

References

1. Penn I. The changing pattern of posttransplant malignancies. Transplant Proc 1991; 23: 1101–03.
2. Opelz G, Henderson R: Incidence of non-Hodgkin lymphoma in kidney and heart transplant recipients. Lancet 1993; 342: 1514–16.
3. Collaborative Transplant Study, Newsletter 2, May 15, 1995.
4. Parkin DM, Muir CS, Whelan SL, Gao YT, et al. Cancer incidence in five continents, vol. VI. Lyon: International agency for research on cancer, 1992.

3. German multicenter analysis of malignancies following renal replacement therapy in children

ANNE-MARGRET WINGEN*

Introduction

The frequency of malignant diseases in adult patients on dialysis figures at about 4% and rises to about 6% after renal transplantation (RTPL) [1–3]. Especially the incidence of lymphomas is augmented: 4 times higher on dialysis and 37 times higher after transplantation as compared to age-matched controls. The risk of patients starting renal replacement therapy (RRT) in childhood to develop a de novo malignancy is less well defined, because the observation period under pediatric care is short as compared to their whole lifetime. While the expected incidence of malignant diseases between the age of 5 and 25 years is 1/10 000 in the normal population, some short-term studies report a frequency of 0.7% of malignancies in children on dialysis and 1–4% after transplantation [4–8]. Among the malignancies in children after transplantation lymphomas were the predominant tumors and comprised 49% of all malignancies in comparison to 11% of tumors in the general pediatric population [4, 7]. To evaluate the frequency of malignancies among patients starting RRT during childhood a retrospective analysis was done with the cooperation of all German pediatric nephrology centers.

Results

1239 children below the age of 15 years started RRT between 1971 and 1993 in Germany. 743 of these patients underwent RTPL during this time. In these children a total of 38 malignancies was recorded, 14 before start of RRT, 5 in patients on dialysis without RTPL and 19 after RTPL.

* For the Arbeitsgemeinschaft Pädiatrische Nephrologie.

J.L. Touraine et al. (eds.), Cancer in Transplantation. Prevention and Treatment, 25–30.

14 children (1%) with malignancies before start of RRT were recorded. In 12/14 children the malignancies were causally related to renal failure: 6 patients with Drash syndrome, 3 patients with bilateral Wilms tumor, 1 patient with M. Bourneville-Pringle and angiomyolipomatosis of the kidneys and renal cancer, 1 patient with neuroblastoma of the kidneys and 1 patient with nephrotoxicity of cytotoxic drugs and retinoblastoma. 6 children were not transplanted, 3 because they died from the tumor and 3 were waiting for a transplant. In 8 children the tumor was diagnosed at the age of 2.0 (1.1–5.5) years, they went to RRT at the age of 5.3 (2.1–12.2) years and were grafted 4.7 ± 2.9 years after the diagnosis of tumor. At last observation, 6.1 ± 4.6 years after RTPL, all were continuously free from malignancy.

In five children (0.7%) malignancies were diagnosed at the age of 7.7 (0.7–13.4) years, 0.3–5.1 years after start of RRT still on dialysis. One boy with secondary polycystic kidney disease and renal carcinoma was cured after bilateral nephrectomy. In one patient with B-cell lymphoma diagnosis was made at autopsy. The second patient with B-cell lymphoma died from his malignancy after 5 months of chemotherapy. In the remaining two children (sarcoma botryoides and dysgerminoma) therapy of the tumor was refused.

Nineteen of 743 children after RTPL (2.6%) developed malignancies. These patients suffered in 58% from glomerular diseases causing RRT. Patients with malignancies after RTPL started RRT at the age of 11.7 ± 3.0 years, went to RTPL 1.4 ± 1.1 years later and the diagnosis of tumor was made 6.9 ± 4.9 years after RTPL at the age of 20.6 (8.3–28,4) years. 3 patients only were below the age of 15 years at the time of occurence of malignant disease. 7 B-cell lymphomas (B-NHL) (3/7 Epstein Barr virus associated), 2 T-cell lymphomas, 2 acute myelocytic leucemias, 2 Kaposi sarcomas, 4 carcinomas and 2 dysgerminomas had been reported. B-NHL had a tendency to occur early after transplantation, while T-cell lymphomas and carcinomas were late complications (Figure 1). 4/7 B-NHL were diagnosed within only 6 months after RTPL. 2/7 B-NHL demonstrated a diffuse spread of monoclonal B-lymphoblasts throughout most organs, including the transplanted kidney, 2 B-NHL were restricted to one tonsil and 3 B-NHL showed massiv tumors in the abdomen. Patients with B-NHL received considerably more immunosuppressive therapy after RTPL as compared to patients with other tumors. While therapy with prednisone and azathioprine did not differ in both groups, all patients with B-NHL were treated with cylosporine A and 86% patients additionally with mono- or polyclonal anti-T-cell antibodies, cyclosporine A was used in 42% and anti-T-cell antibodies in 17% of patients with other tumors only (Figure 2). In 5/11 patients with malignancies of blood cell origin the clinical course was very rapid and diagnosis was made at autopsy (2 B-NHL, 2 T-cell lymphomas, 1 acute myelocytic leucemia). The other patient with acute myelocytic leucemia died after 1 year of chemotherapy from his tumor. Five patients with B-NHL are living 1.1 (0.5–2.3) years after diagnosis and chemotherapy with or without radiotherapy free from signs of

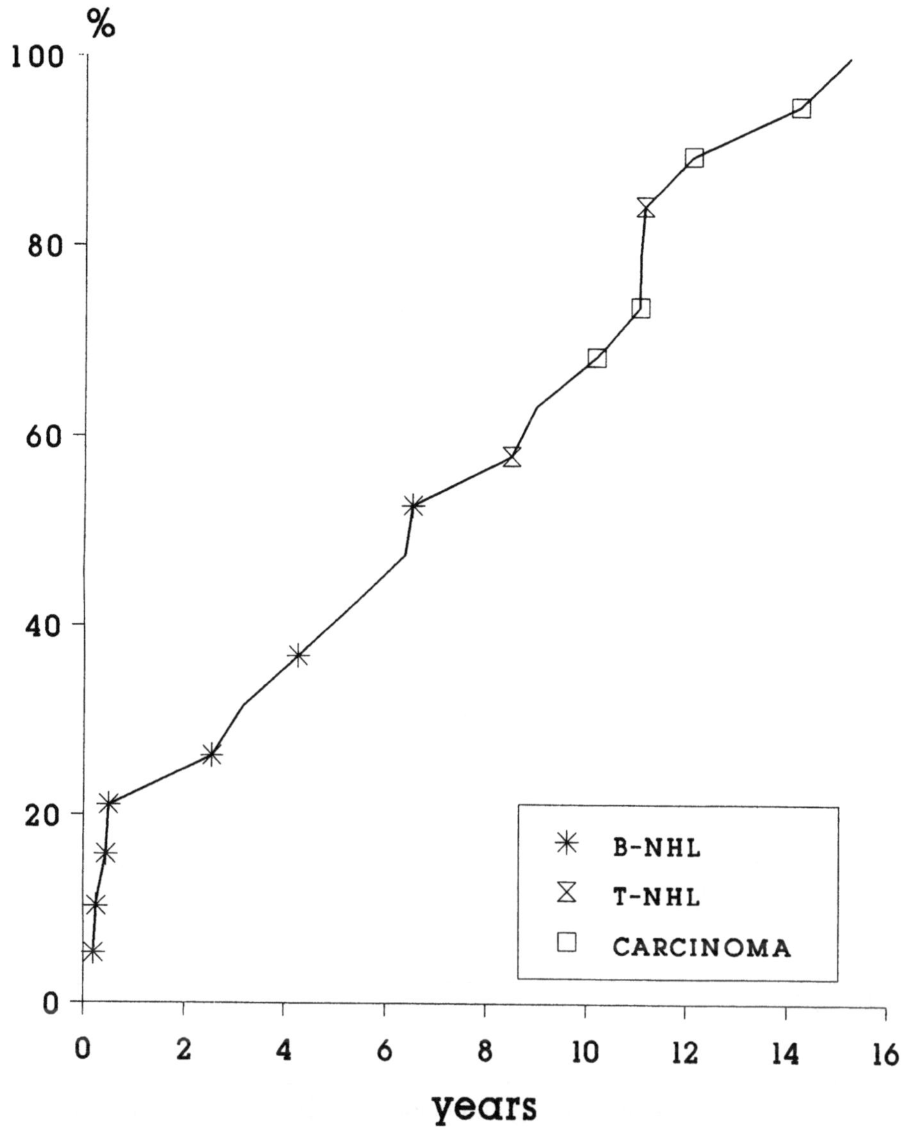

Fig. 1. Cumulative incidence of malignancies during the years after renal transplantation in 19 patients.

malignancy. The 2 patients with Kaposi sarcoma were treated by reduction of immunosuppressive therapy only. One of them died after 3.4 years from the tumor, the other was 1.1 year alive and the tumor still present. From 6 patients with carcinoma and dysgerminoma 5 were surviving 3.4 (2.7–11.9)

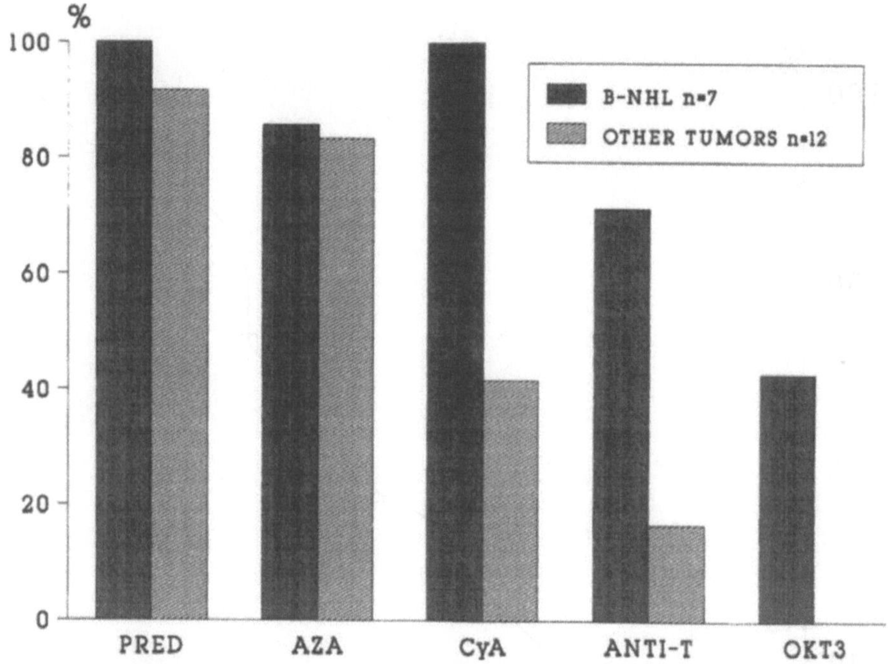

Fig. 2. Frequency of immunosuppressive medications applied after renal transplantation in 7 patients with B-cell lymphomas (B–NHL) compared to 12 patients with other tumors. (PRED = prednisone, AZA = azathioprine, CyA = cyclosporine A, ANTI-T = polyclonal anti-T-cell antibodies, OKT 3 = monoclonal anti-T-cell antibody)

years without signs of malignancy after surgery with or without radiotherapy and 1 patient was still under therapy.

Discussion

The frequency of children with malignancies before RRT was with 1% very low and suggests underreporting and is more likely to be about 3% [5]. But, the types of tumors reported in the present study are representative for these patients. The good outcome supports the usual clinical practise, that children with malignancies before start of RRT should be dialysed, if neccessary, and should be transplanted with a time interval to malignancy which makes recurrence highly unlikely.

Malignancies in children on RRT without RTPL were reported with a frequency of 0.7% (70/10 000) which is considerably higher than 1/10 000 in the general pediatric population. While surgery or radiotherapy can be done as usual, chemotherapy brings a lot of problems. There is little knowledge concerning the dosage of cytotoxic therapy in terminal renal failure. By this, standard chemotherapeutic protocols are not applicable and cytotoxic therapy must be individually designed. In 2 of our patients parents and doctors agreed that the burden of chronic renal failure and dialysis combined with the burden of malignant disease was too high for the children and further therapy was refused.

Frequency of malignancies after renal grafting was with 2.6% definitely higher than in the normal pediatric population. This frequency was in the range of other pediatric publications [5–8] and lower than in adults, who normally have a much higher incidence of malignancies than children. But, many of the malignancies after RTPL may have escaped from the pediatric statistics. These tumors occured in patients starting RRT in childhood, but, most of the tumors developped later, when the patients were grown up and usually nolonger under pediatric care (Figure 1). Therefore, it is highly likely that the total incidence of malignancies after RTPL in childhood is underestimated.

The risk of developing a malignancy after RTPL seems to be related to the renal disease, as glomerular diseases were with 58% among patients with malignancies more common than with 28% in the general pediatric population on RRT [9]. It may be postulated that patients with glomerular diseases have a more profound disturbance of immunesurveillance, permitting glomerular disease as well as malignancy. On the other hand, in many children the glomerular diseases had been treated with immunosuppressive drugs before start of RRT.

Lymphomas were the most common malignancies after RTPL (47%) in children in our study as in others [8]. This rate is higher than in the general pediatric population [4] and higher than in adults after RTPL, where such tumors are seen in 15% only [3]. Lymphomas of B-cell origin developped early after RTPL and their appearance was related to the cumulative amount of immunosuppressive drugs applied (Figure 2). Most pediatric patients with B-NHL were treated after RTPL with prednisone plus azathioprine plus cyclosporine A plus anti-T-cell antibodies. This experience of our study with a small number of patients correlates well with the data published by the collaborative transplant study (CTS) in adults. In the CTS 144 patients with lymphomas in 45141 adults with RTPL were registered. The incidence of lymphomas in adult patients was rising significantly after treatment with anti-T-cell antibodies [10, 11].

While the course of malignancy after RTPL was extremely rapid in 5/19 children (4 with lymphomas and 1 with acute myelocytic leucemia) and their diagnosis was made at autopsy only, 14 patients were available for further therapy of the malignant disease. Looking at the records of these patients, the impression arises, that diagnosis and anti-tumor therapy were delayed and used with caution. But, our data suggest, that 2/3 of malignancies occuring after RTPL are principally treatable diseases. For these patients development of treatment protocols is neccessary and seems promising.

References

1. Robles NR, Calero R, Rengel M, Valderrabano F. Hemodialysis and cancer. Nephron 1990; 54: 271–272.
2. Wilkinson AH, Smith JL, Hunsicker LG et al. Increased frequency of posttransplant lymphomas in patients treated with cyclosporine, azathioprine, and prednisone. Transplantation 1989; 47: 293–296.
3. Penn I. The changing patterns of post-transplant malignancies. Transplant Proc 1991; 23: 1101–1103.
4. Gutjahr P. Epidemiologie. In: Gutjahr P, editor. Krebs bei Kindern und Jugendlichen. Köln: Deutscher Ärzte Verlag, 1993: 20–26.
5. Wingen A-M, Wiesel M, Möhring K, Schärer K, Mehls O. Malignancies in children with renal replacement therapy. Transplant Proc 1994; 26: 5–6.
6. McEnery PT, Stablein DM, Arbus G, Tejani A. Renal transplantation in children. A report of the North American Pediatric Renal Transplant Cooperative Study. New Engl J Med 1992; 326: 1727–1732.
7. Penn I. De novo tumors in pediatric organ transplant recipients. Transplant Proc 1994; 26: 1–2.
8. Penn I. Malignancies in children. In: Tejani AH, Fine RN, editors. Pediatric renal transplantation. New York: Wiley-Liss, 1994: 461–470.
9. Broyer M, Chantler C, Donckerwolcke R, Ehrich JHH, Rizzoni G, Schärer K. The pediatric registry of European Dialysis and Transplant Association: 20 years' experience. Pediatr Nephrol 1993; 7: 758–768.
10. Opelz G, Henderson R for the Collaborative Transplant Study. Incidence of non-Hodgkin lymphoma in kidney and heart transplant recipients. Lancet 1993; 342: 1514–1516.
11. Penn I. Immunosuppression – A contributory factor in lymphoma formation. Clin Transplantation 1992; 6: 214–219.

4. Malignancies transmitted with the transplant

NICOLE LEFRANÇOIS, ANNE CLAIRE MARRAST,
JEANNE-LUCE GARNIER, JEAN-MICHEL DUBERNARD &
JEAN-LOUIS TOURAINE

Introduction

In contrast to patients with normal immune system, tumors can be transmitted to organ transplant recipients due to their immunosuppressive therapy. But in the pioneering years of transplantion, this possibility was regarded as being without foundation. Thus, in the first historic years of transplantation, donors with cancer were accepted for organ donation.

In the first observations by Martin [1], Mac Intosh [2] and Mac Lean [3], cancer has been transmitted by renal allografts, and on these occasions there has been wide dissemination in the host, leading to death of two patients.

Wilson [4] transplanted a kidney from a donor who had died of bronchial carcinoma, in 1968 . Seventeen months later, a metastatic tumor was found to grow in and around the kidney. Withdrawal of immunosuppressive therapy and removal of the graft resulted in rejection of the cancer, with apparent cure. Despite the possibility of cancer rejection after stopping immunosuppressive therapy the risks were considered unacceptable and transplants from cancerous donors were stopped. In 1977, I. Penn [5] suggested guidelines for donor acceptability to avoid cancer transmission. He wrote "accumulated experience has taught us that organs should not be harvested from donors with cancer, except those with low grade malignancies of the skin or with primary neoplasms confined to the brain".

Most malignancies transmitted with the transplant occurred in the early years of transplantation, when the risk of cancer transfer with the transplant was not yet fully appreciated. Currently, despite rigourous medical donor selection, sporadic cases of organ transplants bearing cancer are still encountered in 2 circumstances: when organ transplantation is permormed with a donor with primary central nervous system malignancy or when organ transplantation is performed from a donor with undetected neoplasm before removal.

J.L. Touraine et al. (eds.), Cancer in Transplantation. Prevention and Treatment, 31–38.

Table 1. Malignancies transmitted from donor with primary CNS neoplasm

Authors	Type of CNS tumor	Type of trans-plantation	Time of diagnosis	Outcome
Lefrancois et al. 1987 [6]	Medulloblastoma	Kidney + Pancreas	4 months	Death 5 months Peritoneal metastases
		Kidney	5 months	Alive 12 months Nephrectomy + Chemotherapy
		Heart	6 months	Death 7 months Widespread metastases
Morse et al. (1990) [7]	Glioblastoma	Liver	9 months	Death 10 months – Metastases
		Kidney		Removal 1 month-Alive – no tumor
		Kidney + Heart		Alive 25 months – No tumor
Ruiz et al. 1993 [8]	Glioblastoma multiforme	Kidney	17 months	Removal (2 intrarenal T) Alive 3 months – no tumor
		Kidney	18 months	Removal (1 intrarenal T) Alive 32 months – No tumor
Colquhoun et al. 1994 [9]	Glioblastoma multiforme	Kidney	10 months	Alive – nephrectomy
		Kidney	10 months + irradiation	Alive – nephrectomy

Organ transplantation from donor with primary CNS malignancy

Because primary brain tumors rarely metastasize, brain death secondary to that neoplasms is not considered to be a contraindication to organ donation. Since probabilities are low but not equal to zero, the safety of this practice has always been of some concern. Fortunately, there have been remarkable few reports of documented transmission of primary CNS malignancies to organ recipients. In the literature, we found 4 cases of primary brain transmission (Table 1).

In Lyon, 3 recipients were transplanted with a donor who had a medulloblastoma requiring surgery, chemotherapy, radiotherapy and ventriculo peritoneal derivation 2 weeks before organ removal. Two of the 3 patients died at 5 and 7 months with metastasis despite reduction of immunosuppressive therapy for heart recipient and withdrawal of immunosuppressive therapy, transplant nephrectomy and chemotherapy in the kidney and pancreas recipient. The third patient is alive after nephrectomy and chemotherapy [6]. The case of Morse [7] involved a transmission of glioblastoma to a liver recipient who died with metastasis 10 months later, while the kidney recipient and the kidney plus heart recipient were alive with no tumor. Ruiz [8] described 2 cases of transmission of glioblastoma to two kidney recipients. Seventeen and 18 months after transplantation, they had fever and enlarged kidney transplant. Kidneys were removed and immunocytochemistry showed results consistent with a glioblastoma multiforme. The two patients are alive with no tumor, without any complementary treatment.

Colquhoun [9] in 1994 reported a transmission of glioblastoma to 2 kidney recipients who presented a kidney mass, 10 months after transplantation. The 2 recipients are alive with nephrectomy and radiotherapy.

Among these four donors only our donor had a prior ventriculoperitoneal shunt.

Incidence of various tumor cells types in donors with primary CNS malignancy

The number of donors with primary brain tumors available is uncertain and not reported. Colquhoun [9] reviewed the regional organ procurement agency statistics concerning donors with CNS malignancies from 1986 to 1992 and he reviewed the outcome of all organs used from such donors. He found 34 donors with primary brain tumor supplying 84 organs upon more than 2000 donors. 74% of tumors were glial tumors and the majority of them were of a high grade malignancy. From this group, malignancies developed in 2 renal allograft recipients leaving an overall incidence of transmission from a donor with malignant cerebral histology of 3%. In adults, about 40% of primary brain tumors and glioblastomas represent approximately 50% of all gliomas (10). Glioblastoma multiforme is histologically, with medulloblastoma, the most malignant of glial tumors. Medulloblastoma arises from a more primitive cell line and represents 2% of such tumors in adults but more than 15% in children [11].

Incidence of metastates of primary CNS malignancy

Overall incidence of metastases of malignant brain tumors is low: 0.5% in adult (10) and 2.4% in children [11]. However, in adults, glioblastomas and high grade astrocytomas are among those tumors most likely to be associated with extraneural metastases while in children, medulloblastomas are responsible for 71% of the extracranial metastases. In adult metastasis are mainly pulmonary or pleural, lymph nodes and liver but very rare in the kidney 3%

[10]. Children with medulloblastomas tend to develop bone and bone marrow metastases while those with other brain tumors frequently have invasion of adjacent tissues and then spread to regional lymph nodes and lungs [11].

Risks factors of systemic metastases of primary CNS malignancy

Several factors have been associated with an increased risk of extraneural spread. They include cell type, grade of malignancy and duration of the disease [10]. The generally uncommon extraneural spread of primary brain tumors is due in part to the usually short survival of those patients. As treatments and survival statistics improve, so do the probabilities of systemic spread. Craniotomy is a widely accepted cause of dissemination and was found in 73% of Pasquier cases [10]. Three of ther 4 brain tumor transmissions had craniotomy.

Ventriculosystemic shunts have caused the greatest concern as an intuitive route for metastatic spread but in the series of Pasquier, only 10% of patients had ventricular shunt and 21% had no shunt and no craniotomy. However, in case of medulloblastomas, the role of ventriculosystemic shunt appears to be more evident. It is important to realize that the absence of a shunt should offer no security against the possibility of a metastasing CNS tumor. Lastly, experimentally insufficient radiotherapy, might potentialise malignancy evolution [12].

Organ transplantation from donor with undetected neoplasm before removal

The other current circumstances of donor transmitted cancer is when tumor cells are transplanted accidentally by an organ removed from a cadaveric or living donor who has an unsuspected malignancy. In fact, recently, some cases of cancer transmission from donor with no apparent tumor present at harvesting had been described. Then, we will see the particular case of donors with primary renal tumor. Furthermore, in the literature we found 3 cases of non Hodgkin's lymphomas transmitted from the donor.

Transplantation from donors with no apparent tumor present at harvesting

Table 2 shows the cases of cancer transmission from 9 donors with undetected neoplasms to twenty-one recipients published since 1980. It is important to note that the primary cause of brain death was misdiagnosed in all cases. The initial diagnosis was either primary brain tumor or cerebral haemorrhage. 75% of patients had evidence of malignancy involving the graft. The prognosis was bad and nine recipients died of neoplasia, in a particularly short time in case of liver transplantation with choriocarcinoma [13–19].

Table 2. Patients transplanted from donor with undetected neoplasms

Authors	Presumed cause of brain death	Source of cancer in donor	Organ transplanted	Time mode of diagnosis (months)
Fairman et al.	Male 54 years	Melanoma	Kidney	40.0
1980 [13]	Traffic accident			skin, pulmonary,
				cerebral metastasis
			Kidney	40.0
				Nephrectomy
Marsh et al.	Female 36 years	Choriocarcinoma	Liver	7.0
1987 [14]	cerebral haemorrhage	(no autopsy)	Kidney	?
			Kidney	?
			Kidney	?
			Heart	No tumor
Homburg et al.	Male 43 years	Adenocarcinoma	Kidney	23.0
1988 [15]	Primary brain tumor	of unknown		Kidney,
		origin (autopsy)		regional lymph nodes
Baquero et al.	Female 36 years	Choriocarcinoma	Liver	3.0 (autopsy)
1988 [16]	Cerebra hematoma		Kidney	3.0
			Kidney	3.0
			Heart	No tumor
Oesterwitz et al.	3 Donors	Myeloma Bile dutct and	4 kidneys	No tumor
1991 [17]		Bronchic carcinoma	1 kidney	19.0
Detroz et al.	Female 30 years	Choriocarcinoma	1 kidney	D1-Multiple Intrarenal
1991 [18]	Cerebral haemorrhage	(autopsy)	1 Liver	Tumor
				D39 (BHCG)
		Cervix carcinoma		
		(autopsy)	1 Liver	D1
Bentdal et al.	Male	Renal carcinoma	1 Kidney	3.0 (K bipsy)
1994 [19]	Cerebral haemorrhage		1 kidney	3.0 (K bipsy)

The Cincinnati transplant tumor registry collected data on 161 patients who received organs from donors with neoplasms [20]. Of 142 recipient of cadaver donors 64 (44%) developed tumors involving the graft: 24 were confined to the graft, 4 had local invasion and 36 had metastasis leading to 26 deaths while 9 regressed with treatment and 1 had evolutive cancer. Among 19 recipients of living related donors, 7 developed neoplasms: 4 small tumors were excised at harvesting with no recurrence, 2 were nephrectomized and 1 patient died 10 months later with metastasis. Finally incidence of cancer transmission was 44%.

Table 3. Donor related non Hodgkin's lymphomas

Authors cause of death	Type of organ diagnosis	Time of	Treatment	Outcome
Hjelle et al. 1989 [22]	Kidney Medulloblastoma	4 months Kidney, regional lymph nodes	Reduction of Is, nephrectomy, Acyclovir Radiotherapy Chemotherapy	No EBV serologic markers DNA finger printing analysis + Alive 16 months recurrence
Meduri et al. 1991 [23]	Kidney Cranial trauma	8 months Kidney	Nephrectomy 10 mo. Chemotherapy Radiotherapy	No EBV serologic markers DNA finger printing analysis + Alive 18 months
Schutt et al. 1993 [24]	Kidney Cranial trauma	2 days (2 cms) 9 months	Nephrectomy 9 mo. No other treatment	No EBV infection HLA Lymphocyte of donor origin Alive 33 months

Transplantation from donors with primary renal tumors

I. Penn [21] in a recent publication reported cases of renal carcinomas in the donor, from the CTTR. He found 30 renal tumors present at harvesting, 14 small primary renal carcinomas had good evolution with excision or nephrectomy In 14 instances, a carcinoma of one kidney was found in the cadaver donor: 7 were excised as described above and transplanted, 7 were discarded and among the 7 patients only one had carcinoma but of its own kidney. One renal carcinoma was intentionally transplanted in 1971 and the recipient died 4 months later. One more patient with renal carcinoma and metastasis of adrenal gland was transplanted leading to death of recipient 7 months later. In 17 cases, there was no apparent tumor at harvesting. In 10 cases, transplant nephrectomy was necessary for different reasons and there was no recurrence. The other 7 patients died with metastasis.

There is a relatively low number of carcinomas in donors compared to the high number of preexisting cardinomas in recipients and de novo carcinomas [21].

Donor-transmitted non-Hodgkin's lymphomas

Three patients were described as having donor-transmitted non-Hodgkin's lymphomas from 1989 (Table 3). Of particular interest is the fact that lymphomas occurred in a short time after transplantation (2 days to 8 months) [22, 23, 24]. There was no evidence for EBV infection and the diagnosis of donor origin was unequivocally determined by DNA finger printing analysis in 2 cases and HLA determination in the third case. In the first case, withdrawal of immunosuppressive therapy, nephrectomy, and Acyclovir were unsuccessful, but chemotherapy and radiotherapy resulted in remission ; 16 months later the patient is alive, with recurrence. The second patient is alive at 18 months with nephrectomy, chemotherapy and radiotherapy. The third patient is alive 33 months after transplantation with no other treatment than nephrectomy. These data support the notion that donor cells can undergo malignant transformation in solid organ transplant recipients and such tumors need not carry EBV genetic material.

Conclusion

Patients with past history of cancer are not suitable for organ donation. The incidence of transmission a primary CNS malignancy in a transplanted organ is low but not insignificant. Several factors should be considered before acceptability of a donor: cell type and grade of the tumor, prior history of craniotomy, duration of patient's disease and ventriculo-systemic shunt.

In case of transplantation with a primary CNS malignancy, intensive follow-up of recipients is required. There are some evidences that the risk is higher for liver recipients than for kidney and heart recipients.

Every donor must be carefully screened for possible cancer. A metastasis may masquerade as a primary brain tumor. Especially in cases of choriocarcinoma a post-donation autopsy is recommended. Furthermore organs harvested should be carefully examined and biopsies performed in case of suspicious lesions.

When a kidney has been transplanted from a cadaver donor in whom autopsy revealed cancer, it is recommended to stop immunosuppressive treatment, to perform transplant nephrectomy and in case of residual tumor to apply chemotherapy, radiotherapy and/or immunotherapy. Intensive clinical and radiological follow-up of such patients is necessary. Retransplantation can be discussed in case of complete remission for at least 1 year.

In case of a post-transplant lymphoma, the donor origin of the tumor must be discussed.

References

1. Martin DC, Rubini M, Rosen VJ. Cadaveric renal homotransplantation with inadvertent transplantation of cancer. Jama 1965; 192: 82.
2. McIntosh DA, McPhaul JJ, Peterson EN et al. Homotransplantation of a cadaver neoplasm in a renal homograft. Jama 1965; 192: 1171.
3. Maclean LD, Dossetor JB, Gault MH et al. Renal transplantation using cadaver donors. Arch Surg 1965; 91: 288.

4. Wilson RE, Hager EB, Hampers CL et al. Immunologic rejection of human cancer transplanted with a renal allograft. N Engl J Med 1968; 278: 479.
5. Penn I. Development of cancer as a complication of clinical transplantation. Transplant Proc 1977; XIX: 1121.
6. Lefrancois N, Touraine JL, Cantarovich D et al. Transmission of medulloblastoma from cadaver donor to the organ transplant recipients. Transplant Proc 1987; 19: 2242.
7. Morse JM, Turcotte JG, Merion RM et al. Development of a malignant tumor in a liver transplant graft procured from a donor with a cerebral neoplasm. Transplantation 1990; 50: 875.
8. Ruiz JC, Cotorruelo JG, Tudela V et al. Transmission of glioblastoma multiforme to two kidney transplant recipients from the same donor in the absence of ventricular shunt. Transplantation 1993; 55: 682.
9. Colquhoun SD, Robert ME, Shaked A et al. Transmission of CNS malignancy by organ transplantation. Transplantation 1994; 57: 970.
10. Pasquier B, Pasquier D, N'Golet A et al. Extraneural metastases of astrocytomas and glioblastomas: clinicopathological study of two cases and review of literature. Cancer 1980; 45: 12.
11. Campbell A, Chan HS, Becker LE et al. Extracranial metastases in childhood primary intracranial tumors. A report of 21 cases and review of the literature. Cancer 1984; 53: 974.
12. Zimmerman HM. The natural history of intracranial neoplasms with special references to gliomas. Am J Surg 1957; 93: 913.
13. Fairman RM, Grossman RA, Barker CF et al. Inadvertent transplantation of a melanoma. Transplantation 1980; 30: 328.
14. Marsh JW, Esquirol C, Makowka L et al. Accidental transplantation of malignant tumor from a donor to multiple recipients. Transplantation 1987; 44: 449.
15. Hombourg A, Hofstädter F, Klose KC et al. Regression of an adenocarcinoma transmitted by a cadaver kidney graft. Transplantation 1988; 46: 777.
16. Baquero A, Foote J, Kottle S et al. Inadvertent transplantation of choriocarcinoma into two recipients. Transplant Proc 1988; 19: 98.
17. Oesterwitz ME and Lucius K. Transmission of cancer with cadaveric donor kidneys. Transplant Proc 1991; 23: 2647.
18. Detroz B, Detry M, D'Silva M et al. Organ transplantation with undetected donor neoplasm. Transplant Proc 1991; 23: 2657.
19. Bentdal H, Brekke IB, Lien B et al. Rapid development of cancer in both kidney grafts after transplantation from a donor with undiagnosed malignant disease. Transplant Proc 1994; 26: 1763.
20. Penn I. Donor transmitted disease. Cancer Transplant Proc 1991; 23: 2629.
21. Penn I. Primary kidney tumors before and after renal transplantation. Transplantation 1995; 59: 480.
22. Hjelle B, Evans-Holm M, Yen TSB et al. A poorly differenciated lymphoma of donor origin in a renal allograft recipient. Transplantation 1989; 47: 945.
23. Meduri G, Fromentin L, Viellefond A et al. Donor related non-Hodgkin's lymphoma in a renal allograft recipient. Transplant Proc 1991; 23: 2649.
24. Schutt G, Engemann R, Gassel HJ et al. Donor transmitted non-Hodgkin's lymphoma after renal transplantation a case report. Transplant Proc 1993; 25: 2131.

PART TWO

Malignancies preexisting to transplantation

5. Outcome of preexisting urological tumors in dialysis and in renal transplant recipients

GEORGES KARAM & BENOIT BARROU

Introduction

Urologic tumors in renal failure patients occur in two circumstances: 1) the life expectancy of patients with end stage renal failure increases leading to an increased risk of tumor occurence as this population is aging, 2) renal failure can be the consequence of carcinologic surgery (bilateral renal tumors, nephrectomy of a solitary kidney) or of chemotherapy (platinium for instance). These patients raise the difficult question of whether they should be transplanted and when? To answer this question, one must take in account the risk of recurrence or development of undetected metastasis under immunosuppression as well as the current organ shortage. To better evaluate the results of renal transplantation in those patients, a questionnaire was sent to the French Renal Transplantation Institutions. The results of this survey are presented in this paper.

The main items of the questionnaire were as follows:

- Patient: Social status, underlying nephropathy and renal replacement therapy: hemodialysis or CPAD.
- Tumor: Date of diagnosis, localization, histologic grade, cellular grade, treatment and follow-up.
- Kidney Transplantation: Time interval between tumor diagnosis and transplantation, induction immunosuppressive regimen, maintenance immunosuppressive regimen and graft function.

Results

Twenty two institutions (out of 33) answered the questionnaire. Altogether, there were 33 patients (27 males and 6 females) with a past history of urologic malignancy who either were on dialysis or received a renal transplant. Of those, 4 were children (4–36 months). The median age for the remaining 29 patients was 52 years (19–63 years). The cause of end stage renal failure was a nephropathy in 24 cases, a Drash syndrome in 1 case, and a bilateral

J.L. Touraine et al. (eds.), Cancer in Transplantation. Prevention and Treatment, 41–46.

Table 1. Sites and histological patterns of tumors

Site	Number
Kidney [a]	19
Bladder (Transitionnal carcinoma)	2
Prostate (Adenocarcinoma)	8
Testis [b]	3
Unknown	1
Total	33

[a]: Renal cell carcinoma (11), Wilms' tumor (4), oncocytoma (2), adenoma (2)
[b]: Embryonnal carcinoma (2), seminoma (1)

Table 2. The different treatments of tumors

Kidney	Bladder	Prostate	Testis
Type of treatment and Number			
Bilateral nephrectomy: **6**	Trans urethral resection: **1**	Radical prostatectomy: **6**	Lymph node dissection and chemotherapy: **2**
Nephrectomy (single kidney): **1**	Trans urethral resection and Mitomycine: **1**	Trans urethral resection: **1**	Lymph node dissection, chemotherapy, radiotherapy: **1**
Nephrectomy: **12**		Hormonotherapy: **1**	
Chemo and radiotherapy: **3**			

nephrectomy (or nephrectomy of a solitary kidney) in 8 cases (5 renal cell calcinomas, 3 Wilms' tumors).

In dialysis patients, the circumstances of diagnosis were as follows: gross hematuria (n = 4), abnormal urination (n = 1), abdominal mass (n = 3), testicular mass (n = 2), abdominal pain (n = 1), other pain (n = 2), retroperitoneal enlarged lymph nodes (n = 1). Finally, nineteen patients were symptom free. The median time interval between beginning of dialysis and tumor diagnosis was 11 months (2–170). Sites and histologic patterns of the tumors are listed in Table 1.

Table 3. Patients and graft survivals

Patients: **33**		Grafts: **17**	
Death:	1	Functioning: **15**	
Alive		Lost (chronic rejection):	2
(Disease free):	30		
Unknown:	2	Median creatininemia:	
		130 μmol/l (90–230)	
Median follow-up:		Median follow-up:	
46 (3–303) months		**37 (5–202) months**	

In 27 instances, there was no dissemination. In the remaining cases, the disease spread locally (1 Wilms' tumor), to the regional lymph nodes (1 seminoma and 1 embryonal carcinoma), to lymph nodes and liver (1 embryonal carcinoma), to lungs and testis (1 Wilms' tumor). The different managements of these tumors are listed in Table 2.

Seventeen patients received a cadaveric renal transplant 0 to 150 months after tumor diagnosis (median = 73 months) and 9 to 128 months after dialysis initiation (median = 55 months). Induction immunosuppressive regimen included anti-thymocyte globulines [13] or monoclonal antibodies [3] in 16 out of 17 cases. Cyclosporine A was used as maintenance therapy in 13 cases (in combination with azathioprine and prednisone in 7 cases, azathioprine in 3 cases, and prednisone in 3 cases). Seven recipients experienced no rejection episodes, while 5 experienced 1 and 5 experienced 2 or more. All rejection episodes were treated by bolus of steroides except one treated by ATG. Patient and graft survivals are given in Table 3.

Discussion

Although not all institutions answered the questionnaire, the number of patients is low, making difficult to draw conclusions. In most cases, routine immunosuppressive protocols were used including anti lymphocyte T drugs (induction) and cyclosporine A (maintenance).

Renal tumors

The kidney was the most frequently involved organ, 19 cases out of 33, (57%). This can be explained by: 1) the selection of the patients of the study, all the patients with bilateral renal tumor (or tumor on solitary kidney) have been included. 2) the increased incidence of renal cell carcinoma in dialysis patients with an acquired cystic kidney disease (ACKD). ACKD is frequently encountered in patients on dialysis (35 to 40%). Its incidence increases with dialysis duration to reach 90% after 10 years. The increased risk of renal tumor makes suitable a careful surveillance including a yearly ultrasound imaging of the kidneys. When should these patients be transplanted? In case of symptomatic tumors, a waiting period of at least 2 years is recommended, although preventing only 61% of recurrences (Penn 1993). In contrast, according to the Cincinnati Transplant Tumor registry (CTTR) data (Penn 1993), the risk of recurrence for incidentally found tumors seems very low and a waiting period of one year appears safe enough. In case of Wilms' tumors, an interval of 2 years is also suitable (95% of the recurrences occur within 2 years), although some authors recommend a one year waiting period.

Urothelial tumors

Only 2 cases (low grade) were reported in our survey. The patients received a renal allograft 2.5 and 10 years after. In the second case, we observed a recurrence 4 years posttransplant treated by endoscopic resection and bladder instillation of mitomycine (low grade and superficial tumor). These tumors are known for their high risk of recurrence (50 to 80% after 3 years), even though they are superficial. It is of importance to identify patients with a particularly high risk of recurrence: exposition to carcinogens, multiple tumors, large size of the base of the tumor, dysplasia in other areas, aneuplöd cells. Transplantation must be very carefully considered in these patients and a waiting period of at least 2 years must be observed. After transplantation, a very careful surveillance must be done (native kidneys, native ureters and bladder) including repeated cytologic examination and cystoscopy. In case of invasive tumors, the prognostic remains bad and transplantation should be avoided.

Prostatic carcinoma

It is the most frequent cancer in elderly men. It has been a recent concern since patient life expectancy has increased either in dialysis or in transplantation. Penn, in 1993 reported on 22 cases out of 978 tumors seen prior to or at the time of transplantation. Screening is recommended in men over 50 years for two reasons: 1) to treat them prior to transplantation, 2) to avoid renal transplantation in those whose disease has already disseminated. A waiting time of 2 years prevents only 40% of the recurrences. It should be increased particularly if the Gleason score exceeds 7, the prostatic specific antigen (PSA) exceeds 30 ng/ml. If the tumor is extracapsular or the margins after radical prostatectomy are positive, transplantation should be avoided because of the high risk of recurrency.

Testicular tumors

They mostly occur in young adults (20 to 40 years). Current therapeutic protocols lead to complete remission in almost 90% of the cases. The follow-up care is based on physical examination, tumor markers (alpha FP, bêta HCG) and CT scans (chest and abdomen). Recurrences occur within 2 years in 95% of cases. The relapse rate after transplantation seems as low as 3% (Penn).

Conclusion

The incidence of urologic tumors is increased in dialysis patients as well as in transplant recipients. The role of immunosuppression is still a matter of debate at least for epithelial tumors.

Allograft transplantation raises 3 issues:

1) should the patients with a past history of urologic malignancy be transplantated? The answer is probably yes it they have had a local disease with a short mean relapse time and if they have received an appropriate treatment.
2) How long must be the interval between cancer treatment and transplantation? Theoretically, an interval of 5 years prevents 90% of recurrences of most tumors. This is however a long period of time for people on dialysis awaiting a transplant. Bladder and prostate tumors require often such an interval. However, for Wilms' tumors, asymptomatic small renal tumors and testis tumors it can probably be safely reduced to 2 years.
3) Have the immunosuppression protocols to be modified? The relationship between cancer and immune system remains poorly understood. The role of immunosuppression on virus infections and non Hodgkin's lymphomas is now well established but remains a matter of speculation as long as epithelial tumors are concerned.

Acknowledgments

We would like to thank our colleagues in France for providing us with data on urological tumors in their centers.

References

1. Bretan Pn J R. Acquired renal cystic disease: is there a need for screening for renal cell carcinoma in patients with renal failure? Semin Urol 1994; 12,2: 89–92.
2. Chandhoke P S, Torrence R J, Clayman R V, Rothstein M. Acquired cystic disease of the kidney: a management dilemma. J Urol 1992; 147,4: 969–974.

3. Fairley C K, Sheil A G, McNeil J J, et al. The risk of ano-genital malignancies in dialysis and transplant patients. Clin Nephrol 1994; 41,2: 101–105.
4. Gagnadoux M F, Habib R. Should bilateral nephrectomy be carried out in all children with diffuse mesangial sclerosis prior to renal transplantation in view of the connection with Drash syndrome and therefore the risk of a Wilms' tumor developing? Pediatr Nephrol 1992; 6,3: 266.
5. Heritier P, Bizrane M, Farcot M, et al. Transplantation et tumeurs du rein. J Urol Paris 1990; 96,3: 167–168.
6. Ishikawa I. Acquired cysts and neoplasms of the kidneys in renal allograft recipients. Contrib Nephrol 1992; 100,: 254–268.
7. Ishikawa I. Uremic acquired cystic disease of kidney. Urology 1985; 26,2: 101–108.
8. Khauli R B. Genitourinary malignancies in organ transplant recipient. Semin Urol 1994; 12,3: 224–232.
9. Levine E. Renal cell carcinoma in uremic acquired renal cystic disease: incidence, detection, and management. Urol Radiol 1992; 13,4: 203–210.
10. Levine L A, Gburek B M. Acquired cystic disease and renal adenocarcinoma following renal transplantation. J Urol 1994; 151,1: 129–132.
11. Lien Y H, Hunt K R, Siskind M S, Zukoski C. Association of cyclosporin A with acquired cystic kidney disease of the native kidneys in renal transplant recipients. Kidney Int 1993; 44,3: 613–616.
12. Nakamoto T, Igawa M, Mitani S, et al. Metastatic renal cell carcinoma arising in a native kidney of a renal transplant recipient. J Urol 1994; 152,3: 943–945.
13. Pais E, Pirson Y, Squifflet J P, et al. Kidney transplantation in patients with Wilms' tumor. Transplantation 1992; 53,4: 782–785.
14. Penn I. Dormant metastases [editorial; comment]. Can J Surg 1991; 34,4: 309–310.
15. Penn I. Kidney transplantation in patients previously treated for renal carcinomas [comment]. Transpl Int 1993; 6,6: 350.
16. Penn I. Primary kidney tumors before and after renal transplantation. Transplantation 1995; 59,4: 480–485.
17. Penn I. The effect of immunosuppression on pre-existing cancers. Transplantation 1993; 55,4: 742–747.
18. Penn I. The problem of cancer in organ transplant recipients: An overview. Transplantation Science 1994; 4,1: 23–32.
19. Shoskes D. Urological malignancies in renal transplant repients. Current Opinion in Urology 1995; 5: 91–94.
20. Steinbach F, Novick A C, Shoskes D. Renal transplantation in patients with renal cell carcinoma and von Hippel-Lindau disease. Urology 1994; 44,5: 760–763.
21. Wiggins C, Pontin A R, Manas D, et al. Renal transplantation in patients with bilateral renal carcinoma – How long should we wait? [see comments]. Transpl Int 1993; 6,6: 348–349.
22. Yang C C, Rohr M C, Assimos D G. Pretransplant urologic evaluation. Urology 1994; 43,2: 169–173.

6. Screening for breast and gynecologic carcinomas in transplant patients

PATRICE MATHEVET

1. Screening methods used in gynenocology in the general population

1.1. Breast carcinoma

This carcinoma is in first position for incidence and mortality in french women. About 1 of 11 women is going to have a breast carcinoma. Screening for this cancer was first developped with clinical exam, but currently it is well known that the most profitable method is screening with mammography. Performing mammography each 2 years after the age of 50 years, allows to detect small carcinomas easily curable. Screening with mammography on large populations gives a 30% decrease in breast cancer mortality.

Identification of high-risk population based on epidemiologic results is not easy. Essentially, the most valuable data is the occurence of breast carcinomas in relatives (in particular at a young age). Women with family factors should be screened with mammography at a younger age.

1.2. Cervical carcinoma

Physiopathology of this carcinoma have progressed recently. It has been shown that the vast majority of these cancers is related to the oncogenic effect of human papilloma viruses (HPV), in particular HPV types 16 and 18. Also these carcinomas are preceded by pre-cancerous lesions (cervical intra-epithelial neoplasia (CIN)) which can be detected by cervical cytology (Pap-smear) or colposcopy.

Screening for cervical carcinoma is based on Pap-smear follow-up. Recent guide-lines have been published: screening should be performed between 20 to 65 years, and the interval between 2 cytology should be 3 years (after 2 normal pap-smears). The profit of this program in term of decreased mortality is not well known, but many epidemiologic studies have demonstrated a

J.L. Touraine et al. (eds.), Cancer in Transplantation. Prevention and Treatment, 47–51.

reduction in cervical carcinoma incidence during the last 20 years probably in relation to Pap-smear screening.

Colposcopy as screening method is efficient but too expensive and gives high false-positive rates. HPV typing on cytology has not been evaluated yet, but also seems to be a too expensive method.

1.3. Ano-genital carcinomas (vulvar, vaginal and anal carcinomas)

These cancers are relatively rare in the general population, so they do not benefit from screening programs. Part of vaginal carcinomas could be detected thanks to cervical cytology. Also some ano-genital cancers can be found before they are symptomatic during a routine gynecologic examination.

Recent studies have shown that a large number of these carcinomas are related to HPV.

1.4. Endometrial carcinoma

This cancer occurs in elderly women. Some of the risk factors as estrogens are well known. As the general population get older, the incidence of endometrial cancer increase, but still now there is no screening program.

Usually diagnosis of endometrial carcinoma is made when checking post-menopausal bleeding. Evaluation of endo-vaginal sonography (with pulsed doppler) as a screening method in patients with hormonal replacement therapy is in progress, but no definite recommendation can be made.

1.5. Ovarian carcinoma

Due to the localisation of ovaries, diagnosis of this cancer is often made at advanced stages. The risk factors are not well known (except some cases of family tumors) and the incidence is not important, so elaboration of screening programs seems difficult. Except in cases of family ovarian tumors, endo-vaginal sonography (with pulsed doppler) or serum markers (CA 125, CA 19/9...) are not efficient for ovarian carcinoma screening.

2. Breast and gynecologic carcinomas in transplant recipients

There is an increased incidence of certain cancer in transplant recipients. It seems that this is due to the immuno-suppressive treatments requisite for the transplantation. But epidemiological studies have shown that the incidence of breast, ovarian and endometrial carcinomas are not increased in transplant patients [1].

Femal transplant patients are known to have an increased incidence of HPV associated lesions within the genital region compared with the normal population. In situ and invasive carcinomas of the uterine cervix are 14 fold more frequent in transplant recipients [2]. Also, even if carcinomas of the anogenital area are rare in the general population, there is a 100-fold increased risk of development of these malignancies in transplant patients. It has been emphasized that in immuno-suppressed women, anogenital intraepithelial neoplasia tends to persist, recur, and extend to adjacent areas of the cervix, vagina, vulva and anus in spite of conventional therapy. If not cleared, the lesions can become invasive. This is a "field effect" promoted by HPV infection and leading to multicentric indepedent primary carcinomas involving the ectocervix, vagina, vulva, perineal and perianal skin. Also, it is well known that warts are very frequent in transplant recipients (affecting more than 40% of patients) and recent studies have demonstrated that there is a significantly higher rate of detection of HPV type 16/18 in the women with allografts, in particular in patients who have been immunosuppressed for more than 5 years [3]. All these datas demonstrate that allograft related immune-suppression facilitates the development of epithelial abnormalities in the presence of HPV infection. But other co-factors (as smoking, sexual activity, genital infection with herpes virus...) are involved in the oncogenic effect of HPV infection.

A disturbing feature is that transplant patients with invasive cervical or anogenital lesions, are much younger than their counterparts in the general population. Also it seems that these epithelial abnormalities and invasive lesions are more aggressive in women with allografts [4].

These results should lead to intensification of screening methods for cervical and anogenital lesions in transplant patients whatever their age is.

3. Screening before transplantation

Concerning breast, endometrial and ovarian carcinomas, due to their non-modified incidence in immuno-suppressed patients, the recommendations should be similar to the ones stated for the general population.

For breast cancer screening, a clinical exam is recommended, and if the patient is older than 50 years (or younger with family risk factors) with no mammography performed during the last 2 years, a new bilateral mammography should be realized.

For endometrial cancer, the main point is to ask for post-menopausal bleeding and to risk factors. Also the clinical exam can help to find an enlarged uterus.

For ovarian carcinomas, a clinical exam should try to find enlarged ovaries.

It has to be noticed that, usually during the pre-transplant check-up, a pelvic sonography is performed. This exam can help to screen for endometrial or ovarian carcinoma.

Concerning cervical and ano-genital carcinomas, the problem is different. Due to the increased risk of these malignancies in immuno-suppressed patients, a specific and intensive screening should be performed. Before transplantation, an important gynecologic exam is necessary. This evaluation should try to find any sign of HPV infection and/or genital dysplasia. So a Pap-smear, a colposcopy (with acetic acid and iodine solutions), and an extensive evaluation under colposcopy (with acetic acid and eventually toluidine blue) of all the ano-genital epithelium are required. All abnormal areas should be biopsied. And before transplantation all areas of HPV infection and/or genital dysplasia should be treated adequately (with laser vaporization, resection or 5-fluorouracil vaginal cream). It is recommended to have eradicated all lesions before performing the transplantation. Concerning HPV testing with use of PCR or blotting techniques, its interest in the evaluation of genital HPV infection is poor due to the lack of clinical correlation of these techniques. So they should not be performed routinely.

4. Screening after transplantation

Concerning screening for breast, endometrial and ovarian carcinomas, the recommendations are similar to thoses stated for the general population because the incidence of these malignancies remain the same as the one observed in the general population.

But, concerning cervical and anogenital carcinomas screening, due to their elevated incidence in immuno-suppressed patients in relation to an increased aggressiveness of oncogenic HPV infection, specific prevention methods should be applied. As it has been reported that there is a high rate of false negative results with Pap-smear screening [5], there is a need for colposcopy examination in women with allografts (irrespective of the results of previous cervical smears).Also an extensive evaluation under colposcopy (with acetic acid and eventually toluidine blue) of all the anogenital epithelium is required. All abnormal areas should be biopsied. These evaluations (Pap-smear, colposcopy and 'anogenitoscopy') should be repeated yearly. In case of signs of HPV infection or genital dysplasia, due to the increased risk of progression, all abnormal areas should be adequately treated. The recommended therapy are: laser vaporization or loop electro-resection,and 5-fluorouracil vaginal cream or interferon therapy in case of extensive lesions. Another point of interest is that these epithelial abnormalities occur usually a long time (7–8 years) after the transplantation. So cervical and anogenital screening should be performed yearly whatever is the delay after transplantation.

References

1. Sheil AGR, Flavel S, Disney APS, Mathew TH, Hall BM. Cancer incidence in renal transplant patients treated with Azathioprine or Cyclosporine. Transplantation proceedings 1987; XIX: 2214–2216.
2. Penn I. Cancers of the anogenital region in renal transplant recipients. Cancer 1986; 58: 611–616.

3. Lewenssohn-Fuchs I, Wester D, Bistoletti P, Elfgren K, Ohlman S, Dillner J, Dalianis T. Serological responses to human papillomavirus type 16 antigens in women before and after renal transplantation. J Med Virol 1993; 40: 188–192.
4. Alloub MI, Barr BBB, McLaren KM, Smith IW, Bunney MH, Smart GE. Human papillomavirus infection and cervical intraepithelial neoplasia in women with renal allografts. Br Med J 1989; 298: 153–156.
5. Schield PW, Daunter B, Wright RG. The Pap-smear revisited. Aust NZ J Obstet Gynaecol 1987; 27: 269–282.

7. Results of renal transplantation for Wilms' tumour

MARIE-FRANCE GAGNADOUX, DANIEL BEURTON, DOMINIQUE JAN, YANN RÉVILLON, CLAIRE FÉKÉTÉ, CHANTAL LOIRAT, JEAN-BERNARD PALCOUX, JANINE BEDROSSIAN, DOMINIQUE DURAND, JEAN-MICHEL ZUCKER, JEAN LEMERLE & MICHEL BROYER

Introduction

Wilms' tumour is an uncommon indication for renal transplantation in children. The incidence of end-stage renal failure (ESRF) in Wilms' tumour, indeed, is estimated to be as low as 1% of all Wilms' tumours (10% of bilateral tumours) in two large recent series [1, 2], and is decreasing with better surgical and medical management.

The first attempts to renal transplantation in children with Wilms' tumour, in the 70's, entailed a high mortality rate; however, as early as 1979, PENN [3] showed that transplantation could be safely performed provided a minimal waiting time of 2 years after the treatment of malignancy. The review of 29 published cases by PAIS et al. in 1992 [4] confirmed this finding: mortality was 79% when the waiting time was less than one year whereas it was only 27% when the delay exceeded one year. In a recent study of 76 cases by PENN in 1995 [5], no recurrence was observed in the patients grafted more than 28 months after the removal of tumour. Our series of 17 transplantations in 13 patients confirms this rather optimistic results.

Patients and methods

Our series is comprised of *13 patients* affected with Wilms' tumour during childhood (at 1 to 9 years of age), who received a renal graft in childhood in our hospital (N = 11) or in adulthood in other hospitals (N = 2), between 1979 and 1992. Their age at the first transplantation was 4 to 21 years; 7 were under 10 years of age.

In our series of 806 transplanted children from 1973 to 1993, Wilms' tumour accounts for 1,5% of primary diseases.

J.L. Touraine et al. (eds.), Cancer in Transplantation. Prevention and Treatment, 53–55.

The causes of end-stage renal failure of these patients were the following:

- *bilateral tumours*: 7 patients. In 4, a bilateral nephrectomy had to be performed for an oncological or a technical reason, and ESRF followed immediately the surgery. In the other 3 patients, a progressive sclerosis of the remnant parenchyma occurred 6 to 19 years after a conservative surgery.
- *tumour of a solitary kidney*: 1 patient.
- *associated glomerulopathy*: 4 patients. In 3 cases there was a diffuse mesangial sclerosis, part of the Drash syndrome, which associates nephroblastoma, pseudo-hermaphroditism, and glomerulopathy in very young children. In the 4th patient a focal and segmental hyalinosis developed in the controlateral kidney over 16 years, the relation with Wilms' tumour remaining uncertain.
- *nephrotoxic chemotherapy* in 1 patient who had received an overdose of cisplatinum.

The age at ESRF ranged from 1.5 to 20 years (mean = 8 years).

Two patients had developed metastasis (lung: 2, testicule: 1) shortly after the tumour removal and had been successfuly treated.

The treatment of malignancy in these patients associated chemotherapy pre and/or post-operatively in all cases, radiotherapy in 7 of 13, and surgery in all cases. All remnant renal tissue had been removed before transplantation in all cases except the 2 oldest patients, whose follow-up after the occurrence of malignancy was longer than 15 years.

The minimal delay between the removal of the last malignancy and the transplantation was always longer than 2 years. It was 2 to 3 years in 8 patients, 4 and 7 years in 2 patients, and longer than 15 years in 3 patients. These 13 patients received *17 grafts* (2 grafts in 4 patients). Only one graft was from a living donor and the other 16 were cadaver kidney grafts.

The immunosuppressive regimen was the same as in other patients of the same period (prednisone, azathioprine, ± antilymphocyte serum, ± ciclosporine).

Results

1) Oncological results

With a patients' follow-up after the first transplantation of 0.5 to 15 years (mean = 5.3 years), we observed no recurrence, no metastasis and no second malignancy.

2) Patient survival

The patient survival in these patients is 92% at 2 years, and 83% at 5 years. These values are not different from those observed in the other patients with non-malignant diseases.

Two deaths occurred, one from CMV infection after a failed second graft, and one from unknown cause in the patient's native country.

3) Complications

No specific complication was observed in these patients ; in particular, there were no excessive per-operative difficulties related to previous surgery, no particular sensitivity to immunosuppressive drugs (azathioprine, or antilymphocyte serum), and no excess of infectious complications.

4) Graft survival

There were 8 graft losses, from causes unrelated to primary disease: rejection in 4 patients, graft thrombosis in 2, non fonctioning graft in 1, patient's death in 1. Nine grafts are currently functioning with a follow-up of 2 to 11 years (mean = 4 years).

The graft survival rate of 81% at 1 year, 75% at 2 years, and 60% at 5 years is not significantly different from observed in our whole series.

Commentary

These results are in agreement with the published reports [3, 4, 5], and confirm that, in children previously affected with Wilms' tumour, renal transplantation can be safely performed after 2 years of cancer remission. No recurrence, metastasis or second cancer was observed in our series. No specific complication could be attributed to the primary disease, and, finally the patient survival and the graft outcome were not different of those obtained in patients affected with non malignant primary diseases.

References

1. Tournade MF. Place of kidney transplantation in the treatment of Wilms' tumour. Proceedings of the XXVIth meeting of the International Society of Pediatric Oncology. 1994; Sept. 20–24, Paris.
2. Ritchey ML, Green DM, Thomas P, Haase G, Shochat S. Renal failure in Wilms' tumour. Proceedings of the XXVIth meeting of the International Society of Pediatric Oncology. 1994; Sept. 20–24, Paris.
3. Penn I. Renal transplantation for Wilms' tumour: report of 20 cases. J Urol 1979; 122: 793–794.
4. Pais E, Pirson Y, Squifflet JP et al. Kidney transplantation in patients with Wilms' tumour. Transplantation, 1992; 53: 782–785.
5. Penn I. Primary kidney tumours before and after renal transplantation. Transplantation, 1995; 59: 480–485.

8. Prevention of recurrence after liver transplantation for hepatocellular carcinoma

HENRI BISMUTH, RENÉ ADAM, DENIS CASTAING,
LAURENCE CHICHE & JOSEPH S. RACCUIA

Hepatocellular carcinoma (HCC) when left untreated has an extremely poor prognosis. Liver transplantation in certain situations has proven benefit despite a high incidence of recurrence, although, survival at 5 years, is still the lowest compared to other indications for transplantation. We have, since our initial retrospective report [1], carefully selected patients with a chance for cure based upon the size and number of lesions. Subsequently, in this second prospective period, the results of this new approach were reviewed with emphasis on evaluating factors of recurrence and survival for patients with known HCC in cirrhosis.

Patients and results

Liver transplantation was performed in 92 patients for known HCC in cirrhosis over a 10 year period from 1984 to 1994. Since our initial analysis [1] we have evaluated our morphologic criteria prospectively in 32 (35%) patients selected for treatment with liver transplantation. The etiology of the cirrhoses included post-hepatic (71%), alcoholic (16%), and various (primary biliary cirrhosis, primary sclerosing cholangitis and cryptogenic) other types of cirrhosis (13%). Viral status at the time of liver transplantation was positive for HBS and/or HCV in most patients (78%). The majority of patients (80%) were asymptomatic, with tumors less than 30 mm (56%) and less than 3 nodules (80%). The severity of cirrhosis was divided by grade A (38%), grade B (41%) and grade C (21%). After transplantation postoperative complications occurred in 13 (14%) patients and there were 4 (4%) deaths. Overall survival for all patients for 3, 5, and 7 years was 59, 55 and 51%, while disease-free survival was 55, 46 and 42%. The mean follow-up was 3.6 ± 2.2 years (range from 1 to 10 years).

Prospective application of our initial results [1] was applied (Table 1) and lesions stratified for LT were less numerous and although the majority of tumors were larger than 30 mm there was an obvious increase in the trend

J.L. Touraine et al. (eds.), Cancer in Transplantation. Prevention and Treatment, 57–61.

Table 1. Liver transplantation. Evolution of patient selection.

	n = 60 (1985–1991) Retrospective	n = 32 (1992–1994) Prospective
Number:		
1–2 Nodules	27 (45%)	25 (78%)
≥ 3 Nodules	33 (55%)	7 (22%)
Size:		
≤ 30 mm	21 (35%)	18 (56%)
> 30 mm	39 (65%)	14 (44%)
Size and Number:		
≤ 30 mm, ⩽ 3 Nodules	21(35%)	21(67%)
>30 mm, > 3 Nodules	14 (23%)	5(16%)
3 Year Survival:		
Global	55%	77%
Disease-Free	49%	70%

towards smaller lesions when compared to the first, retrospective period. The salient feature of this prospective application demonstrated a significant increase in the number of patients treated with small (⩽ 30 mm) and less numerous (⩽ 3 nodules) from the first period previously reported (35%) [1] compared to the present second period (67%). This demonstrated a significant increase with both global survival in the first period (55%) [1] versus (77%) prospectively in the second period, and similarly disease-free survival increased from (49%) to (70%) when these factors were analyzed. The influence of tumor size on survival is demonstrated by global survival at 3, 5 and 7 years of 71, 67 and 67% for lesions less than 30 mm, with disease-free survival of 68, 58, and 58%. The lesions which were greater than 30 mm demonstrated global survival at 3, 5 and 7 years of 45, 37 and 28%, with disease free survival of 38, 35 and 24%.

The influence of the number of nodules has demonstrated global survival at 3, 5 and 7 years to be 63, 60 and 60% for 1 to 3 nodules, with a disease-free survival of 60, 58, and 58% respectively. When there were more than 3 nodules the 3, 5 and 10 year global survival was 42, 36 and 36 percent, with a disease-free survival of 35, 35 and 29%.

When these factors were combined survival at 3, 5 and 7 years was 72, 68 and 68% for less than 30 mm and up to three nodules. Tumors greater than 30 mm with up to three nodules demonstrated survivals of 58, 58 and 39%; tumors more than three nodules and less than 30 mm survival was 58, 58 and

58; and if more than three nodules and greater than 30 mm the survival was 32% at 3 years and no survivors at 5 years.

The existence of a portal tumor thrombus revealed a 3 year global survival of 40% and a disease-free survival of 15 percent, and there were no survivors after 5 years. When this is compared to patients without portal tumoral thrombus the global survival at 3, 5 and 10 years was 65, 63 and 56 percent with a disease-free survival of 64, 60 and 52%.

Discussion

The incidence of viral cirrhosis from hepatitis B and C virus is increasing and it is the most common etiologic agent associated with HCC in the world today [2]. The frequency of HCC is steadily multiplying with almost 1 million new cases per year, highest in Africa and increasing in Europe. There is a 6 percent per year conversion rate to HCC in the cirrhotic population [3]. Although alcohol injection and transarterial chemoembolization have been effective adjuvant therapies. Liver resection in mild cirrhosis is applied when resectable, however, this is associated with high rate (70%) of recurrence. Liver transplantation is the only chance for complete and total cure, however, the indications are usually limited to patients with moderate to severe cirrhosis and is most effective when the lesions display morphologic features indicating prolonged global and disease-free survival can be obtained.

In the Paul Brousse series, the size and the number of lesions were substantial factors of recurrence and long-term survival retrospectively [1] and confirmed prospectively (Table 1). The smaller lesions which might represent the only detectable disease at the time of surgery and, therefore, the presence of concomitant unknown lesions is theoretically treated by the total hepatectomy. In our experience at 5 years small tumors had improved survival (67%) over larger lesions (37%), and single known lesions had a better survival (73%) than multiple (> 3) nodules (36%). When both number and size of tumors are examined together, better survival was demonstrated with small (< 30 mm) less numerous (< 3 nodules) tumors. The recurrence-free survival was significantly better with lesions which were smaller (< 30 mm) and less numerous (< 3 nodules) when transplantation (56%) is compared to resection (18%, $p < 0.05$) [1]. Similarly, large (> 30 mm), more numerous (> 3 nodules) lesions have the highest recurrences when compared to smaller, less numerous lesions, and when these factors are combined the prognosis is even worse. Similar results have also been suggested by Iwatsuki [4] and Ismail [5] in series of HCC after liver transplantation.

Tumor thrombi in the portal vein, although not considered a contraindication by many, have demonstrated in our results a disease-free survival dramatically worse in patient with portal tumor invasion. This holds true even when limited to a segment (15% at 3 years) as compared to patients without portal tumor thrombosis (64% at 3 years). We have, therefore, adjusted our policy and now consider this a contraindication for transplantation. Vascular invasion of the tumor into the portal, hepatic vein and artery, was also associated with decreased long-term survival (30%) compared to those without invasion (67%) in our series. This has been confirmed in other series [6].

The tumor morphology at the time of the diagnosis is the best predictor of outcome, and there is no evidence yet indicating that altering the tumor morphology with neoadjuvant chemotherapy positively affects the rate of recurrence or the long-term survival. However, we do initiate chemoembolization [7] once the decision to transplant is made, depending upon the degree of cirrhosis, while patients await liver transplantation.

Complete preoperative evaluation underscores the necessity of strict and frequent follow-up combined with a minimal wait for a liver graft. In the interim, if the situation changes, indications for transplantation should be re-evaluated. The surgery-related factors are related to diligently search for positive lymph nodes and extrahepatic disease at the time of transplantation laparotomy. This cannot be underestimated or overemphasized since treatment strategy can change even at this time. Accordingly, our policy is to perform a complete exploration, including intraoperative ultrasound and to examine suspicious deposits for tumor with multiple frozen-section biopsies just prior to final decision for transplantation.

Ideally, patients with lesions less than 30 mm with a maximum of three nodules, and no evidence of portal tumoral thrombus, are the candidates with the best outcomes in our experience. The formation of this approach stems from the first retrospective study period [1] where we identified factors associated with decreased recurrence and improved overall survival. Presently, in this second prospective period, application of these prognostic elements, in fact, now confirmed these morphologic criteria by demonstrating improved global (77%) and disease-free survival (70%) after liver transplantation for known HCC in cirrhosis at 3 years compared to (55% and 49%) during the first period [1].

In conclusion, prevention of recurrence after liver transplantation for known HCC in cirrhosis begins with proper patient selection. All patients should be offered an in depth array of multimodality therapies up to and including liver resection. Consistent, close and frequent evaluation with re-stratification of therapy reflects the mobility necessary for treating HCC. Presently the prospective application of variables such as tumor size ($\leqslant$30 mm) and number ($\leqslant$3) nodules has been associated with prolonged global and disease-free survival, similar to patients with unknown (< 10 mm) lesions and those without cirrhosis. In the future, application of split-liver grafts in an effort to make transplantation available to more patients with HCC, and the use of tumor markers such as circulating albumin mRNA [8] to aid in predicting the best individual for liver transplantation will be further evaluated.

References

1. Bismuth H, Chiche L, Adam R, et al.: Liver resection versus transplantation for hepatocellular carcinoma in cirrhotic patients. Ann Surg 1993; 218: 145–151.
2. Colombo M: Hepatocellular carcinoma. J Hepatol 1992; 15: 225–236.
3. Carr BI: An assay for micrometastatic hepatocellular carcinoma. Gastroenterology. 1994; 106: 264–267.
4. Iwatzuki S, Starzl TE, Sheahan DG, et al.: Hepatic resection versus transplantation for hepatocellular carcinoma. Ann Surg 1991; 214: 221–229.
5. Ismail T, Angrisani L, Gunson BK, et al.: Primary hepatic malignancy: The role of liver transplantation. Br J Surg 1990; 77: 983–987.
6. O'Grady, JG, Polsen RJ, Rolles K, et al.: Liver transplantation for malignant disease: Results in 93 consecutive patients. Ann Surg, 1988; 207: 373–379; Cancer therapy. Ann Surg 1985; 202: 401–407.
7. Bismuth H, Morino M, Sherlock DG, et al.: Primary treatment of hepatocellular carcinoma by arterial chemoembolization. Ann Surg 1992; 163: 387–394.
8. Matsumura M, Nima Y, Kato N, et al.: Detection of alfafetoprotein mRNA, as an indicator of hematogenous spreading hepatocellular carcinoma, in the circulation: A possible predictor of metastatic hepatocellular carcinoma. Hepatology 1994; 20: 1418–1425.

PART THREE

De novo malignancies after transplantation

9. Skin cancers in organ transplant recipients

SYLVIE EUVRARD, JEAN KANITAKIS, CLAIRE POUTEIL-NOBLE,
YVETTE CHARDONNET, GEORGES DUREAU,
JEAN LOUIS TOURAINE, DANIEL SCHMITT, MICHEL FAURE,
ALAIN CLAUDY & JEAN THIVOLET

Skin cancers

Introduction

Skin cancers especially squamous cell carcinomas (SCC) are the most frequent malignancies in organ transplant recipients; they are often preceded by viral warts and solar keratoses and represent a model of viral carcinogenesis. They appear on sun-exposed areas, tend to be multiple and may have an aggressive course. Human papillomaviruses along with other co-carcinogenic factors such as ultraviolet radiation and immunosuppressive treatment seem to be involved in their development [1, 2].

Because of the long experience with renal transplantation, most publications have been devoted to carcinomas appearing in renal transplant recipients. New data are now available concerning the appearance of these lesions in cardiac [3-6] or hepatic transplant recipients [7].

Epidemiologic factors

The frequency of skin cancers increases with time after transplantation reaching 40%-60% of renal transplant patients after 20 years and also depends on the amount of sun-exposure; the corresponding figures vary from 40% in northern countries [8] to 60% in Australia [9]. In our experience, the development of premalignant and/or malignant epithelial lesions is almost twice as frequent in cardiac than in renal transplant recipients. This difference could be even greater if the shorter follow-up time of cardiac transplant recipients is considered. This is in agreement with a previous series showing that a disproportionately large number of tumours occur in recipients of non-renal organs [10].

Delay: The time lapse from transplantation to the development of skin cancers is on average 7 to 8 years in renal transplant patients [11, 12] and decreases with increasing latitude (less than 3 years in Australia) [13]. For

J.L. Touraine et al. (eds.), Cancer in Transplantation. Prevention and Treatment, 65–72.

patients living in the same latitude, this delay is much shorter after cardiac than renal transplantation (mean 3.9 ± 2.3 vs 8.6 ± 6 years) [6].

Age: The development of the first carcinomas occurs at a significantly younger average age compared with nonimmunosuppressed persons. For example, the mean age for BCC and SCC is 47 and 49.3 years in renal and 59.6 and 58.2 years in cardiac transplant recipients [6] while the corresponding figure for non-immunosuppressed patients is around 70 years [14].

Male sex is a risk factor for the development of carcinomas [12], especially among cardiac transplant recipients [6]. The incidence of skin carcinoma is about 30 times higher in males and 20 times in females when compared with nonimmunosuppressed groups except for the lip where there is a female to male preponderance of 9:1 [15].

Skin type: Patients display a predominance of fair-skinned type and light-coloured eyes (especially those with SCC); this finding is in accordance with previous reports of patients with skin tumours namely SCC [16]- and underlines the role of ultraviolet radiation in cancer development.

Clinical characteristics and course

Location: Carcinomas are mainly located on sun-exposed areas. Patients who receive their transplant before the age of 40 have predominantly extracephalic lesions (80%). In young renal transplant recipients, the dorsum of the hands represents 25% of all locations [6]. By contrast, patients grafted after the age of 40 years develop predominantly cephalic skin carcinomas, as is observed in the general population [17]. Remarkably, basal cell carcinomas are observed either on the cephalic extremity or the upper trunk [6].

Carcinomas are often associated with warts and various epithelial lesions such as premalignant keratoses, Bowen's disease and keratoacanthomas (KA). The clinical aspects are often confusing: SCC may simulate warts or KA. The differential diagnosis between KA and SCC is sometimes difficult; therefore the development of KA must be considered as important as that of SCC since they may have an aggressive course [13].

Carcinomas are predominantly SCC; the SCC/BCC ratio is reversed as compared to that of the general population: 0.1:1 [11] and varies from 1.2:1 to 15:1 [1, 9–11]. This reversal – which is much more prominent in renal than in cardiac transplant recipients (2.3 *vs* 1.08:1) – seems less pronounced in Scandinavian countries.

Course: All lesions tend to be multiple, and after several years some patients may develop over 50 tumours. SCC sometimes show a very rapid growth enlarging within a short time and may be complicated by repeated local recurrences after surgical treatment. The risk of metastasis per patient (6 to 8%) [4, 9] appears higher than in control groups where it varies from 3.6% [17] to 5.2% [18]. An older age at the time of appearance of SCC, the multiplicity of SCC and the cephalic location seem to be factors of poor prognosis [19]. From an histological point of view a prevailing feature of aggressive SCC seems to be their thickness, inasmuch as most lesions reach at least the subcutaneous adipose tissue.

Pathogenic factors

The role of HPV is suggested clinically by the presence of warts in the same locations as carcinomas and histologically by the presence of intermediate forms from common warts to invasive carcinoma. There are now several virological studies on large series of tumours which have shown HPV DNA in about 50% of premalignant lesions and carcinomas from renal graft patients [1, 2, 20, 21]. This is in contrast with the results obtained in similar lesions from the general population.

Virological studies have been carried out on the distribution of HPV types in renal graft patients by molecular biology methods. The usual tissue-specific distribution of HPV is switched in transplant recipients; hence mucosal types can be found on exposed areas. Types that are known to be oncogenic have been detected in benign lesions and benign types may be found within malignant lesions. Epidermodysplasia verruciformis (EV)-associated HPV types or related types have been detected by several authors [1, 21, 22]. Other HPV types may also be present since a limited number of HPV types were tested out of over 70 distinct types that have now been identified. However, although most studies report concordant results despite the heterogeneity of the technique used for HPV detection (PCR, *in situ* hybridization or Southern blot), some authors failed to detect HPV DNA within carcinomas [23, 24]; these discrepancies could be due to a varying sensitivity of the methods used or to the choice of the HPV types sought. The role of the virus remains unclear: HPV necessitate other cocarcinogenic factors; they could be implicated in the initiation of carcinomas by activation of c-*myc* and/or c-Ha-*ras* oncogenes [25] or interaction with UV-induced p53 gene mutations [26].

Immunodepression itself is certainly involved since an increase of cutaneous cancers has been reported in patients undergoing hemodialysis [27], renal failure being accompanied by cellular immune deficiency; on the other hand carcinomas associated with multiple warts have also been reported in AIDS patients [28].

The role of a graft-antigenic stimulation is suggested by the fact that graft recipients develop more cancers than other subjects under immunosuppressive treatment.

The specific role of each drug is still debated [29, 30]; there is also varying individual sensitivity to immunosuppressive treatment so that the role of the mean doses of the drugs is difficult to assess. Renal graft recipients with dysplastic lesions have significantly higher levels of the active azathioprine metabolite 6-thioguanine in their red blood cells than do matched controls without lesions [31]. Several cases of carcinoma development following cyclosporine introduction have been reported [32, 33]; in two patient groups matched as to age and number of years after transplantation, Shuttleworth et al [30] found more dysplastic lesions in the cyclosporine group. The higher incidence of tumours in cardiac transplant recipients can tentatively be explained by the greater intensity of the immunosuppressive treatment. On the whole, the length and intensity of immunosuppressive treatment is probably more important than the nature of the drug.

Ultraviolet radiation: the most decisive factor for the development of skin carcinomas is probably ultraviolet radiation since warts and carcinomas appear on sun-exposed areas and in light-skinned patients. UV light produces a decrease in the number of epidermal Langerhans cells. Although contradictory results have been reported [34], Langerhans cells may be also altered by the immunosuppressive treatment. UVB radiation converts Langerhans cells from immunogenic to tolerogenic antigen-presenting cells. This induces a local immunodeficiency that may facilitate HPV proliferation and tumour promotion. Sun exposure before transplantation has to be considered [16].

Genetic factors could also intervene in the progression towards malignancy. It was found that renal transplant patients with skin cancer presented no switch of the humoral response (IgM to IgG) to EV-associated HPV and were predominantly HLA-DR7 [35]. The results of various studies concerning the influence of HLA antigen (distribution or matching) in organ transplant recipients with skin cancer are contradictory [5, 15, 35, 36]; however, an increased frequency of HLA-DR7 among patients with skin cancers as compared with the remaining ones was reported in two independent studies [35, 36].

Age at transplantation: the greater frequency of skin cancer that we observed in cardiac compared with renal transplant patients could at least in part be accounted for by their older age at transplantation (average 16 years); this is in disagreement with the results of Birkeland on the risk of cancers at all sites which was reported to be increased for patients grafted before the age of 45 years [15].

The reason why cardiac transplant recipients develop proportionally more BCC than renal transplant recipients is not clear. The fact that they are older at the time of transplantation could be a possible explanation. In favour of this contention is the fact that the SCC/BCC ratio was reported to be much higher in pediatric organ transplant recipients than in adults [37]; furthermore, our patients who had both types of lesions tended to develop BCC later than SCC. Nevertheless, renal and cardiac transplant recipients with BCC were not significantly older than those with SCC.

Finally, the possibility that the nature of the organ grafted could influence the type of (cutaneous) tumours cannot be ruled out. Liver transplant recipients also seem to develop more frequently BCC than SCC [7].

Treatment

Most SCC are successfully treated by surgical excision. Topical retinoids can be helpful to treat multiple premalignant lesions and prevent the occurrence of carcinomas [38]. Resurfacing the back of the hands may be useful in renal transplant patients having multiple lesions over this area [39]. When carcinomas become numerous or aggressive a reduction of the immunosuppressive treatment should be attempted [40]. Systemic retinoids alone [41] or in combination with topical treatment [42] can also be used since they slow down the development of carcinomas and dysplastic lesions without inducing graft rejection; unfortunately, their action is merely suspensive and their long-term use is limited by the frequent increase of serum lipids and hepatic intolerance. Hence, systemic retinoids should be reserved to the most severe cases either during one or two years if the immunosuppressive treatment can be substantially reduced or definitively when tapering of immunosuppressive treatment is not feasible. If tumoural progression is not abrogated by these methods and metastases develop, chemotherapy or interferon α could be added; however, the risk of acute rejection of the graft due to interferon should be seriously considered. Radiotherapy seems ineffective; we have followed patients who developed recurrences while receiving this treatment.

Anogenital cancers

Carcinomas of the anogenital region (anus, perianal skin and external genitalia) are rare in the general population. The risk for their development is one of the most increased in transplant patients [43]. For instance, vulvar cancer is 30 times more frequent than in control groups [15, 44]. The detailed study of Penn [45] reveals an average time interval after transplantation of 7 to 8 years and a female preponderance. The anus and perianal area represent 60% of locations in males and 30% in females whereas in females, vulva is involved in 80% of the cases, in males, genitalia are involved in only 40% of patients. Regional lymph-node involvement occurs in 11% of patients. Lesions tend to be multiple especially in female patients who may present simultaneous or successive involvement of the anogenital area, the cervix (30%), vagina or urethra.

HPV are probably involved since about one third of patients have a past history of condylomata acuminata. However, studies concerning HPV infection in genitalia were performed in most cases on cervix and recently on anus and showed frequently the presence of oncogenic types [46–48]; they confirmed that renal allograft recipients are at high risk of developing anal and genital HPV infection and neoplasia [49]. Similarly to non immunosuppressed groups, risk factors include other infections (especially chlamydia and herpes simplex), number of partners and cigarette smoking.

Treatment includes surgery, decrease of the immunosuppressive treatment, and applications of 5 fluoro-uracile for *in situ* lesions.

In conclusion, carcinomas in graft patients represent a model of viral carcinogenesis. HPV probably act synergistically with other cocarcinogenic factors, UV radiation and immunosuppressive treatment being the most decisive ones. Therefore, patients should be advised to avoid sun exposure as soon as they apply for grafting. The presence of warts in graft recipients must lead to a careful dermatologic surveillance; treatment of aggressive SCC in transplant recipients may be very difficult and therefore efforts must be carried out towards prevention through regular dermatological examination and early destruction of premalignant lesions. The comparative study of cutaneous premalignant and malignant epithelial lesions in renal and cardiac transplant patients brings reflexion on the biologic behaviour of BCC and SCC in the course of immunodepression. Further studies are required to assess the respective role of the grafted organ, immunosuppressive treatment and age in the occurrence of cutaneous malignancies.

References

1. Barr BBB, Benton EC, Mc Laren K, et al. Human papillomavirus infection and skin cancer in renal allograft recipients. Lancet 1989; i: 124–9.
2. Euvrard S, Chardonnet Y, Pouteil-Noble C, et al. Association of skin malignancies with various and multiple carcinogenic and non carcinogenic human papillomaviruses in renal transplant recipients. Cancer 1993; 72: 2198–2206.
3. O'Connell BM, Abel EA, Nickoloff BJ, et al. Dermatologic complications following heart transplantation. J Heart Transplant 1986; 5: 430–6.
4. Penn I. Tumors after renal and cardiac transplantation. Hematol Oncol Clin North America 1993; 7: 431–45.
5. Espana A, Redondo P, Fernandez AL, et al. Skin cancer in heart transplant recipients. J Am Acad Dermatol 1995; 32: 458–465.
6. Euvrard S, Kanitakis J, Pouteil-Noble C, et al. Comparative epidemiologic study of premalignant and malignant epithelial cutaneous lesions developing after renal and cardiac transplantation. J Am Acad Dermatol 1995 33, 222–9.
7. Levy M, Backman L, Husberg B et al. De novo malignancy following liver transplantation: a single-center study. Transplant Proc 1993; 25: 1397–9.
8. Hartevelt MM, Bouwes-Bavinck JN, Koote A, Vermeer BJ, Vandenbroucke JP. Incidence of skin cancer after renal transplantation in the Netherlands. Transplantation 1990; 49: 506–9.
9. Sheil AGR. Development of malignancy following renal transplantation in Australia and New Zealand. Transplant Proc 1992; 24: 1275–9.
10. Penn I, Brunson M.E. Cancers after cyclosporine therapy. Transplant Proc 1988; 20: suppl.3, 885–92.
11. Gupta AK, Cardella CJ, Habermann HF. Cutaneous malignant neoplasms in patients with renal transplants. Arch Dermatol 1986; 122: 1288–93.
12. Liddington M, Richardson AJ, Higgins RM, et al. Skin cancer in renal transplant recipients. Br J Surg 1989; 76: 1002–5.
13. Hardie IR, Strong RW, Hartley LCJ, et al. Skin cancer in causacian renal allograft recipients living in a subtropical climate. Surgery 1980; 87: 177–83.

14. Cohen E, Komorowski RA, Clowry LJ. Cutaneous complications in renal transplant recipients. Am J Clin Pathol 1987; 88: 32–7.
15. Birkeland S, Storm HH, Lamm LU et al: Cancer risk after renal transplantation in nordic countries. Int J Cancer 1995; 60: 183–9.
16. Bouwes Bavinck JN, De Boer A, Vermeer BJ, et al. Sunlight, keratotic skin lesions and skin cancer in renal transplant recipients. Br J Dermatol 1993; 129: 242–9.
17. Chuang TY, Popescu NA, Su WPD, Chute CGE. Squamous cell carcinoma: a population-based incidence study in Rochester, Minn. Arch Dermatol 1990; 126: 185–8.
18. Rowe DE, Carrol RJ, Day C. Prognostic factors for local recurrence, metastasis, and survival rates in squamous cell cerccinom of the skir., ear and lip. J Am Acad Dermatol 1992; 26: 976–90.
19. Euvrard S, Kanitakis J, Pouteil-Noble C, et al. Aggressive Squamous Cell Carcinomas in Organ Transplant Recipients. Transplant Proc 1995; 27: 1767–8.
20. Stark LA, Arends MJ, McLaren KM, et al. Prevalence of human papillomavirus DNA in cutaneous neoplasms from renal allograft recipients supports a possible viral role in tumour promotion. Br J Cancer 1994; 69: 222–9.
21. Shamanin V, Glover M, Rausch C, et al. Specific types of human papillomavirus found in benign proliferations and carcinomas of the skin in immunosuppressed patients. Cancer Res 1994; 54: 4610–3.
22. Tieben LM, Berkhout RJM, Smits HL, et al. Detection of epidermodysplasia verruciformis-like human papillomavirus types in malignant and pre-malignant skin lesions of renal transplant recipients. Br J Dermatol 1994; 131: 226–230.
23. Smith SE, Davis IC, Leshin B, Fleischer AB, White, WL, Feldman R. Absence of human papillomavirus in squamous cell carcinomas of non genital skin from immunocompromised renal transplant patients. Arch Dermatol 1993; 129: 1585–8.
24. McGregor JM, Farthing A, Crook T, et al. Post-transplant skin cancer: A possible role for p53 gene mutation but not for oncogenic human papillomaviruses. J Am Acad Dermatol 1994; 30: 701–6.
25. Pelisson I, Soler C, Pechoux C, et al: c-*myc* and c-Ha-*ras* cellular oncogenes and human papillomaviruses in benign and malignant cutaneous lesions. J Dermatol Sci 1992; 3: 56–67.
26. Pelisson I, Chardonnet Y, Euvrard S, Schmitt D. Immunohistochemical detection of p 53 protein in cutaneous lesions from transplant recipients harbouring human papillomavirus DNA. Virchows Archiv 1994; 424: 623–630.
27. Sheil AGR, Flavel S, Disney APS, Mathew TH. Cancer in dialysis and transplant patients. Transplant Proc 1985; 17: 195–8.
28. Milburn PB, Brandsma JL, Goldsman Cl, Teplitz ED, Herlman EI. Disseminated warts and evolving squamous cell carcinoma in a patient with acquired immunodeficiency syndrome. J Am Acad Dermatol 1988; 19: 401–5.
29. Calne RY. Cyclosporin in cadaveric renal transplantation: 5 year follow up of a multicentre trial. Lancet 1987; ii: 506–7.
30. Shuttleworth D, Marks R, Griffin PJA, Salaman JR. Epidermal dysplasia and cyclosporine therapy in renal transplant patients: a comparison with azathioprine. Br J Dermatol 1989; 120: 551–4.
31. Lennard L, Thomas MJ, Harrington CI, Maddocks JL. Skin cancer in renal transplant recipients is associated with increased concentrations of 6-thioguanine nucleotide in red blood cells. Br J Dermatol 1985; 113: 723–9.
32. Thompson JF, Allen R, Morris PJ, et al. Skin cancer in renal transplant patients treated with cyclosporin. Lancet 1985; i: 158–9.
33. Price ML, Tidman MJ, Young RW, Mac Donald DM. Cyclosporin A and cutaneous malignancy. Br J Dermatol 1985; 113 (suppl 29): 37.

34. Servitje O, Seron D, Ferrer I, Carrera M, Pagerols X, Peyri J. Quantitative and morphometric analysis of Langerhans cells in non-exposed skin in renal transplant patients. J Cutan Pathol 1991; 18: 106–11.
35. Bouwes Bavinck JN, Gissmann L, Claas FHJ, Van der Woude FJ, Vermeer BJ, et al. Relation between skin cancer humoral responses to human papillomaviruses, and HLA Class II Molecules in renal transplant recipients. J Immunol 1993; 151: 1579–86.
36. Czarnecki D, Watkins F, Leahy S, et al. Skin cancers and HLA frequencies in renal transplant recipients. Clin Lab Invest 1992; 185: 9–11.
37. Penn I. De novo malignancy in pediatric organ transplant recipients. J Pediat Surg 1994; 29: 221–8.
38. Euvrard S, Verschoore M, Touraine JL, et al. Topical retinoids for warts and keratoses in transplant recipients. Lancet 1992; 340: 48–9.
39. Van Zuuren EJ, Posma AN, Scholtens REM, Vermeer BJ, van der Woude FJ, Bouwes Bavinck. Resurfacing the back of the hand as treatment and prevention of multiple skin cancers in kidney transplant recipients. J Am Acad Dermatol 1994; 31: 760–4.
40. Euvrard S, Pouteil-Noble C, Kanitakis J, et al. Successive occurrence of T-cell and B-cell lymphomas after renal transplantation in a patient with multiple cutaneous squamous cell carcinomas. N Engl J Med 1992; 327: 1924–7.
41. Shuttleworth D, Marks R, Griffin PJA, Salaman JR. Treatment of cutaneous neoplasia with Etretinate renal transplant recipients. Quart J Med 1988; 68: 717–25.
42. Rook AH, Jaworsky C, Nguyen T, Grossman RA, Wolfe JT, Witmer WK, Kligman AM. Beneficial effect of low-dose systemic retinoid in combination with topical tretinoin for the treatment and prophylaxis of premalignant and malignant skin lesions in renal transplant recipients. Transplantation 1995; 59: 714–9.
43. Blohme I. Carcinoma of the vulva in renal transplant patients. Transplant Science 1994; 4: 6–8.
44. Sheil AGR, Flavel S, Disney APS, Mathew TH, Hall BM. Cancer incidence in renal transplant patients treated with Azathioprine or Cyclosporine. Transplant Proc 1987; 19: 2214–6.
45. Penn I. Cancers of the anogenital region in renal transplant recipients. Cancer 1986; 58: 611–6
46. Blessing K, McLaren KM, Morris R, et al. Detection of human papillomavirus in skin and genital lesions of renal allograft recipients by in situ hybridization. Histopathology 1990; 16: 181–5
47. Lewensohn-Fuchs I, Wester D, Bistoletti P, et al. Serological responses to human Papillomavirus type 16 Antigens in women before and after renal transplantation. J Med Virol 1993; 40: 188–192.
48. Ogunbiyi OA, Scholefield H, Raftery AT, et al. Prevalence of anal human papillomavirus infection and intraepithelial neoplasia in renal allograft recipients. Br J Surg 1994; 81: 365–7.
49. Touraine JL, Lavagna-Maurice C, Dargent D. Infections à HPV, dysplasies et néoplasies intra-épithéliales du col utérin chez les femmes immunodéprimées. Gynécologie 1990; 41: 323–6

10. Kaposi's sarcoma in organ transplantation (Lyon Experience, 1965–1995)

JEAN-LOUIS TOURAINE, PABLO RAFFAELE, JULES TRAEGER, JEANNE-LUCE GARNIER, NICOLE LEFRANCOIS, CLAIRE POUTEIL-NOBLE, ANNE-CLAIRE MARRAST, SAMEH DAOUD & SYLVIE EUVRARD

Introduction

Kaposi's sarcoma (KS) or Kaposi's disease has been especially observed in certain groups of patients: elderly individuals from Mediterranean countries or Central Europe, young Black Africans ("endemic forms"), AIDS patients (with a possibility of rapidly severe evolution of Kaposi's disease), homosexual males without HIV infection, transplant patients treated with immunosuppressive therapy. The frequency of this disease, formerly relatively rare, and its evolutive course, comparatively slow in the past, have been significantly modified with the emergence of the AIDS epidemic and with the rapidly increasing number of patients subjected to prolonged immunosuppressive therapy to prevent transplant rejection.

Among *de novo* cancers which occur in organ allograft recipients, KS ranked fifth on the frequency list, after cancers of skin and lips, lymphomas, carcinomas of lung and carcinomas of uterus, and before carcinomas of colon and rectum, carcinomas of kidney and carcinomas of breast [1]. In some countries such as Saudi Arabia it was even found to be the most common of all malignancies which develop in patients with a kidney transplant [2]. An epidemiologic study of KS incidence among renal transplant recipients was carried out in comparison with controls of the same ethnic origin. A 400-500 fold increase was found in the transplant population [3]. These data were confirmed by the analysis of I. Penn who observed that KS accounted for 4.13% of all cancers among organ transplant patients whereas it only represented 0.02-0.07% of all cancers in the general population of United States [1].

In Lyon we have observed 12 cases of KS among renal transplant patients over the last 30 years, a period during which 2500 transplants of the kidney or the pancreas have been performed. The six initial cases have been previously

J.L. Touraine et al. (eds.), Cancer in Transplantation. Prevention and Treatment, 73–80.

Table 1. Characteristics of patients who developed Kaposi's sarcoma

Characteristics	Number of patients or period of time
Male: Female ratio	11 pts: 1 pt
Origin:	
Italian	9/12 pts
Armenian	1/12 pts
French	2/12 pts
Mean age at KS detection	43.1 ± 8.9 yrs
Mean time on hemodialysis	42.8 ± 29.8 mos
Delay between transplant and KS detection	37.2 ± 26.7 mos (range 3* – 204 mos)
Previous blood transfusions (2–10)	12/12 pts
Positive HIV serology	0/12 pts
Positive HBV serology	3/12 pts
Positive HCV serology	2/12 pts
Positive CMV serology	11/12 pts
Reactivation of CMV infection	7/12 pts

* Limited KS (very low grade) was possibly present at the time of transplantation in 2 patients although it was detected 3 months later.

reported in a brief communication [4] and we now describe the whole group of 12 patients with KS.

Patients who developed KS

As shown in Table 1, the male predominance is significant. KS was found in only 1 female patient of our group, a finding in accordance with the very rare occurrence of KS among females of the general population, but with a larger desequilibrium than that noticed by I. Penn in the transplant population where the recorded male to female ratio was 3:1 [5].

The predominance of certain ethnic groups which are more susceptible to KS development was obvious in our experience: 9 of the 12 KS patients were of Italian origin although Italian patients only accounted for 20% of all our transplant population. The 3 non-Italian patients who developed KS were 2 French patients and 1 Armenian patient (Table 1).

The mean age of the patients at the time of KS detection was 43.1 years (Table 1). These patients had remained on hemodialysis for a varied period of time which averaged 42.8 months. The delay between transplantation and

Table 2. Characteristics of transplantation in patients who later developed Kaposi's sarcoma

Characteristics	Number of patients or number of cells
Transplants of:	
kidney alone	10 pts
kidney + pancreas	2 pts
Donors: unrelated cadaver	11 pts
related living donor	1 pt
Immunosuppressive treatment:	
ALG + AZA + CS	4 pts
CYS + AZA + CS	1 pt
ALG + CYS + AZA + CS	6 pts
OKT3 + CYS + AZA + CS	1 pt
CD4+ lymphocytes at the time of KS detection in transplant patients:	755 ± 214 cells/μl of blood

the identification of the first KS manifestations ranged from 3 to 204 months, with a mean of 37.2 months. It is very likely that the 2 patients with an obvious KS detected at 3 months could have a very low grade disease at the time of transplantation itself, prior to immunosuppressive treatment; one of these 2 patients has noted a very small purple spot of flat appearance at the time of surgery and it progressed to complete KS lesions in 3 months, probably due to immunosuppression.

All our patients had received blood transfusion in the past but it is fair to mention that a large majority of our transplant patients had been transfused since, until a recent period, we had a systematic transfusion protocole prior to transplantation. None of these 12 patients had positive HIV serology. Most of them, as in the general population, had positive CMV serology and 7 patients had a demonstrable reactivation of CMV infection during the period of time between transplantation and KS detection (Table 1). Three patients had a positive hepatitis B virus serology and 2 patients had a positive hepatitis C virus serology.

Immunosuppressive treatment

Our patients were treated with a variety of immunosuppressive drugs to prevent rejection of their kidney transplant (12 patients), associated with a pancreas transplant in 2 of them.

The transplanted kidney was provided by a related living donor in 1 case and by cadaveric donors in all other circumstances.

As shown in Table 2, the immunosuppressive treatment involved the association of anti-lymphocyte globulins (ALG), Azathioprine and Corticosteroids in 10 patients (4 patients with this treatment alone and 6 patients with this treatment associated with Cyclosporin A). Another patient had a triple therapy with Cyclosporin A, Azathioprine and corticosteroids while the last patient had a quadruple therapy with OKT3, Cyclosporin A, Azathioprine and Corticosteroids. These various treatments merely reflect our modifications of immunosuppressive regimen with time. The patients with a quadruple therapy received OKT3 or ALG for a limited number of weeks, a period during which Cyclosporin A was given at comparatively low dose.

Especially during the ALG or OKT3 treatment, the number of peripheral blood $CD4^+$ lymphocytes was significantly decreased, but in most patients it progressively increased thereafter. At the time of KS detection, only 2 patients had a $CD4^+$ lymphopenia below 400 cells/μl of blood. The mean $CD4^+$ cell count, at this time, was found to be 755/μl of blood in our group of 12 patients (Table 2).

Tissues invaded by KS

All our patients, except one, had skin lesions and this cutaneous involvement was diffused to several foci in 10 cases while it was restricted to 1 lesion of the leg in 1 case (Table 3).

In these 11 patients, KS was diagnosed in face of purple macules or elevated lesions that were located at the site of the surgical scar, on the legs, the back, the thorax or the face of the patients. Histology was confirmatory in all cases.

Three of these patients also had mucosa lesions in the oropharyngeal sphere. Some of these 11 patients with cutaneous lesions additionally had gastro-intestinal involvement (3 KS of the stomach) or invasion of the lungs and/or of the lymph nodes (Table 3). The 12th patient had an apparently isolated KS of lymph nodes.

As expected, and as also mentioned in other reports [5], visceral disease proved to be more severe and more resistant to therapy than in the purely cutaneous KS.

Treatment of KS

Immunosuppressive therapy was tapered in all patients to allow restoration of immune function to a large degree. Depending on the severity of KS at the time of diagnosis, the immunosuppression was either completely discontinued for a transient period, or it was only reduced by at least half (Table 4).

Table 3. Tissues involved by Kaposi's sarcoma in transplant patients

Tissue involvement	Number of patients	Characteristics of lesions
Skin lesions	11/12	– Morphology: elevated or flat, purple
		– Histologic confirmation in every case
		– Diffuse localisation with at least 2 separate foci in all patients but one:
		– abdomen (surgical scar)
		– back
		– legs
		– face (nose, ears)
		– thorax
Oropharyngeal mucosa lesions	3/12	– Morphology: slightly elevated and purple
		– Associated to skin and/or visceral lesions
Visceral lesions:		
– stomach	3/12	Associated to skin and/or
– lung	1/12	mucosa lesions
– lymph nodes	2/12	One of the two patients had an isolated lymph node involvement

Table 4. Treatment of Kaposi's sarcoma in transplant patients

Treatment	Number of patients
Discontinuation or significant reduction of immunosuppressive therapy	12
Chemotherapy (Vindesine, Vinblastine or Bleomycine)	7
rIFN-α (3×10^6 u 3 times weekly)	2
Local treatment:	
– surgical excision of some lesions	4
– radiotherapy	2

Seven of these patients received an additional treatment with chemotherapy in the form of Vindesine, Vinblastine or Bleomycine, depending on the year when KS appeared.

Table 5. Results of treatment and follow-up of patients with Kaposi's sarcoma

Patient condition	Number of patients
Disappearance or significant reduction of KS lesions	12
Patient alive	11
Renal transplant function:	
– satisfactory (blood creatinine < 200 μmol/l)	5
– intermediate (blood creatinine = 300 μmol/l)	1
– deteriorated (back to hemodialysis treatment 2–36 months later)	5

Recombinant interferon α was given to 2 patients at the dose of 3×10^6u three times per week, but it accelerated the unfavorable evolution of chronic rejection in both cases.

In addition to the systemic treatment, local radiotherapy or surgical excision of some lesions was occasionally used.

Results of KS treatment

As a result of the dramatic reduction of immunosuppressive therapy, KS lesions regressed in all 12 patients (Table 5). The improvement was rapid and complete in some patients, almost complete and slower in a few others.

Eleven of the patients are alive and the 12th patient died of unrelated myocardial infarction after KS lesions had regressed.

The function of the renal transplant could be considered as satisfactory in 5 patients, intermediate in 1 patient and poor in 5 patients (Table 5). Due to discontinuation of immunosuppression and/or interferon therapy, 5 patients developed acute or chronic rejection and they had to start again hemodialysis 2 to 36 months after identification of KS lesions. The patient with intermediate renal function had already elevated blood creatinine prior to KS and the very slow deterioration did not appear to be affected by this episode since blood creatinine remains close to 300 μmol/l over the last 3 years, without significant progression when immunosuppression was reduced.

On the whole, KS is less severe than in AIDS patients, possibly because immune restoration is possible thanks to tapering of immunosuppressive drugs. The price to pay for cure of Kaposi's sarcoma in transplant patients is an increased risk of transplant loss, as a consequence of reduced immunosuppression. Elevation of blood creatinine does not occur systematically in such circumstances, showing a better than expected tolerance of the transplant and a possibility to decrease the "over immunosuppression". Several months later, when all KS lesions have regressed, it is possible to slightly increase again the immunosuppressive therapy without resuming drugs at the same level as previously, to avoid recurrence of KS.

Virological origin of KS

For a long time, a virologic etiology to KS has been suspected [6, 7] and epidemiological studies in AIDS patients have indicated that one important condition of infection with such a putative virus might be sexual transmission [8, 9].

Recently, Y. Chang and co-workers have identified herpesvirus-like DNA sequences in AIDS-associated KS [10]. These data have been confirmed by a number of studies showing that a newly discovered herpesvirus is specifically found in KS patients, whether KS occurs in AIDS patients, HIV negative male homosexuals, Mediterranean or "classic" KS [11-14] and in some body-cavity-based lymphomas of AIDS patients [15]. Although this is the 9th human herpesvirus, this agent has been designated HHV-8 for "human herpesvirus 8" [16]. Current virological studies will soon determine whether HHV-8 is present in our transplant patients with KS as well as in other comparable patients from transplant centers of various countries.

Conclusion

Kaposi's disease appears to be approximately 500 fold more frequent in the transplant population than in the general population, mainly due to immunosuppressive therapy. It is especially found in transplant patients of certain ethnic groups. We have observed 12 such cases, some of which having merely a cutaneous involvement, others comprising visceral lesions. In all cases, tapering of immunosuppressive drugs resulted in improvement of Kaposi's disease and eventually in full disappearance of the lesions. Such a result sometimes required additional chemotherapy. Several patients had rejection of the transplanted kidney when the treatment was reduced, the others have maintained a good renal function. HHV-8 is a likely cause for the various types of Kaposi's sarcoma occurring in different groups of patients.

References

1. Penn I. Post-transplant kidney cancers and skin cancers (including Kaposi's sarcoma). In: D. Schmähl & I. Penn, editors. Cancer in Organ Transplant Recipients.Springer-Verlag, Berlin, 1991: 46–53.
2. Al-Sulaiman MH, Al-Khader AA. Kaposi's sarcoma in renal transplant recipients. Transplant Science 1994; 4: 46–60.

3. Harwood AR, Osaba D, Hofstader SL et al. Kaposi's sarcoma in recipients of renal transplants. Am J Med 1979; 67: 759–765.
4. Touraine J-L, Garnier JL, Lefrançois N et al. Severe lymphoproliferative disease and Kaposi sarcoma in transplant patients. Transpl Proc 1989; 21: 3197–3198.
5. Penn I. Epidemiology of cancer in transplant patients. 1995 This issue.
6. Giraldo G, Beth E, Haguenau F. Herpes-type virus particles in tissue culture of Kaposi's sarcoma from different geographic regions. J Nat Cancer Inst 1972; 49: 1509–1513.
7. Beral V, Peterman TA, Berkelman RL, Jaffe HW. Kaposi's sarcoma among persons with AIDS: a sexually transmitted infection ? Lancet 1990; 335: 123–128.
8. Peterman TA, Jaffe HW, Beral V. Epidemiologic clues to the etiology of Kaposi's sarcoma. AIDS 1993; 7: 605–611.
9. Franceschi S, Rezza G, Serraino D, Cozzi Lepri A, Geddes M, Cote T. Risk for Kaposi's sarcoma among Italian women with AIDS. J Acquir Immune Defic Syndr 1995; 9: 313–314.
10. Chang Y, Cesarman E, Pessin MS et al. Identification of Herpesvirus-like DNA sequences in AIDS-associated Kaposi's sarcoma. Science 1994; 266: 1865–1869.
11. Huang YQ, Li JJ, Kaplan MH et al. Human herpesvirus-like nucleic acid in various forms of Kaposi's sarcoma. Lancet 1995; 345: 759–761.
12. Dupin N, Grandadam M, Calvez V et al. Herpesvirus-like DNA sequences in patients with Mediterranean Kaposi's sarcoma. Lancet 1995; 345: 761–762.
13. Moore PS, Chang Y. Detection of Herpesvirus-like DNA sequences in Kaposi's sarcoma in patients with and those without HIV infection. N Engl J Med 1995; 332: 1181–1185.
14. Ambroziak JA, Blackbourn DJ, Herndier BG et al. Herpes-like sequences in HIV-infected and uninfected Kaposi's sarcoma patients. Science 1995; 268: 582–583.
15. Cesarman E, Chang Y, Moore PS, Said JW, Knowles DM. Kaposi's sarcoma-associated Herpesvirus-liked DNA sequences in AIDS-related body-cavity-based lymphomas. N Engl J Med 1995; 332: 1186–1191.
16. Roizman B. New viral footprints in Kaposi's sarcoma. N Engl J Med 1995; 332: 1227–1228.

11. Human T-cell leukemia virus type I (HTLV-I) and transplantation

ALI BAZARBACHI & ANTOINE GESSAIN

Human T-cell leukemia virus type I (HTLV-I) [1] is a retrovirus unevenly distributed around the World. The main endemic regions are southwestern Japan, intertropical Africa, the Caribbean and South America [2, 3]. HTLV-I is the causative agent of Adult T cell leukemia/lymphoma (ATL) [4] and of Tropical spastic paraparesis/ HTLV-I associated myelopathy (TSP/HAM) [5]. However, only a small proportion (1 to 5%) of HTLV-I infected individuals will develop an ATL or a TSP/HAM, and the majority of the infected patients remain asymptomatic for their entire life. The biological features of HTLV-I associated syndromes are summarized in Table 1.

ATL is an aggressive malignancy of mature activated CD4 positive T-cells, with a poor prognosis, mainly due to its resistance to conventional chemotherapy [6, 7]. The circulating leukemic cells are abnormal CD4+, CD25+ lymphocytes with indented or convoluted nuclei ("Flower cells"). Patients with ATL have serum antibodies to HTLV-I (4) and monoclonal integration of HTLV-I provirus(es), often defective, in the malignant cells [8]. Principal clinical features of ATL [9] include lymphadenopathy, hepatosplenomegaly, specific skin lesions, and hypercalcemia. The immune system is severely compromised giving rise to opportunistic infection. Variation in clinical presentation has led to the classification of ATL into four different clinical subtypes: smouldering ATL, chronic ATL, acute ATL, and the lymphomatous type [10]. These are usually, but not necessarily, sequential. The mechanism of HTLV-I induced leukemogenesis is not fully elucidated. HTLV-I infection is considered to be the first event of a multistep oncogenic process whose later steps are unknown [11].

TSP/HAM is a chronic progressive demyelinating disease that affects predominantly the thoracic spinal cord. Clinically, TSP/HAM is characterized by a paraparesis or a paraplegia with gradual onset and variable degrees of sensory loss, without evidence of motor neuron involvement, spinal cord compression, or supramedullary disseminated lesions [12]. Serum and cerebrospinal fluid (CSF) contain high level of HTLV-I antibodies, exhibit an intrathecal synthesis of specific anti-HTLV-I immunoglobulins with oligoclonal bands.

J.L. Touraine et al. (eds.), Cancer in Transplantation. Prevention and Treatment, 81–87.

Table 1. Biological features of HTLV-I associated syndromes

		ATL			Intermediate	Healthy
		Leukemic form	"Smoldering" form	TSP/HAM	state	carriers
Lymphocytosis/mm^3		$10^4 - 5 \times 10^5$	Normal	Normal	Normal	Normal
ATL cells (%)		10–99	0.5–5	0–20	0–2	Absent – rare
CD4/CD8 ratio		↑++	↑+/-	↑+	Normal	Normal
CD25 (TAC) +ve cells		↑++	↑+/-	↑+	↑+/-	Normal
HLA.DR, DP, DQ +ve cells		↑++	↑+/-	↑++	↑+/-	Normal
Hypercalcemia (% of cases)		50	–	–	–	–
Specific cutaneous lesions		Frequent	Very frequent	Absent	Absent	Absent
Immunodeficiency		++	+	++	+/-	–
Anti HTLV-I antibodies						
Serum		+	+	++ (high titer)	+	+
CSF		–	–	+	–	–
Intrathecal synthesis of IgG		–	–	+	–	–
CSF IgG oligoclonal bands		–	–	+	–	–
Soluble serum IL2 receptor		++++	+++	++	+	+
HTLV-I[a] proviral integration	Mode	Monoclonal	Monoclonal	Polyclonal[b]	Polyclonal	Non detectable
	Site	leukemic, lymphnode, pleural, ascitic fluid cells,	leukemic cells, cutaneous infiltrate	PBMCs[c]	PBMCs[c]	PBMCs[c]
	% of cases	100	100	85	100	0
PCR[d] HLTV-I		+++	++	++	++	+
Viral load in PBMC		Very high	High	High	High	Low
T cell receptor (α, β and γ)		Clonal, rearranged	Clonal, rearranged	Non rearranged	Non rearranged	Non rearranged

[a] Determined by Souther Blot analysis.
[b] In 10/20% of cases a clonal integration of HTLV-I is present in the PBMCs.
[c] PBMCs: peripheral blood mononuclear cells.
[d] PCR: polymerase chain reaction.

A high frequency of cytotoxic CD8 cells is observed in the blood and the CSF. Even if the association of HTLV-I infection and TSP/HAM outcome is well established, the pathogenesis of this disease remains unknown. Two main hypothesis exist: direct infection of some cells in the central nervous system with a subsequent cytotoxic immune response resulting in demyelination, versus the existence of an autoimmune process due to the activation of autoreactive T cell clones by HTLV-I.

Transmission of HTLV-I infection occurs through sexual contact, (chiefly from men to women), from mother to child by breast feeding, shared contaminated needles among drug abusers, and blood transfusion of infected cells [3]. The intravenous route of infection by blood transfusion appears as the most efficient mode of HTLV-I transmission with a 15 to 60% risk of infection for the transfused persons by a contaminated cellular blood product [13–15]. HTLV-I infection by blood transfusion is cell associated (presence of infected lymphocytes in whole blood, platelets and red cells concentrates). This has been well documented by the fact that freshly frozen plasma without live cells is not infectious [13–16]. Furthermore, platelets transfusion appears more likely to transmit HTLV-I infection than red blood cells because they are more likely contaminated by lymphocytes. In endemic areas, multitransfused patients have a high HTLV-I seroprevalence rate [17]. In the USA, among 211 adults with leukemia who received multiple transfusions, 6 were found to be seropositive for HTLV-I and seroconversion could be documented in three patients [18]. However, the long latent period between HTLV-I infection and the occurrence of an ATL or a TSP/HAM has led to uncertainty about the practical benefits of screening blood donors in area of low prevalence of HTLV-I. It is worth mentioning that several cases of subacute myelopathy have been reported after the transfusion of a blood product contaminated with HTLV-I, either in areas of high or low HTLV-I endemicity, and this led several countries to the screening for HTLV-I infection of all blood or organ donors, in order to prevent disease as well as the transmission of the virus. Screening of blood donations was first implemented in Japan, starting in 1986 [14], in French West Indies in 1989, in the USA in 1989 [15], in Canada in 1990, in France in 1991 [19], and in Denmark and Netherlands in 1994, but is still not compulsory in the UK, Italy and the other European countries. In France, screening for HTLV-I infection is also obligatory for organ or bone marrow donors.

A few cases of HTLV-I infection have been reported after bone marrow or organ transplantation. A clinical description of the typical case has been reported in detail [20]. Briefly, a 41 year old Caucasian man of French origin presented a rapidly progressive paraplegia, four months after cardiac transplantation for hypertrophic cardiomyopathy. Clinical, radiological and biological signs led to the diagnosis of TSP/HAM with specific IgG antibodies to HTLV-I detected in his serum and cerebrospinal fluid. During transplantation, he received 21 units of packed red cells, 30 units of random platelets,

8 units of fresh frozen plasma and cryoprecipitates. Before and at the time of the cardiac transplantation, the patient had no detectable HTLV-I antibodies. Evidence of HTLV-I seroconversion was observed 14 weeks after he received blood contaminated with HTLV-I. At this time, HTLV-I IgM antibodies were detected in his serum while assays for HTLV-I IgG were negative. Nine months after transplantation, peripheral blood smears showed 4% of ATL like abnormal lymphocytes with hyperconvoluted nuclei. At this time, southern blot analysis revealed clonal integration of HTLV-I provirus in about 10% of his fresh peripheral blood mononuclear cells. The heart donor was seronegative for HTLV-I. Of the 59 blood donors, one healthy woman from the French West Indies was strongly HTLV-I seropositive. In a similar way, a rapid progressive HTLV-I associated myelopathy has been reported after blood transfusion in two immunosuppressed patients, one of whom had aplastic anemia and the other was the recipient of a renal transplant receiving immunosuppressive chemotherapy [21]. These three cases suggest that the coexistent drug-induced immunosuppression may play a role in the rapid developement of the myelopathy, and emphasize the clonal expansion of HTLV-I infected T-cells.

In Japan, transmission of HTLV-I by blood transfusion has been virtually eliminated by screening of blood donations for antibody to the virus. As a consequence, Japanese studies also indicate a marked reduction (about 15%) in the incidence of new cases of TSP/HAM after initiation of blood screening [22].

The seroprevalence of HTLV-I infection among recipients of organ transplants, and in particular renal transplants was investigated in different areas. In fact, HTLV-I infection may be acquired after transplantation either from the donor kidney or from blood transfusion given during the perioperative period. In Brazil, a relatively endemic region for HTLV-I infection, 11.1% of the renal transplanted patients were seropositive for HTLV-I by enzyme-linked immunosorbant assay (ELISA), while only 1.34% of the native inhabitants and 0.73% of the descendants from Japanese living in Brazil were seropositive [23]. In the USA, the prevalence of HIV-1 and HTLV-I infection has been investigated retrospectively by ELISA test and Western blot confirmation, on 224 sera from patients undergoing renal transplantation between 1979 and 1985 [24]. Six patients (2.7%) were found to have retroviral infection, four with HIV-1 and two with HTLV-I. All these retroviral infections were acquired after transplantation except for one patient who was seropositive for HTLV-I before transplantation.

Seroprevalence of HTLV-I and HTLV-II has also been investigated in patients about to undergo bone marrow transplantation (BMT) in a single referral center in the USA [25]. The authors found one of 317 (0.3%) marrow transplant patients to be HTLV-I positive, and none to be HTLV-II positive before transplant. However, the incidence of HTLV-I infection after BMT was not reported.

Ljugman et al. [26] recently reported the infection of donor lymphocytes with HTLV-I following allogenic bone marrow transplantation for acute ATL. The donor was an HTLV-I negative identical sibling. The patient died of an acute encephalitis and HTLV-I could be detected in autopsy material from the brain. The use of allogenic BMT in the treatment of ATL has been reported in a very few number of patients. One patient died 3 months after BMT for acute ATL from a cytomegalovirus pneumonitis with no evidence of relapse at post mortem analysis, suggesting a possible cure effect of this procedure in ATL [27]. However, in a second patient, relapse of ATL occurred 25 days after BMT [28].

Treatment of HTLV-I associated diseases remains disappointing. Corticosteroids and immunosuppressor treatment usually result in only short-term improvement in TSP/HAM, and symptomatic therapy is useful in decreasing the spasticity and painful paresthesias as well as in improving sphincter dysfunction. ATL has a very poor prognosis, mainly due to its resistance to conventional chemotherapy. Antiretroviral therapy associating alpha-interferon and zidovudine seems to induce a rapid and durable responses in ATL [29, 30].

Conclusion

Human T cell Leukemia virus type I (HTLV-I) is the causative agent of Adult T cell leukemia/lymphoma (ATL) and Tropical spastic paraparesis/HTLV-I associated myelopathy (TSP/HAM). HTLV-I can be transmitted through infected cells in blood transfusion or organ transplant, with several reported cases of rapid occurrence of subacute TSP/HAM after contamination, mainly in the situations of immunocompromised recipients. In contrast, the development of an ATL after contamination by these ways seems extremely rare, if it exists [31]. ATL probably requires HTLV-I infection during the childhood by breast feeding. Bone marrow transplantation has been proposed in the treatment of ATL, with however a high toxicity of this procedure and some reported very early relapses after transplantation. Moreover, BMT from HTLV-I negative donor into HTLV-I positive recipients may lead to the infection of donor lymphocytes. Finally, a careful screening for HTLV-I infection in blood and organ donors is required, even in low HTLV-I endemic areas, to avoid the dissemination of the virus and the occurrence of more aggressive HTLV-I related diseases in immunocompromised recipients.

References

1. Poiesz BJ, Ruscetti FW, Gazdar AF, Bunn PA, Minna JD, Gallo RC. Detection and isolation of type C retrovirus particles from fresh and cultured lymphocytes of a patient with cutaneous T-cell lymphoma. Proc Natl Acad Sci USA 1980; 77: 7415–7419.

2. Müeller N. The epidemiology of HTLV-I infection. Cancer Causes and Control 1991; 2: 37–52.
3. Kaplan JE, Khabbaz RF. The epidemiology of Human T-lymphotropic virus Types I and II. Medical Virology 1993; 3: 137–148.
4. Hinuma Y, Nagata K, Hanaoka M et al. Adult T-cell leukaemia: Antigen in an ATL cell line and detection of antibodies to the antigen in human sera. Proc Natl Acad Sci USA 1981; 78: 6476–6480.
5. Gessain A, Barin F, Vernant JC et al. Antibodies to human T-lymphotropic virus type-I in patients with tropical spastic paraparesis. Lancet 1985; 2: 407–410.
6. Bunn PA Jr, Schechter GP, Jaffe E et al. Clinical course of retrovirus-associated adult T cell lymphoma in the United states. N Engl J Med 1983; 309: 257–264.
7. Shimoyama M. Treatment of patients with adult T-cell leukemia-lymphoma: An overview. Gann Monograph on Cancer Research 1992; 39: 43–56.
8. Seiki M, Eddy R, Shaws TB, Yoshida M. Non specific integration of the HTLV-I provirus genome into adult T cell leukemia. Nature 1984; 309: 640–642.
9. Takatsuki F, Yamaguchi K, Hattori T. Adult T-cell leukemia/lymphoma. In: Gallo RC, and Wong-Staal F, editors. Retrovirus Biology and Human Disease. New York: Marcel Decker, 1990; 147–159.
10. Shimoyama and members of the Lymphoma study group. Diagnostic criteria and classification of clinical subtypes of adult T-cell leukemia-lymphoma. Br J Hem. 1991; 79: 428–437.
11. Höllsberg P, Hafler D. Pathogenesis of diseases induced by human lymphotropic virus type I infection. N Engl J Med 1993; 328: 1173–1182.
12. Gessain A, Gout O. Chronic myelopathy associated with human T-lymphotropic virus type I (HTLV-I). Annals of Internal Medicine 1992; 117: 933–946.
13. Okochi K, Sato H, Hinuma Y. A retrospective study on transmission of adult T-cell leukemia virus type I (HTLV-I) by blood transfusion: seroconversion in recipients. Vox sang 1984; 46: 245–253.
14. Inaba S, Sato H, Okochi K et al. Prevention of transmission of human T-lymphotropic virus type 1 (HTLV-I) through transfusion, by donor screening with antibody to the virus. One year experience. Transfusion 1989; 29: 7–11.
15. Sandler S, Fang CT, Williams AE. Human T-cell lymphotropic virus type I and II in transfusion medicine. Transfusion Medicine Reviews 1991; 5: 93–107.
16. Lairmore MD, Jason JM, Hartley TM, Khabbaz RF, Evatt BL. Absence of human T-cell lymphotropic virus type I coinfection in human immunodeficiency virus-infected hemophilic men. Blood 1989; 74: 2596–2599.
17. Gessain A, Gazallo L, Yoyo M, Fortier L, Robert Guroff M, De Thé G. Scickle cell anemia patients from Martinique have an increased prevalence of HTLV-I antibodies. Lancet 1984; 2: 1155–1156.
18. Minamoto G, Gold J, Scheinberg D et al. Infection with human T-cell leukemia virus type I in patients with leukemia. N Engl J Med 1988; 318: 219–222.
19. Pillonel J, Lemaire JM, Courouce AM. Epidemiologie de l'HTLV-I chez les donneurs de sang domiciliés en France métropolitaine (Juillet 1991–Juin 1993). Med Mal infect 1994; 24: 548–552.
20. Gout O, Baulac M, Gessain A et al. Rapid development of myelopathy after HTLV-I infection acquired by transfusion during cardiac transplantation. N Engl J Med 1990; 322: 383–388.
21. Kuroda Y, Takashima H, Yukitake M, Sakemi T. Development of HTLV-I associated myelopathy after blood transfusion in a patient with aplastic anemia and a recipient of a renal transplant. J Neurol Sci 1992; 109: 196–199.
22. Osame M, Janssen R, Kubota H, et al. Nationwide survey of HTLV-I associated myelopathy in Japan: association with blood transfusion. Ann Neurol 1990; 28: 50–56.

23. Linhares MI, Eizuru Y, de Andrade GP et al. Human T cell leukemia virus type I (HTLV-I) antibodies in healthy populations and renal transplanted patients in the north-east of Brazil. Microbiol Immunol 1994; 38: 475–478.
24. Perez G, Ortiz-Interian C, Bourgoignie J et al. HIV-1 and HTLV-I infection in renal transplant recipients. J. Acquired Immune Deficiency Syndromes 1990; 3: 35–40.
25. Loughran TP. Seroprevalence of HTLV-I and HTLV-II in marrow transplant recipients. Bone marrow transplantation 1994; 14: 433–436.
26. Ljungman P, Lawler M, Asjo B et al. Infection of donor lymphocytes with human T lymphotropic virus type I (HTLV-I) following allogenic bone marrow transplantation for HTLV-I positive adult T-cell leukemia. British J Haematol 1994; 88: 403–405.
27. Sobue R, Yamauchi T, Miyamura K, et al; Treatment of adult T-cell leukemia with mega-dose cyclophosphamide and total body irradiation followed by allogenic bone marrow transplantation. Bone marrow transplantation 1987; 2: 441–444.
28. Rio B, Louvet C, Gessain A et al. Adult T cell leukaemia and non malignant adenopathies associated with HTLV-I in patients from the Carribean and Africa. Presse Med 1990; 19: 746–751.
29. Gill P, Masood R, Cai J et al. Novel antiviral therapy for adult T-cell leukemia secondary to HTLV-I infection. Blood 1992; 80 suppl/1: 74a.
30. Hermine O, Bouscary D, Gessain A, Turlure P, LeBlond V, Franck N, Buzyn-Veil A, Rio B, Macintyre E, Dreyfus F, Bazarbachi A. Treatment of HTLV-I associated adult T-cell leukemia-lymphoma with a combination of zidovudine and alpha-interferon. N Eng J Med 1995 (In press).
31. Williams NP, Tsduda H, Yamagushi K et al. Blood transfusion induced opportunistic Adult T-cell leukemia/lymphoma after Hodgkin's disease. Leukemia and Lymphoma 1991; 5: 435–439.

12. Hepatitis B virus and primary liver cancer in Hepatitis B surface antigen positive and negative patients

PATRICIA PATERLINI & CHRISTIAN BRÉCHOT

Introduction

The review by Dr Johnson clearly indicates the strength of the epidemiological association between chronic infection by HBV and hepatocellular carcinoma (HCC), the most frequent histological form of primary liver cancer (PLC). However, the mechanisms involved in liver carcinogenesis still remain a matter of debate. Cirrhosis, which is present in around 90% of patients with HCC tumors in most areas, has long been recognized as an important risk factor. Early clinical observations in Africa showed the evolution of acute hepatitis (AH) to chronic active hepatitis (CAH), cirrhosis and, eventually, liver cancer [1, 2]. The importance of this association has since been confirmed but its prevalence is considered to be lower in Africa (around 50% of cases) than in Asia, Europe, and America (80–100%). The molecular basis of the promoting effect of cirrhosis is far from clear but generally related to "liver cell regeneration".

There are two likely modes of hepatocyte regeneration (see reviews from Drs Michalopoulos and Carr). After partial hepatectomy the liver regains its normal size and weight, under the influence of balance between positive and negative regulatory factors. During cirrhosis, irreversible nodular changes appear, in which hepatocytes lose their normal plate arrangement, are surrounded by extensive fibrosis, and show evidence of increased DNA synthesis [3]. The pattern of growth regulating molecules in cirrhosis is thus likely to be very different to those known to be involved after partial hepatectomy. Unfortunately, there is a lack of accurate animal models of liver cirrhosis, even though baboons chronically intoxicated with alcohol can show some characteristic features. The liver lesions observed in rats after carbon tetrachloride (CCL4) treatment bear little resemblance to cirrhosis. As discussed in Dr Buendia's paper, woodchucks and ground squirrels chronically infected

J.L. Touraine et al. (eds.), Cancer in Transplantation. Prevention and Treatment, 89–113.

by the woodchuck hepatitis virus (WHBV) and the ground squirrel hepatitis virus (GHBV), respectively, develop CAH without cirrhosis and ducks infected by the duck hepatitis virus (DHBV) rarely show features of chronic liver disease. Other models can, however, be useful for studying the molecular mechanisms of liver cell regeneration secondary to chronic hepatocyte necrosis. In particular, the liver of some transgenic mice expresses a large amount of the large envelope protein encoded by the PreS1/S2/S sequences of HBV. The accumulation of this viral protein in hepatocytes has a direct toxic effect and leads to cell necrosis; liver cancer develops after an average of 18 months, probably as a consequence of the continuous cell regeneration [4]. This is one case in which liver cancer cells emerge in the apparent absence of genetic priming events such as those involved in chemical carcinogenesis. In addition, these mice show increased sensitivity to chemical carcinogenes, a situation reminiscent of human exposure to both HBV and chemical carcinogenes.

Although there is general agreement on the importance of cirrhosis in the carcinogenic process, the existence of a direct effect of HBV in liver cell transformation is still controversial. The demonstration in 1980 that HBV DNA integrated into the DNA of tumor cells from patients with HCC led to attempts to identify the cellular sequences adjacent to the sites of HBV DNA integration [5–12]: by analogy with tumors induced by retroviruses, it was expected that HBV DNA would be integrated in the vicinity of oncogenes, which had recently been identified. In fact, this was not the case in sharp contrast with results subsequently obtained in woodchuck HCC (see review by Dr Buendia). While this is now often taken as evidence against a direct role of HBV and for the sole responsibility of cirrhosis in liver cancer, there are in fact several lines of evidence that HBV is directly involved in HCC. Indeed, integration of HBV DNA can lead to chromosomal rearrangements at the site of integration [13], and evidence of insertional mutagenesis has been obtained in some humans HCC and around half of woodchuck HCC. Integration of the viral DNA also frequently leads to the synthesis of truncated envelope viral proteins which have been shown to possess transactivating effects on oncogenes such as *fos* [14, 15]; furthermore, the transactivating X viral protein, which is probably involved in the transformation process, can be synthesized from both free and integrated HBV DNA sequences [16,17]. It is thus very likely that liver cancer results from an accumulation of several events, viz. chronic active hepatitis and cirrhosis due to environmental factors (alcohol, HBV, and HCV; see reviews by Dr Nishioka and Colombo), together with genetic effects on liver cells of HBV DNA replication and integration, as well as chemical carcinogenes (e.g. aflatoxin B1: see reviews by Dr Montesano and Ozturk).

This review will focus on the role of HBV in liver cancer in patients with and without serological evidence of chronic HBV infection, together with the potential implications of the integration of HBV DNA sequences into hepatocyte DNA. The review by Dr Kékulé specifically deals with the potential oncogenic effects of the HBV X and PreS2/S proteins, while that of Dr Buendia shows the interest of animal models for studies on Hepadna virus related-liver carcinogenesis.

HBV DNA sequences in the liver of Hepatitis B surface antigen-positive HBV carriers

HBV DNA was initially characterized by means of the Southern blot procedure. Viral DNA sequences were then cloned to define their structure more accurately, and viral RNAs were analysed in detail. The distinction between free and integrated HBV DNA in the Southern blot procedure is based on the use of different restriction enzymes which either do not cut most HBV genomes, or cut at one or two sites.

Using this strategy, it has been shown that HBV DNA sequences are integrated into cellular DNA in most (around 90%) but not all liver tumor samples from hepatitis B surface antigen (HBsAG) – positive patients [18]. The Southern blotting usually suggested monoclonal or oligoclonal proliferation of the cells containing HBV DNA [18–20]. Discrete bands were obtained after digestion of tumor cell DNA by restriction enzymes such as Hind III (which usually do not cut cloned HBV genomes) but were absent from the undigested-DNA pattern. The restriction DNA profile differs from one tumor to the next and generally reveals several different integration sites; however, clonally expanded cells containing a single integration site are found in some cases [18]. It is noteworthy that, even in HBsAg positive PLCs, HBV DNA is sometimes not detectable in all tumor cells, suggesting that integration in some HBsAg-positive patients, is not always necessary to maintain a transformed phenotype (Bréchot & Paterlini, unpublished observations). Integration of HBV DNA is not restricted to tumor cells: clonally expanded cells containing integrated HBV DNA molecules can be identified in the non-tumorous, cirrhotic, livers of patients with HCC [21, 22]. However, the restriction profile differs from that of tumor, suggesting the coexistence of different clones in the liver prior to tumor development; alternatively, secondary chromosomal rearrangements might have occurred during the tumor growth [23].

Integration has also been demonstrated in chronic HBV carriers (both adults and children) with no evidence of HCC [21, 24–29]. Although the restriction profiles in these cases can be consistent with clonal expansion of infected cells, another pattern is more frequent. As HBV DNA integrates at sites varying from one cell to the next, the length of the Hind III-digested DNA fragments which include the viral and adjacent cellular DNA always differ, and only a smear thus appears on the autoradiogram. In this situation, the use of enzymes which cut restriction sites located within the viral genome can reveal "internal" HBV-specific bands. This suggests either little or no proliferation of cells containing HBV sequences [18]. Some studies have even suggested that such a restriction profile consistent with HBV DNA integration can be observed at the acute stage of HBV infection and in subjects with a severe form of acute hepatitis [30].

In short, integration precedes the development of the tumor. Comparative analysis of the various restriction profiles at different times in the course of HBV infection suggests a progressive clonal expansion of some infected cells which is only detectable in patients infected for a long time. Integration of HBV DNA is not necessary for its replication, but occurs when cellular DNA replicates during liver cell proliferation secondary to necrosis of adjacent hepatocytes [31].

Free viral DNA is also frequently detected by Southern blotting [13, 21, 23, 32, 33]. The presence of HBV DNA replicative intermediates is generally associated with an HBV viremia, although in some patients (particularly those with HCC) replicative forms can be detected in the liver while HBV DNA is undetectable (by dot blot) in the serum; this suggests defective viral encapsidation and/or release [34]. Free monomeric HBV DNA can also be detected, mostly at the end of viral multiplication in acute or chronic infection. Finally, free oligomeric HBV DNA forms with complex structures have been evidenced in a few acutely infected patients; their significance is not known, but they could feasibly be intermediates in the integration process [30, 35]. Viral oligomers have been detected in woodchucks infected by WHV [36].

It is, however, important to note the technical limitations of the Southern blot assay for the analysis of HBV DNA status; in particular, it is often difficult to detect integrated sequences in hepatocytes which have undergone little or no clonal expansion when free viral DNA is also present [18, 37]. Furthermore, the Southern technique provides no information as to the identity of the infected cells.

A combination of immunohistochemical and in situ hybridisation procedures has been used to settle this latter point. HBV DNA replication, as shown by the detection of HBV DNA replicative forms (in the cytoplasm) and HBcAg (mostly in the nucleus), as well as HBsAg synthesis, are generally found in different hepatocytes [38–41]. At the time of tumor development, the degree of viral DNA replication has usually decreased and HBsAg can be detected in around 20% of cases in tumor cells [42]; HBcAg is very rarely detectable [34, 42]. In contrast, in the adjacent non-tumor cirrhotic liver, both HBsAg and HBcAg are detectable. These observations have led to suggestions that different cell populations are infected by HBV: the differentiating status of some hepatocytes might be compatible with HBV DNA replication and HBcAg expression and would thus be targets for the immune response; in contrast, other liver cells might not support a complete replicative cycle, only express HBsAg, and be progressively selected during chronic HBV carriage [43]. When HCC occurs, the tumor cells are no longer permissive for the viral DNA replication and do not express HBcAg; however, recent evidence suggests that they frequently (up to 80% in one study) express the viral X protein [42].

The availability of the HBV DNA probes, together with improvements in serological tests for hepatitis e antigen (HBeAg), has allowed a precise appraisal of the course of HBV infection to be made (see review from DR Kremsdorf). During chronic HBV infection, one can schematically distinguish two phases: the viral multiplication phase, as shown by the detection of serum HBeAg and HBV DNA, is highly variable from one patient to the next, and is followed by an HBV carriage phase, as shown by HBsAg positivity and the absence of markers of HBV multiplication. Reactivation of viral multiplication may, however, occur, together with an exacerbation of liver cell necrosis. As mentioned earlier, HBV multiplication has generally declined markedly when HCC develops, at least in Western countries, Africa, and Japan; in Taiwan, HBV multiplication persists when HCC occurs [44, 45]. In Western countries and Africa, some investigators have shown the persistence of replicative intermediates in the tumor liver cells of patients with HCC and suggested that they might not be normally encapsidated [34]; it is not, however, known if this leads to further integration of viral DNA into cellular DNA and thereby modifies the course of tumor development.

HBV DNA can be detected in cell types other than hepatocytes; classical Southern blot analysis, PCR, and in situ hybridisation have revealed it in mononuclear blood cells [46–50] , biliary and smooth muscle cells [51], as well as in the pancreas, kidney [52–58] and sperm cells [49, 59]. The most frequently identified viral DNA form is a 3.2 kb DNA molecule whose migration in agarose gels is consistent with a linear structure; viral oligomers have been also shown in mononuclear blood cells, but the integration of HBV DNA suggested by some Southern Blot analyses has not been clearly established. Infection of mononuclear blood cells is an early event in the course of HBV infection: indeed, a combination of classical Southern blot analysis and PCR has been used to detect viral DNA (together with HBV transcripts) in both acutely [48, 60] and chronically [61] infected subjects. In woodchucks, mononuclear bone marrow cells are the first to show evidence of WHV DNA in an experimental acute infection [62–66]. In humans, CD4+ and CD8+ T lymphocytes, B lymphocytes, macrophages and polymorphonuclears cells score positive for HBV DNA (Calmus et al.; in preparation) [67].

Taken together, these results show that the tropism of the virus is broader than previously thought, but that replication of HBV DNA mostly occurs in liver cells. Viral DNA replication has been however identified in the peripheral mononuclear blood cells (PBMNC) of a few patients and also in chronically infected woodchuck [64]. HBV DNA replication can be stimulated by addition of the mitogens Lipopolysaccharide and Phytohemagglutinin to short-term culture of woodchuck and human PBMNC, respectively [61, 63, 64, 68, 69]. Evidence of HBV multiplication has been found in bone marrow cells from an HBV-infected subject and immortalised by Epstein Barr virus infection [50], as well as in the monocytic cell line U937 [70]; *in vitro* infection of normal bone marrow cells has been also reported which might be associated to cytopathic effects on the infected cells [71, 72]. Infection of mononuclear cells might have important implications. First, they might constitute a "reservoir" for HBV DNA, as shown for several other viruses, and this could account for some reinfections after liver transplantation [73]. There is also indirect evidences of a selection of HBV DNA mutants in these cells [74]. Finally, infection of PBMNC may contribute to the immunological defect in chronic HBV carriers, and lead to interact with other lymphotropic viruses such as HIV [75].

It is important to note that, in 1993, the physiological implications of the presence of HBV DNA in these various cell types are unknown; the stage of cell differentiation at which viral infection occurs and the nature of the receptor that binds HBV particles are also unclear. It has even been hypothesized that direct transfer of HBV DNA from one mononuclear blood cell to another might occur, independently of viral multiplication [76].

Structure of integrated HBV and flanking cellular DNA sequences

Integrated HBV DNA sequences have been characterized in cell lines derived from hepatocellular carcinomas, and directly in tumor tissues. However, the total number of independent HCCs so far analyzed is still limited.

Structure of integrated viral DNA

There is no single structure, but some common features can be seen in independent cases. At least one region of the viral genome is preferentially involved in integration: the region of the cohesive end part of HBV DNA and the direct repeats DR1 and DR2, at which synthesis of the minus and plus DNA strands, respectively, are initiated [9, 52, 53, 77–82]. In a survey of 17 clones [78], half the integrations occurred in the cohesive end overlap or in sequences close to or included in DR1 and DR2. When duplicated HBV DNA sequences are identified (in a "head-to-tail" or "tail-to-tail" arrangement) the viral-viral junctions are also frequently located in this cohesive end region of the genome. In PLC/PRF5 cells integration was reported to occur frequently in the single-stranded part of the HBV DNA [9], but this result was subsequently challenged by the analysis of other integrants from the same cell line.

Uninterrupted linear HBV DNAs, with insertions in the X and C open Reading Frames (ORFs) and small deletions (10–100 bp) at the viral/host junction, have been shown in some tumors, but this is a rather rare event; in the PLC/PRF5 cell line, for example, none of the 7 integrants yielded such structures. More frequently, complex rearrangements of the viral sequences occur in tumors, with deletions, insertions or duplications [28, 83]. Short HBV sequences or, in contrast, greater-than-unit-length genomes can be shown. It is important to note that such rearrangements are not specific to tumor samples but can also be detected in liver samples from patients with chronic active hepatitis and apparently free off HCC [84].

The S ORF is often conserved and its integrity has been confirmed in a few cases by the expression of HBsAG upon transfection of the clones containing the integrated HBV DNA [52, 53, 85]. In contrast, the core gene is frequently deleted [22, 79, 86–92] while the X ORF is frequently truncated by insertion in the cohesive end region of the viral genome. A frequent observation is therefore insertion in the cohesive end on one side while the other junction is located between the C and the PreS genes and integration of an HBV DNA molecule extending from PreS to X genes has been observed in several cases. Another relatively common feature of independent HCCs is the apparent conservation, even in complex HBV DNA structures, of PreS2/S ORFs truncated at the 3′ part of the S gene, possibly leading to truncated PreS2/S proteins with a transactivating effect [14, 78, 93] (see review by Dr Kékulé). The sequences located 5′ to the PreS and S genes might therefore also be prone to recombination with the host genome, possibly in correlation with transcriptional activity.

It is interesting that none of the integrated HBV genomes so far reported have structures which would allow them to be transcribed into pregenomic RNA, the template for HBV DNA replication.

Finally intriguing results have been reported for the PLC/PRF5 cell line: for example, a 182 bp sequence detected at one of the virus/host junctions is only 40% homologous to HBV, is apparently not a cellular sequence, and might be implicated in several independent integrations [94]. Furthermore, one analysis suggested integration of four different adw HBV DNA molecules in this one cell line. While these are potentially very interesting observations, their implications are unclear as similar results have not been reported *in vivo*. Along the same line, evidence have been presented *in vivo* for recombination between free and integrated viral DNA together with multiple integration events [95].

Structure of the viral/cellular DNA junctions

Again there is no single pattern. Most results are consistent with an illegitimate recombination event between the viral and cellular DNA, frequently associated with a short deletion of cellular DNA at the site of integration [17, 94, 96, 97]. In some integrants there is partial sequence homology between the deleted cellular DNA and the viral genome close to the integration site, and it might be involved in this process [83, 87, 88, 98–101]. In contrast, integration of an uninterrupted linear HBV DNA led to duplication of a 12 bp cellular DNA segment at the integration site, a feature reminiscent of retrovirus integration [101], but this observation has remained anecdotal. There is so far no evidence of a single cell sequence being a target for HBV DNA integration. In several integrants, however, integration frequently occurs in repeat sequences (Alu or satellite III DNA sequences) [94, 102, 103] possibly implicated in non-homologous recombination. In this regard, a detailed analysis of the PLC/PRF5 cell line has shown that 8 of the 9 integrated HBV DNAs are present in the H3 component of the human genome; it represents about 4% of total cellular DNA, has a base composition (51% GC) close to that of HBV DNA (49% GC), and includes Alu repeats [104]. This observation suggests preferential targeting of HBV DNA integration as is the case of some retroviruses, but has not yet been extended to HBV DNA sequences from other HCCs.

Duplication and inversion of integrated HBV DNA can also involve adjacent cells DNA in some tumors [13, 78]. An amplification and translocation of the HBV DNA sequence, together with the adjacent host cell DNA, from one cellular domain to another has also been shown in PLC/PRF5 cells [105, 106.

Mechanisms possibly involved in HBV DNA integration

Taken together, the results presented above are consistent with several different modes of viral integration; in some tumors, where the cohesive end and the core sequences are located on the two extremities of the integrant, one of the viral/host junction is generated by insertion of the 5′ end of the linear minus-strand replicative intermediate, while the other junction shows either no specific location in the viral genome or is preferentially inserted in the PreS ORFs; whether the location of this second junction in the HBV DNA is a secondary recombination event (deletion ?) or rather reflects integration of subgenomic replicative intermediates is not known [28, 78, 101, 107]. Alternatively, the substrate for the integration may be an opened relaxed circular or linear form of HBV DNA [77, 108], the insertion being generated by strand invasion and displacement. In other cases, rearrangements creating complex oligomeric HBV DNA structures may have occurred before integration, and free oligomers have been detected in the liver of woodchucks with HCC, humans with acute hepatitis, and in mononuclear blood cells (see previous section).

Whatever the substrate for integration, non-homologous recombination probably involves topoisomerase I which has cleavage sites near DR1 in HBV and WHV [42, 109–111].

The frequent insertion of HBV DNA in the cohesive overlap might have important consequences for molecular events occurring after integration. It has indeed been proposed that, once integrated, the cohesive end of the viral genome might be "reactivated" by proteins such as the terminal DNA-binding protein [78]. This might generate further rearrangements of the integrated

HBV sequences as well as recombination between HBV genomes inserted on different chromosomes, resulting in chromosomal translocation [31]. In line with this hypothesis, an *in vitro* assay showed indirect evidence of increased recombination events due to HBV DNA in the presence of liver cell protein extracts from patients with HCC [31, 98, 108, 112–114]. If these molecular events are relevant *in vivo*, "reactivation" of HBV recombination should be prevented by the immediate encapsidation of the viral polymerase. At this purpose, it has been hypothesized that, abnormal encapsidation of the replicative HBV DNA may occur in tumors [34, 45, 115].

Consequences of HBV DNA integration

Chromosomal DNA instability

HBV DNA integration sites have been mapped to different chromosomes, although an increased rate of insertions on chromosomes 11 and 17 has been observed [14, 78, 98, 99, 116, 117]. Integration can lead to small deletions (a few base pairs) in the cellular DNA but, several large chromosomal deletions (chromosome 11p14, 4q32, 11q13 in particular [118, 119] have been shown. Translocations have been also described at the site of HBV DNA integration (chromosomes: 17/X; 5/9; 17/18 (17q21-22/18q11.1-q11.2) [60, 98, 100]. In one tumor, integrated HBV sequences were found to be co-amplified with the *hst-1* oncogene [120].

These results, combined with those concerning the modes of HBV DNA integration, have led to suggestions that HBV DNA integration might increase the likelihood of chromosomal rearrengements [31], possibly with a contribution by tumor suppressor genes or oncogenes. However, there has been no direct evidence so far of such a gene at a deletion site or at a translocation breakpoint.

On the same line, integrated HBV DNA sequence have been shown to coamplify with the transforming gene *hst-1* in a human HCC [120].

Synthesis of the X and truncated PreS2/S proteins

Despite the frequent rearrangements of integrated HBV DNA sequences, an intact X protein or a truncated form retaining a transactivating effect on cellular oncogenes can be potentially synthetized in several tumors. In addition, as pointed out earlier, a PreS2/S ORF truncated at the 3′ part of the S gene is present in around 25% of tumors and this may lead to the synthesis of a transactivating protein. These observations may have very important implications for liver carcinogenesis and are discussed in the review by Dr Kékulé.

Insertional mutagenesis

Two different situations must be distinguished: in HCCs in woodchucks infected by WHV, insertion of the WHV DNA into the *c-myc* or *N-myc* oncogenes is frequent (identified in half the tumors so far analysed) [80, 121, 122]. In contrast, in human tumors, a direct cis-acting promoter insertion mechanism has only been definitely shown in two cases, and both tumors developed on a histologically non-cirrhotic liver with evidence of clonal proliferation of cells containing a single HBV integration site. In the first case, HBV DNA integration occurred in an exon of the retinoic acid receptor B gene (RAR B); 29 aminoacids of the viral PreS1 gene were fused to the DNA-binding and hormone-binding domains of the RAR, which is a member of the steroid-thyroid receptor gene family [107, 123]. The major role of retinoic acid and retinoids in cell differentiation and proliferation is well established and it is plausible that viral insertion, by generating a chimaeric HBV/RAR B protein, was involved in the liver cell transformation. The transformation of erythrocytic progenitor cells by retrovirus carrying the hybrid HBV RAR B contract is indeed consistent with this hypothesis [124]. In addition, the identification of RAR B led to the detection of a family of genes encoding, in particular, the RAR A receptor. The chromosomal translocation t [15, 17] in the promyelocytic form of acute leukemia has now been shown to fuse RAR A to a new cellular gene (PML) [125, 126].

In the second case, the human cyclin A-encoding gene was identified by our group in an early liver cancer developing on a histologically normal liver [127, 128]. We have now cloned and sequenced the entire normal cyclin A gene and shown that integration of HBV DNA occurs in the second intron. We have also recently demonstrated that the insertion of HBV DNA markedly modifies the cyclin A expression pattern. Northern Blot analysis of the original tumor (referred to as "HEN") showed an intense accumulation of cyclin A and HBV transcript (1). A cDNA library was generated from the original tumor tissue, and this allowed us to determine the structure of the two (1.7 and 2.7 kb) RNAs identified in this tissue with both HBV and cyclin A probes. They are both synthesized from the HBV PreS2/S promoter and, after splicing in the middle of the S gene, joined the exon 3-8 of the cyclin A gene [129]. The Pres2/S promoter is known to drive the expression of the middle and large proteins of the viral surface antigen (AGHBs). It functions constitutively (in contrast to the core gene promoter), and expression of HBsAg is often maintained in liver cancers despite dedifferentiation of the transformed hepatocyte. Northern blots showed no evidence of transcription of the unoccupied cyclin A allele in the tumor but there was no sign of a gross rearrangement at the cyclin A locus; this might therefore solely reflect a low rate of cyclin A RNA transcription in a tumor with a low proliferation index [129].

Cyclin A plays a major role in both the G2/M and G1/S check-points of the cell cycle, binding to the E2F transcription factor which activates the transcription of genes involved in cell proliferation [130–133]. In fact, cyclin A is included in multimeric complexes including (besides E2F) the retinoblastoma protein related p107 protein, and P33 CDK2 kinase [134].

Analysis of the protein potentially encoded in the tumor by the hybrid RNAs yielded several points of interest: they code for a 430-aminoacid chimeric protein, in which the N-terminal 152 aminoacids of cyclin A are replaced by 150 aminoacids from the PreS2 and S viral proteins, while the C-terminal two-thirds of cyclin A, including the cyclin box, remain intact. The cyclin A degradation sequences located in the N-terminal part of the protein are therefore deleted. Using an *in vitro* degradation assay with frog oocytes, we verified that HBV/cyclin A is not degradable [129]. It is, however, striking that despite the large amount of HBV/Cyclin RNAs in tumor tissue, we failed to detect hybrid protein in these samples by means of Western blotting. This might be due to modifications in the structure of the protein to low-level expression in tumor cells (possibly necessary to avoid a cytotoxic effect of cyclin A) [129].

Several hypotheses can be proposed to account for its potential role in cell transformation: the absence of degradation of a molecule retaining the ability to complex to and activate cdk kinases might lead to unregulated and premature DNA synthesis and thus to cell proliferation. In *S. cerevisiae*, expression of an undegradable CLN3 G1 cyclin advances the START and renders cells unresponsive to negative regulation by mating pheromones. It is also quite plausible that the location of the HBV/cyclin A protein is changed, given the membrane location of PreS2/S molecules in HBV-infected cells. Finally, it is noteworthy that the PreS2/S viral sequences present in HBV/cyclin A are deleted in their C-terminal part and thus have a similar structure to the PreS2/S proteins known to transactivate the *c-myc* and *c-fos* proto-oncogenes [130]. We are now investigating its effect on the cell phenotype *in vitro* and *in vivo*. The results obtained with this tumor contrast with those obtained with liver cancers, in which no HBV DNA integrated in the cyclin A gene: only 6/43 showed a significant increase in the amount of cyclin A transcripts and none yielded evidence of a rearrangement of the cyclin A gene (Paterlini, unpublished observations). This phenomenon must therefore be viewed as a rare event, at least in liver cancer. On the other hand, our group has shown that the expression of cyclin A RNA or protein is an interesting marker of tumor cell proliferation *in vivo* [135, 136].

Two further cases of cis activation of a cellular gene have recently been shown; in one of the integration sites, in the PLC/PRF/5 cell line, HBV DNA inserted into the gene encoding human mevalonate kinase; the results are reminiscent of those obtained with the cyclin A gene since hybrid transcripts are synthesized from the PreS2/S promoter and fused to the cellular sequence. Mevalonate kinase had previously only been identified in the rat; by phosphorylating cholesterol, it regulates the synthesis of isoprenoid compounds which are involved in cell proliferation [137]. In addition, it has been recently shown in a human HCC that HBV DNA has inserted into a gene homologous to the epidermal growth factor receptor encoding gene [138].

It is interesting to note that in the four cases so far reported the study of integrated HBV DNA has led to the identification a new gene encoding a protein with a major role in cell proliferation or differentiation. In addition, in three of these samples, sufficient material was available to demonstrate that the viral insertion modified the expression of the gene, with synthesis of hybrid transcripts potentially encoding fusion proteins. While this result strongly argues for a role of HBV DNA insertion in liver cell transformation these findings have remained isolated.

Why insertional mutagenesis is frequent in woodchuck HCCs and rare in human tumors is not clear. It is, however, important to bear in mind that human HCC is a heterogeneous group of tumors; in particular, the small subgroup of patients with tumors arising on non-cirrhotic livers may differ with regard to the sites of HBV DNA integration, from those with tumor developing on a cirrhotic liver. As a result, the number of tumors so far analysed in detail may still be too limited.

Escape of cells containing the integrated HBV DNA from the immune response

Besides the direct effects of HBV on the hepatocyte, integration frequently interrupts the HBcAg gene; in addition, viral DNA replication usually markedly decreases at the time of tumor development, leading to a fall in HBcAg synthesis [34, 45, 115]. In view of the role of HBc and HBe epitopes in the immune response to infected cells, it is plausible that cells containing integrated HBV DNA might "escape" immune destruction, thus conferring a selective growth advantage in the chronic course of infection.

Hepatacellular carcinoma in Hepatitis B surface antigen-negative patients

As discussed, there are striking geographical variations in the association between HCC and chronic infection by HBV. In Western countries (i.e Northern Europe, USA), and in Japan only 15 to 20% of tumors occur in HBsAg-positive patients, and other environmental factors such as alcohol and infection by hepatitis C virus (HCV) are clearly major risk factors. A number of epidemiological studies have shown a high prevalence of anti-HBs and anti-HBc antibodies in HBsAg-negative subjects (around 40 to 50% in France), indicating exposure to the virus [2, 18, 139]. These antibodies generally reflect resolved HBV infection; in HBsAg-negative subjects with HCC, however, HBV DNA sequences can be detected in the tumors, demonstrating the persistence of the viral infection and suggesting its implication in liver carcinogenesis [18]. It is important to realise that the improvement in the sensitivity of tests for HBsAg, together with the introduction of sensitive tests for HBV DNA, has modified the criteria for the diagnosis of HBV infection;

there is indeed a spectrum of chronic HBV infections with a low replication rate which, might also be a risk factor for liver cancer [140–144].

In this section, we will review the main issues raised by these observations.

The prevalence of HBV DNA in liver tumors of HBsAg-negative patients

The actual prevalence of these HBV DNA-positive HCCs in HBsAg-negative subjects has been a matter of debate, due to the low copy number per cell of viral DNA sequences (estimated at 0.1 to 0.01). Studies performed in different geographical areas have given very different results, probably because of different technical conditions (specificity and sensitivity) as well as distinct epidemiological situations. Thanks to the sensitivity of the Polymerase Chain Reaction (PCR) the previous observations have been confirmed. In addition, PCR has been used to demonstrate transmission of HBV particles present in the serum of these HBsAg-negative patients to chimpanzees, and to determine the nucleotidic sequence of the HBV genomes. For example, in a study performed in patients from areas of high (South Africa) and low (France, Italy) HBV prevalence, HBV DNA was detected in 37/63 HBsAg negative patients, including 15 of 24 serologically recovered and 13 of 32 patients with no detectable HBV serological markers [135, 145, 146]. Similar results were also recently obtained in Spain, Africa, and in the United States. It is striking that there was no real correlation between the serological HBV profiles and the presence or absence of HBV DNA in serum or tumor specimens. Taken together, these studies show that HBV infection persists in a large number of subjects with HBsAg-negative HCCs.

Structure of HBV DNA in tumors

With regard to the state of HBV DNA, its low copy number per cell has hampered the interpretation of the results of Southern blotting. However, using our PCR test and distinct primers distributed on the S, PRE/S, C, and X HBV genes, we were able to provide further information. For several patients, a positive result was only obtained with some of the HBV primers, a finding consistent with the presence of defective HBV DNA. In other cases, the tumor DNA scored positive with all the HBV primers, a fact consistent with the presence of free or integrated HBV DNA and no gross rearrangements. Interestingly, defective HBV genomes have been identified more frequently in tumors than in non tumor tissues. In addition, they also have been shown more frequently in completely seronegative individuals than in anti HBs and anti HBc positive subjects; this observation likely reflects a technical point since the presence of defective HBV DNA can be obscured by concomitant complete viral genomes.

The PCR profiles obtained with DNA from tumor, non-tumor, and serum samples from the same European patients showed marked differences. In the serum and non tumor samples, amplification was achieved with all the primers tested; in contrast, tumor DNA repeatedly gave negative results with at least one primers. These findings demonstrate that the HBV DNA sequences in the tumor do not derive from contaminating nontumor cells or serum-derived particles. They are also consistent with the clonal expansion of cells containing defective and integrated HBV DNA [135].

Among the factors which might account for the negativity of serological HBsAg tests are a low level of infectious HBV particles at the time of contamination, an abnormal host immune response to the virus, and genetic variations of the HBV genomes. These possibilities are discussed in Chapter X on the genetic variations of HBV.

Transcription of the HBV DNA sequences

Northern blot analysis has not proven sensitive enough for the detection of HBV RNAs in these tumors. In contrast, cDNA synthesis followed by PCR with primers on the S gene (RT-PCR) revealed HBV RNA sequences in most of HBV DNA-positive tumors from HBsAg-negative patients. Owing to the compact organisation of the HBV genome it was, however, not possible to determine precisely which viral transcripts were synthesized. In a recent study [136], we investigated the HBV RNAs with primers located on the S, C, and X encoding sequences. X, but not C and S, transcripts were identified in tumor tissues from 7 of the 9 HbsAg (-) HBV DNA (+) patients studied [136]. This may provide a clue to the pathogenesis of these tumors in view of the potential transforming properties of the X protein envisaged in HBsAg-positive liver cancers (see review by Dr Kékulé).

Potential role of HBV in the pathogenesis of HBsAg-negative HCC

Taken together, the results demonstrate a high rate of persistent HBV infection in patients negative for serum-HBsAg, many of whom also lack detectable antibodies to the virus. They also show clonal expansion of the tumor cells containing the integrated viral DNA and the preferential transcription in these cells of HBV RNA sequences encoding the viral X protein. While these findings strongly argue for a role for HBV in the development of these tumors, one highly paradoxical result still remains to be explained: why is the copy number of HBV DNA per cell so low if clonal expansion of infected cells occurs? One hypothesis is that HBV might act as an "initiating" agent, and that maintenance of the transformation process does not require the persistence of HBV DNA; in addition, there may be chromosomal rearrangements which eliminate the viral DNA from the tumor clones. This explanation has also been forwarded to account for human and bovine papillomavirus- and some retrovirus-related tumors [147–149].

The involvement of HBV in HBsAg negative liver cancers is also reinforced by two lines of evidences. In the woodchuck model of HCC, 17% of animals infected by the WHV developed primary liver cancers despite negativation of the assay for WHV surface antigen in the serum and appearance of antibodies to the surface and capsid viral antigenes; in addition, WHV DNA was detected in the tumor tissues of these animals with a much lower copy per cell number than in WHsAg-positive woodchucks (around 1 and 1000 molecules per cell, respectively) [65, 66, 150], an observation quite similar to that we have discussed in previous sections in human HCCs. Ground squirrel might also turn out to be an interesting model for this issue since GSHV DNA sequences have been identified in HCCs developing in completely seronegative animals [151]. Another line of evidence for a direct role of HBV in the liver cancer stands from the detection of HBV DNA in a significant number (7/12) of HCCs in HBsAg negative patients, developing on non cirrhotic, histologically close to normal livers: thus, cirrhosis cannot solely account for the induction of the cancer in these cases [146].

Interaction between HBV, HCV and alcohol

HBV and HCV can interact with chronic alcoholic consumption and there is circumstantial evidence of a high prevalence of HBV and HCV infection in alcoholics. The high prevalence of anti-HCV in alcoholics with cirrhosis (40–50%), relative to those with minimal liver damage (around 20%) suggests that HCV infection might be involved in the development of cirrhosis in some of these patients. This might also account for the high prevalence of anti-HCV (50%) in alcoholics with HCC [139, 152–156]. In contrast, there is no evidence of a role of HBV in the development of alcoholic cirrhosis, since the prevalence of anti-HBs and anti-HBc, although higher than in the general population, does not significantly differ with regard to the presence or absence of cirrhosis (diagnosed in around 20% of cases). There is, however, evidence of a role of HBV in liver cancers in alcoholics since the prevalence of serological HBV markers is significantly increased in these patients (around 50%) and the tumors frequently contain HBV DNA sequences [156-160]. Regardless of chronic alcohol consumption, it is clear that chronic infection by HCV is an important etiological factor in HBsAg-negative HCCs although the prevalence of anti-HCV antibodies varies considerably from one part of the world to the next (80% in Japan, 60–70% in Southern Europe, 40–50% in France and 10–30% in Africa) [139, 154, 161–166]. The presence of HCV RNA sequences has been demonstrated in tumor tissue and there is evidence of an ongoing HCV multiplication concomitant with tumor development; as with HBV, the number of HCV RNA copies per cell is apparently low but, in contrast to HBV, no HCV DNA sequences are detected and the virus does not thus integrate into cellular DNA [135,167,168]. A recent study conducted in France showed that most of HBsAg-negative liver cancer tissues (from alcoholics and non-alcoholics) contained HCV RNA (7/22), HBV DNA (7/22), or both (4/22) [135]. Similar results have been obtained in the USA (169, 170) and in Spain [171]. Primary liver cancer in low endemic areas thus shows a strong association with both viral infections, a fact that has important implications for prevention campaigns.

Conclusion: HBV in HBsAg positive and negative primary liver cancers: Hypothetical mechanisms

We have presented, in the previous sections, evidences for the involvement of HBV in both HBsAg positive and negative liver cancers. Obviously, other factors (such as HCV, alcohol, chemical carcinogenes and hormonal factors) should be also included in the multifactorial process involved in liver carcinogenesis.

A major difference between HBsAg positive and HBsAg negative HBV DNA positive PLCs is related to the number of viral DNA sequence per cell and the rate of HBV DNA replication.

In HBsAg positive chronic carriers, HBV multiplication is sustained for enough time to induce liver cell necrosis and thus secondary proliferation of adjacent liver cells (ie: regeneration). In these subjects, HBV may therefore act at two complementary steps of liver cell transformation: it might exert a direct role by a combination of transactivation and integration; in addition, it can induce promotion and clonal expansion of the initiated "cells" by inducing liver cell necrosis and regeneration.

In contrast, in HBsAg negative HBV DNA positive patients, the number of HBV DNA copy per cell is low and viral DNA replication is barely detectable. In most of these cases, therefore, it is unlikely that HBV is solely involved in liver cell necrosis, chronic active hepatitis and cirrhosis. Instead, other factors such as HCV, alcohol or other still unrecognized agents might be responsible for cirrhosis and thus promotion of the neoplastic transformation. On the other hand, we have presented evidences for the persistence of integrated viral DNA which may exert a direct effect via integration and/or transactivation. HBV might, therefore, be able to initiate liver cell transformation in a limited number of clonally extended cells; the subsequent development of an HCC would be dependent of the effect of co-factors able to promote liver cell regeneration via development of cirrhosis.

In conclusion: epidemiological molecular and experimental animals studies strongly support a role for HBV DNA persistence in the development of hepatocellular carcinoma. The experimental data indicate that liver cell proliferation is necessary for the integration of HBV DNA; in term, HBV integration of the HBV genome can exerce a direct mutagenetic effect which will be fixed by the liver cell regeneration and eventually amplified.

References

1. Kew MC. Role of cirrhosis in hepatocarcinogenesis. In Liver cell carcinoma, Bannasch, P, Keppler, D, Weber, G, Kluwer Academic Publishers, Dordrecht, The Netherlands 1989; 37.
2. Kew MC, Popper H. Relationship between hepatocellular carcinoma and cirrhosis. Sem Liver Dis 1984; 4: 136.
3. Tarao K, Shimizu A, Ohkawa S, Harada M, Ito Y, Tamai S, Kuni Y, Okamoto N, Inoue T, Kanisawa M. Development of hepatocellular carcinoma associated with increases in DNA synthesis in the surrounding cirrhosis. Gastroenterology 1992; 103: 595.
4. Chisari FV, Klopchin K, Moriyama T, Pasquinelli C, Dunsford HA, Sell S, Pinkert CA, Brinster RL, Palmiter RD, Molecular pathogenesis of hepatocellular carcinoma in hepatitis B virus transgenic mice. Cell 1989; 59: 1145.
5. Bréchot C, Pourcel C, Louise A, Rain B, Tiollais P, Presence of integrated hepatitis B virus DNA sequences in cellular DNA of human hepatocellular carcinoma. Nature 1980; 286: 533.
6. Edman JC, Gray P, Valenzuela P, Rall LB, Rutter WJ, Integration of hepatitis B virus sequences and their expression in a human hepatoma cell. Nature 1980; 286: 535.
7. Marion PL, Oshiro LS, Regnery DC, Scullard GH, Robinson WS, A virus in beechey ground squirrels that is related to hepatitis B virus of humans. Proc Natl Acad Sci USA 1980; 77: 2941.
8. Chakraborty PR, Ruiz Opazo H, Shouval D, Shafritz DA. Identification of integrated hepatitis B virus DNA and expression of viral RNA in an HBsAg-producing human hepatocellular carcinoma cell line. Nature 1980; 286: 531.
9. Koshy R, Koch S, Freytag von Loringhoven A, Kahmann R, Murray K, Hofschneider PH. Integration of hepatitis B virus DNA: evidence for integration in the single-stranded gap. Cell 1983; 34: 215.
10. Koshy R, Meyer M, Kékulé A, Lauer U, Caselmann WH, Hofschneider PH. Altered functions of hepatitis B virus proteins as a consequence of viral DNA integration may lead to hepatocyte transformation, in Hollinger FB, Lemon SM, Margolis H, Viral Hepatitis and Liver Disease, Williams and Wilkins, USA, 1991; 566.
11. Koshy R, Wells J, Deregulation of cellular gene expression by HBV transactivators in hepatocarcinogenesis. Adv Appl Biotechnol Ser 1991; 13: 159.
12. Monjardino JP, Fowler MJF, Thomas HC, Defective hepatitis B virus DNA molecules detected in a stable integration pattern in a hepatoma cell line, and in induced tumours and derived cell lines. J Gen Virol 1983; 64: 2299.
13. Matsubara K, Tokino T, Integration of hepatitis B virus DNA and its implications for hepatocarcinogenesis. Mol Biol Med 1990; 7: 243.
14. Meyer M, Caselman W, Schlüter V, Schreck R, Hofschneider P, Baeuerle P, Hepatitis B virus transactivator MHBst: activation of NF-KB, selective inhibition by antioxidants and integral membrane localization. The EMBO Journal 1992; 11: 2991.
15. Kekulé AS, Lauer U, Meyer M, Caselmann WH, Hofschneider PH, Koshy, R, The pre-S2/S region of integrated hepatitis B virus DNA encodes a transcriptional transactivator. Nature 1990; 43: 457.
16. Twu JS, Schloemer RH, Transcriptional trans-activating function of hepatitis B virus. J Virol 1987; 61.
17. Takada S, Koike K, Trans-activation function of a 3′ truncated X gene-cell fusion product from integrated hepatitis B virus DNA in chronic hepatitis tissues. Proc Natl Acad Sci USA 1990; 87: 5628.
18. Bréchot C, Hepatitis B virus (HBV) and hepatocellular carcinoma. HBV DNA status and its implications. J Hepatology1987; 4: 269.
19. Blum HE, Offensperger W-B, Walter S, Offensperger A, Wahl C, Zeschnigk C, Gerok W, Hepatocellular carcinoma and hepatitis B virus infection: molecular evidence for

monoclonal origin and expansion of malignantly transformed hepatocytes. J Cancer Res Clin Oncol 1987; 113: 466.
20. Miller RH, Robinson WS, Common evolutionary origin of hepatitis B virus and retroviruses. Proc Natl Acad Sci USA 1986; 83: 2531.
21. Bréchot C, Hadchouel M, Scotto J, Degos F, Charnay P, Trépo C, Tiollais P, Detection of hepatitis B virus DNA in liver and serum: a direct appraisal of the chronic carrier state. Lancet 1981; ii: 765.
22. Takada S, Yaginuma K, Arii M, Nakamura I, Shirakata Y, Kobayashi M, Koike K, Molecular biology of hepatitis B virus and hepatocellular carcinoma, in Primary Liver Cancer in Japan, (eds.), T. T. et al., Springer-Verlag, Tokyo 1992; 75.
23. Robinson WS, Hepadnaviridae and their replication, in Fields Virology, Fields BN, Knipe DM, Chanock RM, Hirsch MS, Melnick JL, Monath TP, Roizman B, Raven Press, New York 1990; 2137.
24. Bréchot C, Hadchouel J, Scotto M, Fonck F, Potet G, Tiollais P, State of hepatitis B virus DNA in hepatocytes of patients with HbsAg positive and HbsAg negative liver diseases. Proc Natl Acad Sci USA 1981; 78: 3906.
25. Shafritz DA, Shouval D, Sherman H, Hadziyannis S, Kew, MC, Integration of hepatitis B virus DNA into the genome of liver cells in chronic liver disease and hepatocellular carcinoma. New Engl J Med 1981; 305: 1067.
26. Kam W, Rall LB, Smuckler EA, Scmid R, Rutter WJ, Hepatitis B viral DNA in liver and serum of asymptomatic carriers. Proc Natl Acad Sci USA 1982; 79: 7522.
27. Hadziyannis SJ, Lieberman HM, Karvountzis GG, Shafritz, DA, Analysis of liver disease, nuclear HBsAg, viral replication, and hepatitis B virus DNA, in liver and serum of HBeAg vs. anti-Hbe positive carriers of hepatitis B virus. Hepatology1983; 3: 656.
28. Yaginuma K, Kobayashi H, Kobayashi M, Morishima T, Matsuyama K, Koike K, Multiple integration site of hepatitis B virus DNA in hepatocellular carcinoma and chronic active hepatitis tissues from children. J Virol 1987; 61: 1808.
29. Yasui H, Hino O, Ohtake K, Machinami R, Kitagawa T, Clonal growth of hepatitis B virus integrated hepatocytes in cirrhotic liver nodules. Cancer Research 1992; 52: 6810.
30. Lugassy C, Bernuau J, Thiers V, Krosgaard K, Degott C, Wantzin P, Schalm SW, Rueff B, Benhamou JP, Tiollais P, Bréchot C, Sequences of hepatitis B virus DNA in the serum and liver of patients with acute benign and fulminant hepatitis. J Infect Dis 1987; 155: 64.
31. Hino O, Tabata S, Hotta Y, Evidence for increased *in vitro* recombination with insertion of human hepatitis B virus DNA. Proc Natl Acad Sci USA 1991; 88: 9248.
32. Scotto J, Hadchouel M, Wain-Hobson S, Sonigo P, Couroucé A-M, Tiollais P, Bréchot C, Hepatitis B virus DNA in Dane particules: Evidence for the presence of replicative intermediates, J Infect Dis 1985; 151: 610.
33. Matsubara K, Chromosomal changes associated with hepatitis B virus DNA integration and hepatocarcinogenesis, in Molecular Biology of the Hepatitis B Virus, McLachlan, A, CRC Press, Inc, Boca Raton, Florida 1991; 245.
34. Raimondo G, Burk R, Lieberman H, Muschel J, Hadziyannis S, Will H, Kew M, Dusheiko G, Shafritz D, Interrupted replication of hepatitis B virus in liver tissue of HBsAg carriers with hepatocellular carcinoma. Virology 1988; 166: 103.
35. Bréchot C, Lugassy C, Dejean A, Pontisso P, Thiers V, Berthelot P, Tiollais P, Hepatitis B virus DNA in infected human tissues viral hepatitis 1984; 395.
36. Rogler CE, Summers J, Novel forms of woodchuck hepatitis virus DNA isolated from chronically infected woodchuck liver nuclei. J Virol 1982; 44: 852.
37. Bowyer S, Dusheiko G, Schoub B, Kew M, Expression of the hepatitis B virus genome in chronic hepatitis B carriers and patients with hepatocellular carcinoma. Proc Natl Acad Sci 1987; 84: 847.

38. Fournier J-G, Kessous A, Richer G, Bréchot C, Simard R, Detection of hepatitis B viral RNAs in human liver tissues by in situ hybridization. Biol Cell 1982; 43: 225.
39. Burrell J, Gowans E, Rowland R, Correlation between liver histology and markers of hepatitis B virus replication in infected patients: a study by "*in situ* hybridization". Hepatology 1984; 4: 20.
40. Alberti A, Trevisan A, Fattovich G, The role of hepatitis B virus replication and hepatocytes membrane expression in the pathogenesis of HBV-related hepatic damage 1984; 134.
41. Mondelli M, Naumov N, Eddleston A, The immunopathogenesis of liver cell damage in chronic infection, in Advances in hepatitis Research, Chisari, F, Masson, New York 1984; 144.
42. Wang W, London WT, Lega L, Feitelson MA, HBxAg in the liver from carrier patients with chronic hepatitis and cirrhosis. Hepatology 1991; 14: 29.
43. London WT, Blumberg BS, Acellular model of the role of hepatitis virus in the pathogenesis of primary hepatocellular carcinoma. Hepatology1982; 2: 105.
44. Chen C, Diani A, Brown P, Kaluzny M, Epps D, Detection of hepatitis B virus DNA in hepatocellular carcinoma 1986; 67: 1868.
45. Loncarevic IF, Zentgraf H, Schröder CH, Sequence of a replication competent hepatitis B virus genome with a preX open reading frame. Nucl Acids Res 1990; 18: 4940.
46. Elfassi E, Romet-Lemonne JL, Essex M, Frances-McLane M, Haseltine WA, Evidence of extrachromosomal forms of hepatitis B viral DNA in a bone marrow culture obtained from a patient recently infected with hepatitis B virus. Proc Natl Acad Sci USA 1984; 81: 3526.
47. Pontisso P, Poon MC, Tiollais P, Bréchot C, Detection of HBV DNA in mononuclear blood cells. British Medical Journal 1984; 288: 1563.
48. Pasquinelli C, Lauré F, Chatenaud L, Beauvin G, Gazengee C, Bismuth H, Degos F, Tiollais P, Bach JF, Bréchot C, Hepatitis B virus DNA in mononuclear blood cells. J Hepatology1986; 3: 95.
49. Hadchouel M, Scotto J, Huset C et al, Presence of HBV DNA in spermatozoa – A possible vertical transmission of HBV via the germ line, J Med Virol 1985; 16: 61.
50. Romet-Lemonne JL, McLane MF, Elfassi E et al, Hepatitis B virus infection in cultured human lymphoblastoid cells. Science 1983; 221: 667.
51. Blum H, Stowring L, Figus A, Montgomery C, Haase A, Vyas G, Detection of hepatitis B virus DNA in hepatocytes, bile duct epithelium, and vascular elements by in situ hybridization. Proc Natl Acad Sci 1983; 81: 6685.
52. Dejean A, Sonigo P, Wain-Hobson S, Tiollais P, Specific hepatitis B virus integration in hepatocellular carcinoma DNA through a viral 11 base pair direct repeat. Proc Natl Acad Sci USA 1984; 81: 5350.
53. Dejean A, Lugassi C, Zafrani S, Tiollais P, Bréchot C, Detection of hepatitis B virus DNA in pancreas, kidney and skin of two human carriers of the virus. J Gen Virol 1984; 65: 651.
54. Yoffe B, Burns DK, Bhatt HS, Combes B, Extrahepatic hepatitis B virus DNA sequences in patients with acute hepatitis B infection. Hepatology1990; 12: 187.
55. Omata M, Significance of extrahepatic replication of HBV, Hepatology1990; 12: 364.
56. Shimoda T, Shikata T, Karasawa T, Tsukagoshi S, Light microscopic localization of hepatitis B virus antigens in the human pancreas. Gastro 1981; 81: 898.
57. Yoffe B, Noonan C, Melnick J, Hollinger F, Hepatitis B virus DNA in mononuclear cells and analysis of cell subsets for the presence of replicative intermediates of viral DNA. J Infect Dis 1986; 153: 471.
58. Galun E, Offensperger W-B, Von Weizsäcker F, Offensperger S, Wands JR, Blum HE, Human non-hepatocytes support hepadnaviral replication and virion production. J Gen Virol 1992; 73: 173.

59. Naumova AK, Kisselev LL, Biological consequences of interactions between hepatitis B virus and human nonhepatic cellular genomes. Biomed Sci 1990; 1: 233.
60. Pasquinelli C, Garreau F, Bougueleret L, Cariani E, Grzeschik KH, Thiers V, Croissant O, Hadchouel M, Tiollais P, Bréchot C, Rearrangement of a common cellular DNA domain on chromosome 4 in human primary liver tumors. J Virol 1988; 62: 629.
61. Baginski I, Chemin I, Bouffard P, Hantz O, Trepo C, Detection of polyadenylated RNA in hepatitis B virus-infected peripheral blood mononuclear cells by polymerase chain reaction. J Infect Dis 1991; 163: 996.
62. Korba BE, Wells F, Tennant BC, Cote PJ, Gerin JL, Lymphoid cells in the spleens of woodchuck hepatitis virus-infected woodchucks are a site of active viral replication. J Virol 1987; 61: 1318.
63. Korba BE, Gowans EJ, Wells FV, Tennant BC, Clarke R, Gerin JL, Systemic distribution of woodchuck hepatitis virus in the tissue of experimentally infected woodchucks. Virology 1988; 165: 172.
64. Korba BE, Cote PJ, Gerin JL, Mitogen-induced replication of woodchuck hepatitis virus in cultured peripheral blood lymphocytes. Science 1988; 241: 1213.
65. Korba BE, Wells FV, Baldwin B, Cote PJ, Tennant BC, Popper H, Gerin JL, Hepatocellular carcinoma in woodchuck hepatitis virus-infected woodchucks: presence of viral DNA in tumor tissue from chronic carriers and animals serologically recovered from acute infections. Hepatology 1989; 9: 461.
66. Korba BE, Cote PJ, Wells FV, Baldwin B, Popper H, Purcell RH, Tennant BC, Gerin JL, Natural history of woodchuck hepatitis virus infections during the course of experimental viral infection: Molecular virologic features of the liver and lymphoid tissues. J Virol 1989; 63: 1360.
67. Lie-Injo L, Balasegaray M, Lopez C, Herrera A, Hepatitis B virus DNA in liver and white blood cells of patients with hepatoma. DNA 1983; 2: 301.
68. Bouffard P, Lamelin J-P, Zoulim F, Lepot D, Trépo C, Phytohemagglutinin and concanavalin A activate hepatitis B virus in peripheral blood mononuclear cells of patients with chronic hepatitis B virus infection. J Med Virol 1992; 37: 255.
69. Bouffard P, Hayashi PH, Avecedo R, Levy N, Zeldis JB, Hepatitis C virus is detected in a monocyte/macrophage subpopulation of peripheral blood mononuclear cells of infected patients. J Infect Dis 1992; 166: 1276.
70. Müller C, Bergmann K, Gerin J, Korba B, Production of hepatitis B virus by stably transfected monocytic cell line U-937: a model for extrahepatic hepatitis B virus replication. J Infect Dis 1992; 165: 929.
71. Zeldis JB, Mugishima H, Steinberg HN, Nir E, Gale RP, *In vitro* hepatitis B virus infection of human bone marrow cells. J Clin Invest 1986; 78: 411.
72. Steinberg HS, Bouffard P, Trépo C, Zeldis JB, *In vitro* inhibition of hemopoietic cell line growth by hepatitis B virus. J Hepatology1990; 64: 2577.
73. Féray C, Zignego A, Samuel D, Bismuth A, Reynes A, Bismuth H, Bréchot C, Persistent hepatitis B virus liver infection: the liver transplantation model. Transplantation 1990; 49: 1155.
74. Gerken G, Kremsdorf D, Capel F, Petit MA, Dauguet C, Manns MP, Meyer zum Büschenfelde KH, Bréchot C, Hepatitis B defective virus with rearrangements in the preS gene during chronic HBV infection. Virol 1991; 183: 555.
75. Lauré F, Zaguri D, Saimot A, Gallo R, Hahn B, Bréchot C, Hepatitis B virus DNA sequences in lymphoid cells for patients with AIDS and AIDS-related complex. Science 1985; 229: 561.
76. Colucci G, Lyons P, Beazer Y, Waksal SD, Production of hepatitis B virus infected human B-cell hybridomas: transmission of the viral genome to normal lymphocytes in cocultures. Virol 1988; 238.

77. Shih C, Burke K, Chou MJ, Zeldis JB, Yang CS, Lee CS, Isselbacher KJ, Wands JR, Goodman H, Tight clustering of human hepatitis B virus integration sites in hepatomas near a triple-stranded region. J Virol 1987; 61: 3491.
78. Nagaya T, Nakamura T, Tokino T, Tsurimoto T, Imai M, Mayumi T, Kamino K, Yamamura K, Matsubara K, The mode of hepatitis B virus DNA integration in chromosomes of human hepatocellular carcinoma. Genes Dev 1987; 1: 773.
79. Zhou YZ, Butel JS, Li PJ, Finegold MJ, Melnick JL, Integrated state of subgenomic fragments of hepatitis B virus DNA in hepatocellular carcinoma from mainland China. JNCI 1987; 79: 223.
80. Buendia MA, Hepatitis B viruses and hepatocellular carcinoma. Adv Cancer Res 1992; 59: 167.
81. Fowler M, Thomas H, Monjardino J, Cloning and analysis of integrated hepatitis B virus DNA of the adr suntype derived from a human primary liver cell carcinoma. J Gen Virol 1986; 61: 771.
82. Quade K, Saldanha J, Thomas H, Monjardino J, Integration of hepatitis B virus DNA through a mutational hot spot within the cohesive regio in a case of hepatocellular carcinoma. J Gen Virol 1992; 73: 179.
83. Mizusawa H, Taira M, Yaginuma K, Kobayashi M, Yoshida E, Koike K, Inversely repeating integrated hepatitis B virus DNA and cellular flanking sequences in the human hepatoma-derived cell line huSP. Proc Natl Acad Sci USA 1985; 82: 208.
84. Tanaka Y, Esumi M, Shikata T, Frequent integration of hepatitis B virus DNA in noncancerous liver tissue from hepatocellular carcinoma patients. J Med Virol 198; 26: 7.
85. Freytag von Loringhoven A, Koch S, Hofschneider PH, Koshy R, Co-transcribed 3′ host sequences augment expression of integrated hepatitis B virus DNA. EMBO J 1985; 4: 249.
86. Chang MH, Chen PJ, Chen JY, Lai MY, Hsu HC, Lian DC, Liu YG, Chen DS, Hepatitis B virus integration in hepatitis B virus-related hepatocellular carcinoma in childhood. Hepatology 1991; 13: 316.
87. Koch S, Freytag von Loringhoven A, Kahmann R, Hofschneider PH, Koshy R, The genetic organization of integrated hepatitis B virus DNA in the human hepatoma cell line PLC/PRF/5. Nucl Acids Res 1984; 12: 6871
88. Koch S, Freytag von Loringhoven A, Hofschneider PH, Koshy R, Amplification and rearrangement in hepatoma cell DNA associated with integrated hepatitis B virus DNA. EMBO J 1984; 3: 2185.
89. Koike K, Kobayashi M, Mizusawa H, Yoshida E, Yaginuma K, Taira M, Rearrangement of the surface antigen gene of hepatitis B virus integrated in the human hepatoma cell lines. Nucl Acids Res 1983; 11: 5391.
90. Choo K-B, Liu M-S, Chang P-C, Wu S-M, Su M-W, Pan C-C, Han S-H, Analysis of six distinct integrated hepatitis B virus sequences cloned from the cellular DNA of a human hepatocellular carcinoma. Virol 1986; 154: 405.
91. Shaul Y, Ziemer M, Garcia PD, Crawford R, Hsu H, Valenzuela P, Rutter WJ, Cloning and analysis of integrated hepatitis virus sequences from a human hepatoma cell line. J Virol 1984; 51: 776.
92. Takada, Takase S, Enomoto N, Takada A, Date T, Clinical backgrounds of the patients having different types of hepatitis C virus genomes. J Hepatology1992; 14: 35.
93. Meyer M, Wiedorn KH, Hofschneider PH, Chromosome 17:7 translocation is associated with hepatitis B virus DNA integratioon in human hepatocellular carcinoma DNA. Hepatology 1992; 15: 665.
94. Berger I, Shaul Y, Integration of hepatitis B virus: analysis of unoccupied sites. J Virol 1987; 61: 1180.

95. Georgi-Geisberger P, Berns H, Loncarevic IF, Yu Z-Y, Tang Z-Y, Zentgraf H, Schröder CH, Mutations on free and integrated hepatitis B virus DNA in a hepatocellular carcinoma: footprints of homologous recombination. Oncol 1992; 49: 386.
96. Takada S, Gotoh Y, Hayashi S, Yoshida M, Koike K, Structural rearrangement of integrated hepatitis B virus DNA as well as cellular flanking DNA is present in chronically infected hepatic tissues. J Virol 1990; 822.
97. Nakamura T, Tokino T, Nagaya T, Matsubara K, Microdeletion associated with the integration process of hepatitis B virus DNA. Nucleic Acids Res 1988; 16: 4865.
98. Hino O, Shows TB, Rogler CE, Hepatitis B virus integration site in hepatocellular carcinoma at chromosome 17;18 translocation. Proc Natl Acad Sci USA 1986; 83: 8338.
99. Rogler CE, Sherman M, Su CY, Shafritz DA, Summers J, Shows TB, Henderson A, Kew M, Deletion in chromosome 11p associated with a hepatitis B integration site in hepatocellular carcinoma. Science 1985; 230: 319.
100. Tokino T, Fukushige S, Nakamura T, Nagaya T, Murotsu T, Shiga K, Aoki N, Matsubara K, Chromosomal translocation and inverted duplication associated with integrated hepatitis B virus in hepatocellular carcinomas. J Virol 1987; 61: 3848.
101. Yaginuma K, Kobayashi M, Yoshida E, Koike K, Hepatitis B virus integration in hepatocellular carcinoma DNA: duplication of cellular flanking sequences at the integration site. Proc Natl Acad Sci USA 1985; 82: 4458.
102. Shaul Y, Garcia PD, Schonberg S, Rutter WJ, Integration of hepatitis B virus DNA in chromosome-specific satellite sequences. J Virol 1986; 59: 731.
103. Matsumoto H, Yoneyama T, Mitamura K, Osuga T, Shimojo H, Miyamura T, Analysis of integrated hepatitis B virus DNA and cellular flanking sequences cloned from a hepatocellular carcinoma. Int J Cancer 1988; 42: 1.
104. Zerial M, Salinas J, Filipski J, Bernardi G, Genomic localization of hepatitis B virus in a human hepatoma cell line. Nucl Acids Res 1986; 14: 8373.
105. Ziemer M, Gàrcia P, Shaul Y, Rutter WJ, Sequence of hepatitis B virus DNA incorporated into the genome of a human hepatoma cell line. J Virol 1985; 53: 885.
106. Bowcock A, Pinto M, Bey E, Kuyl J, Dusheiko G, Bernstein R, The PLC/PRF/5 human hepatoma cell line. II. Chromosomal assignment of hepatitis B virus integration sites. Cancer Gent. Cytogenet 1985; 18: 19.
107. Dejean A, Bougueleret L, Grzeschik KH, Tiollais P, Hepatitis B virus DNA integration in a sequence homologous to v-erbA and steroid receptor genes in a hepatocellular carcinoma. Nature 1986; 322: 70.
108. Hino O, Ohtake K, Rogler CE, Features of two hepatitis B virus (HBV) DNA integrations suggest mechanisms of HBV integration. J Virol 1989; 63: 2638.
109. Wang HP, Rogler CE, Topoisomerase I-mediated integration of hepadnavirus DNA *in vitro*. J Virol 1991; 65: 2381.
110. Wang W-P, Myers RL, Chiu I-M, Single primmer-mediated polymerase chain reaction: application in cloning of two different 5′-untranslated sequences of acidic fibroblast growth factor mRNA. DNA and Cell Biology 1991; 10: 771.
111. Wang W, London T, Feitelson M, Hepatitis B x antigen in hepatitis B virus carrier patients with liver cancer. Cancer Research 1991; 51: 4971.
112. Hino O, Kitagawa T, Koike K, Kobayashi M, Hara M, Mori W, Nakashima T, Hattori N, Sugano H, Detection of hepatitis B virus DNA in hepatocellular carcinomas in Japan 1984; 4: 90.
113. Hino O, Kitagawa T, Sugano H, Relationship between serum and histochemical markers for hepatitis B virus and rate of viral integration in hepatocellular carcinomas in Japan. Int J Cancer 1985; 5.
114. Hino O, Kitagawa T, Nomura K, Ohtake K, Yasui H, Okamoto N, Hirayama Y, Comparative molecular pathogenesis of hepatocellular carcinomas. In Comparative molecular

carcinogenesis, Klein-Szanto AJP, Anderson MW, Barrett JC, Slaga TJ, Wiley Liss, Inc 1992; 173.
115. Loncarevic I, Schrantz P, Zentgraf H, Liang X, Herrman G, Tang Z, Schröder C, Replication of hepatitis B virus in a hepatocellular carcinoma. Virology 1990; 174: 158.
116. Tokino T, Matsubara K, Chromosomal sites for hepatitis B virus integration in human hepatocellular carcinoma. J Virol 1991; 65: 6761.
117. Slagle BL, Zhou YZ, Butel JS, Hepatitis B virus integration event in human chromosome 17p near the p53 gene identifies the region of the chromosome commonly deleted in virus-positive hepatocellular carcinomas. Cancer Res 1991; 51: 49.
118. Wang HP, Rogler CE, Deletions in human chromosome arms 11p and 13 p in primary hepatocellular carcinomas 1988; 48: 72.
119. Urano Y, Watanabe K, Lin C, Hino O, Tamaoki T, Interstitial chromosomal deletion within 4q11-q13 in a human hepatoma cell line. Cancer Research 1991; 51: 1460.
120. Hatada I, Tokino T, Ochiya T, Matsubara K, Co-amplification of integrated hepatitis B virus DNA and transforming gene hst-1 in a hepatocellular carcinoma. Oncogene 1988; 3: 537.
121. Fourel G, Tiollais P, Buendia MA, Nucleotide sequence of the woodchuck N-myc gene (WN-myc1). Nucl Acids Res 1990; 18: 4918.
122. Fourel G, Trépo C, Bougueleret L, Henglein B, Ponzetto A, Tiollais P, Buendia MA, Frequent activation of N-myc genes by hepadnavirus insertion in woodchuck liver tumours. Nature 1990; 347: 294.
123. Dejean A, De Thé H, Hepatitis B virus as an insertional mutagen in a human hepatocellular carcinoma. Mol Biol Med 1990; 7: 213.
124. Garcia M, De Thé H, Tiollais P, Samarut J, Dejean A, A hepatitis B virus pre-S-retinoic acid receptor béta chimera transforms erythrocytic progenitor cells *in vitro*. Cell Biology 1993; 90: 89.
125. De Thé H, Chomienne C, Lanotte M, Degos L, Dejean A, The t(15;17) translocation of acute promyelocytic leukemia fuses the retinoic acid receptor alpha gene to a novel transcribed locus. Nature 1990; 347: 558.
126. De Thé H, Lavau C, Marchio A, Chomienne C, Degos L, Dejean A, The PML-RAR-alpha fusion mRNA generated by the t(15,17) translocation in acute promyelocytic leukaemia encodes a functionally altered retinoic acid receptor. Cell 1991; 66: 675.
127. Wang Y, Chen P, Wu X, Sun AL, Wang H, Zhu YA, Li ZP, A new enhancer element, ENII, identified in the X gene of hepatitis B virus. J Virol 1990; 64: 3977.
128. Wang J, Chenivesse X, Henglein B, Bréchot C, Hepatitis B virus integration in a cyclin A gene in a hepatocellular carcinoma. Nature 1990; 343: 555.
129. Wang J, Zindy F, Chenivesse X, Lamas E, Henglein B, Bréchot C, Modification of cyclin A expression by hepatitis B virus DNA integration in a hepatocellular carcinoma. Oncogene 1992; 7: 1653.
130. Bréchot C, Oncogenic activation of cyclin A. Cur Op Gen Dev 1993; 3.
131. Pines J, Hunter T, Human cyclin A is adenovirus E1A-associated protein p60 and behavves differently from cyclin B. Nature 1990; 346: 760.
132. Nurse P, Universal control mechanism regulating onset of M-phase. Nature 1991; 344: 503.
133. Zindy F, Lamas E, Chenivesse X, Sobczak J, Wang J, Fesquet D, Henglein B, Bréchot C, Cyclin A is required in S phase in normal epithelial cells. Bioch. Biophys. Res Com 1992; 182: 1144.
134. Nevins J, E2F: link between the Rb tumor suppressor protein and viral oncoproteins. Science 1992; 258: 424.
135. Paterlini P, Driss F, Pisi E, Franco D, Berthelot P, Bréchot C, Persistence of hepatitis B and hepatitis C viral genomes in primary liver cancers from HBsAg negative patients: a study of a low endemic area. Hepatology 1993; 17: 20.

136. Paterlini P, Poussin P, D'Errico A, De Mitri S, Kew M, Grigioni W, Franco D, Bréchot C, Rate of persistence, structure and expression of HBV genome in HCC developing in HBsg negative patients. In: Nishioka K, Suzuki H, Mishiro S, Oda T. Eds, Viral Hepatitis and liver diseases, Springer Verlag, in press.
137. Graef E, Caselmann W, Wells J, Koshy K, Activation of cellular genes by hepatitis B virus in hepatocellular carcinogenesis, International Symposium on Viral Hepatitis and Liver Disease, Tokyo 1993; 58.
138. Zhang X-K, Egan JO, Huang D-P, Sun Z-L, Chien VKY, Chiu J-F, Hepatitis B virus DNA integration and expression of an Erb B-like gene in human hepatocellular carcinoma. Biochem Biophys Res Com 1992; 188: 344.
139. Colombo M, Hepatocellular carcinoma. J Hepatology1992; 15: 225.
140. Bréchot C, Degos F, Lugassy C, Thiers V, Zafrani S, Franco D, Bismuth H, Trépo C, Benhamou JP, Wands J, Isselbacher K, Tiollais P, Berthelot P, Hepatitis B virus DNA in patients with chronic liver disease and negative test for hepatitis B surface antigen, NEJM 1985; 312: 270.
141. Bréchot C, Housset C, Traitements antiviraux des hépatites chroniques. Encyclopédie Médico-chirurgicale 1990; 11: 11.
142. Bréchot C, Polymerase chain reaction. A new tool for the study of viral infections in hepatology. J Hepatology1990; 11: 124.
143. Kremsdorf D, Prochon C, Kim JP, Reyes GR, Bréchot C, Partial nucleotide sequence analysis of a french hepatitis C virus: implications for HCV genetic variability in the E2/NS1 protein. J Gen Virol 1991; 72: 2557.
144. Liang T, Baruch Y, Ben-Porath E, Hepatitis B virus infection in patients with idiopathic liver disease. Hepatology 1991; 13: 1044.
145. Paterlini P, Gerken G, Nakajima E, Terré S, D'Errico A, Grigioni W, Nalpas B, Franco D, Wands J, Kew M, Pisi E, Tiollais P, Bréchot C, Polymerase chain reaction to detect hepatitis B virus DNA and RNA sequences in primary liver cancers from patients negative for hepatitis B surface antigen 1990; 323: 80.
146. Paterlini P, Gerken G, Khemeny F, Franco D, D'Errico A, Grigioni W, Wands J, Kew M, Pisi E, Tiollais P, Bréchot C, Primary liver cancer in HBsAg negative patients: a study of HBV genome using the polymerase chain reaction, in Viral hepatitis and liver disease, Hollinger FB, Lemon SM, Margolies HS, Williams and Wilkins, Baltimore 1991; 222.
147. Galloway DA, McDougall JK, The oncogenic potential of herpes simplex virus: evidence for a "hit and run" mechanism. Nature 1983; 302: 21.
148. Smith KT, Campo MS, "Hit and run" transformation of mouse C127 cells by bovine papillomavirus type 4: the viral DNA is required for the initiation but not for maintenance of the transformed phenotype. Virol 1988; 64: 39.
149. Morgan D, Pecararo G, Rosenberg I, Defendi V, Human papillomavirus type 6b DNA is required for initiation but not maintenance of transformation of C127 mouse cells. J Virol 1990; 64: 969.
150. Gerin JL, Cote PJ, Korba BE, Miller RH, Purcell RH, Tennant BC, Hepatitis B virus and liver cancer: the woodchuck as an experimental model of hepadnavirus-induced liver cancer, in Viral Hepatitis and Liver Disease, Hollinger FB, Lemon SM, Margolis H, Williams and Wilkins, Baltimore 1991; 556.
151. Transy C, Fourel G, Robinson WS, Tiollais P, Marion PL, Buendia MA, Frequent amplification of c-myc in ground squirrel liver tumors associated with past or ongoing infection with a hepadnavirus. Proc Natl Acad Sci USA 1992; 89: 3874.
152. Parés A, Barrera JM, Caballeria J, Ercilla G, Bruguera M, Caballeria L, Castillo R et al, Hepatitis C virus antibodies in chronic alcoholic patients: association with severity of liver injury. Hepatology1990; 12: 1295.
153. Mendenhall CL, Seeff L, Diehl AM, Ghosn SJ, French SW, Gartside PS, Rouster SD, Buskell-Bales Z, Grossman CJ, Roselle GA, Weesner RE, Garcia-Pont P, Goldberg SJ,

Kiernan TW, Tamburro CH, Zetterman R, Chedid A, Chen T, Rabin L, Group TVCS, Antibodies to hepatitis B virus and hepatitis C virus in alcoholic hepatitis and cirrhosis: their prevalence and clinical relevance. Hepatology1991; 14: 581.

154. Nalpas B, Driss F, Pol S, Hamelin B, Housset C, Bréchot C, Association between HCV and HBV infection in hepatocellular carcinoma and alcoholic liver disease. J Hepatology1991; 12: 70.

155. Nalpas B, Thiers V, Pol S, Driss F, Thepot V, Berthelot P, Bréchot C, Hepatitis C viremia and anti-HCV antibodies in alcoholics. J Hepatology1992; 14: 381.

156. Nalpas B, Bréchot C, The role of hepatitis virusees in the Genesis of hepatocellular carcinoma in alcoholic cirrhotics, in Alcohol and cancer, Watson, R, CRC 1992.

157. Nalpas B, Berthelot P, Thiers V, Duhamel G, Courouce A, Tiollais P, Bréchot C, Hepatitis B virus multiplication in the absence of usual serological markers – A study of 146 alcoholics. J Hepatology1985; 1: 89.

158. Saunders J, Wodak A, Morgan-Capner P, Whyte Y, Portmann B, Davis M, Williams R, Importance of mmarkers of hepatitis B virus in alcoholic liver disease. Brit Med J 1983; 286: 1851.

159. Poynard T, Aubert A, Lazizi Y, Bedona P, Hamelin B, Tenis B, Naveau S, Dubreuil P, Pillot J, Chaput J, Independent risk factors for hepatocellular carcinoma in French drinkers. Hepatology 1991; 13: 896.

160. Attali P, Thibault N, Buffet C, Briantais M, Papoz L, Chaput J, Etienne J, Les marqueurs du virus B chez les alcooliques chroniques. Gastroenterol. Clin Biol 1981; 5: 1095.

161. Nishioka K, Watanabe J, Furata S, Tanaka E, Iino S, Suzuki H, Tsuji T, Yano M, Kuo G, Choo Q-L, Houghton M, Oda T, A high prevalence of antibody to the hepatitis C virus in patients with hepatocellular carcinoma in Japan 1991; 67: 429-433.

162. Bruix J, Banera J, Calvet X, Ercilla G, Costa J, Sanches-Tapias J, Ventura H, Vall M, Brughera M, Bru C, Castillo R, Rodes J, Prevalence of antibodies to hepatocellular carcinoma and hepatic cirrhosis. Lancet 1989; 2: 1004.

163. Simonetti RG, Cammà C, Fiorello F, Cottone M, Rapicetta M, Marino L, Fiorentino G, Craxì A, Ciccaglione A, Guiseppetti R, Stroffolini T, Pagliaro L, Hepatitis C virus infection as a risk factor for hepatocellular carcinoma in patients with cirrhosis. Ann Int Med 1992; 116: 97.

164. Hasan F, Jeffers L, De Modina M, Reddy K, Parker T, Schiff E, Houghton M, Choo Q, Kuo G, Hepatitis C associated hepatocellular carcinoma. Hepatology 1990; 12: 589.

165. Kew M, Houghton M, Choo Q, Kuo G, Hepatitis C virus antibodies in Southern African blacks with hepatocellular carcinoma. Lancet 1990; 1: 893.

166. Dazza MC, Meneses LV, Girard PM, Paterlini P, Villaroel C, Bréchot C, Larouzé B, Polymerase chain reaction for detection of hepatitis B virus DNA in HBsAg seronegative patients with hepatocellular carcinoma from Mozambique 1991; 85: 277.

167. Ohkoshi S, Detection of HBV DNA in non-A, non-B hepatic tissues using the polymerase chain reaction assay. Gastroenterol. Jpn 1991; 26: 728.

168. Yoneyama T, Takeuchi K, Watanabe Y, Harada H, Ohabyashi A, Tanaka Y, Yuasa T, Saito I, Miyamura T, Detection of hepatitis C virus cDNA sequence by the polymerase chain reaction in hepatocellular carcinoma tissues. Jpn J Med Sci Biol 1990; 43: 89.

169. Liang T, Jeffers L, Cheinquer H, Reddy R, Idrovo I, Parker T, Rabassa A, De Medina M, Schiff E, Viral etiology of hepatocellular carcinoma in United States. Hepatology 1992; 16: 128.

170. Gerber MA, Shieh YSC, Shim K-S, Thung SN, Demetris AJ, Schwartz M, Akyol G, Dash S, Detection of replicative hepatitis C virus sequences in hepatocellular carcinoma. Am J Pathol 1992; 141: 1271.

171. Ruiz J, Sangro B, Guende JI, Beloqui O, Riezu-Boj JI, Herrero JI, Prieto J, Hepatitis B and C viral infections in patients with hepatocellular carcinoma. Hepatology 1992; 3: 637.

13. Malignancies in patients with pancreas and kidney transplants

DIEGO CANTAROVICH, JACQUES DANTAL & J.P. SOULILLOU

Introduction

It is well known that the incidence of malignancies is greatly increased in patients receiving biological and/or chemical immunosuppression for maintenance of their allo-transplants. Data concerning renal transplant patients is well documented throughout the world. However, little is known among diabetic patients undergoing pancreas/renal transplantation.

It has been claimed that the incidence of pancreatic cancer, lymphoma and some skin cancers is increased among diabetic patients [1–12]. However, whether diabetes mellitus could indeed be a risk factor for malignancy is unknown. In 1970, Kessler proposed a genetic relationship between diabetes and cancer [13]. More recently, Gruber et al. found that nondiabetic status was an independent prognostic indicator in developing cancer following adult primary renal transplantation [14].

In an attempt to answer the question of whether pancreas/renal transplant patients are more or less exposed to cancer than renal transplant ones, we carried out a retrospective study of our single centre transplant patient population who received either combined pancreas/renal or isolated renal transplants.

Patients and immunosuppression

A total of 107 combined pancreas/renal transplantations was performed between November 1987 and April 1995. All pancreatic grafts were segmental and the exocrine tissue was occluded with neoprene. Diabetic patients were 20 to 61 years at the time of transplantation (mean 39); 58% were men and all but one were white. Regarding renal transplant patients, a total of 1,643 patients (mean age 39, 2–73) was transplanted in our unit since the beginning of our clinical transplant program in 1970. The great majority of patients were white and 61% were males.

J.L. Touraine et al. (eds.), Cancer in Transplantation. Prevention and Treatment, 115–119.

Table 1. Number of malignancies reported among pancreas/renal and renal transplant patients at the University of Nantes

	Pancreas/renal	Renal
number of pts.	107	1643
PTLD	1	21
myeloma	1	0
skin cancer	2	75
pancreas cancer	1	0
pancreas cancer notive allograft	1	/
testis cancer	1	0
other	0	46
Total (incl. skin)	7 (6.5%)	142 (8.6%)
Total (excl. skin)	5 (4.7%)	71 (4.3%)

PTLD denotes post-transplant lympho-proliferative disorder.

Pancreas/renal transplant patients received either sequential quadruple (ciclosporine, azathioprine, steroids and antithymocyte globulin or an anti-IL2-R monoclonal antibody) or triple (ciclosporine, steroids and azathioprine or antithymocyte globulin, azathioprine and steroids) therapy as induction immunosuppression, and ciclosporine plus azathioprine therapy as maintenance immunosuppression. In case of an acute rejection episode, OKT3 was given.

Renal transplant patients received conventional (azathioprine and steroids) immunosuppression until 1980. Antithymocyte globulin (Pasteur/Mérieux, France) was thereafter associated to the conventional treatment. Ciclosporine was introduced in 1981. Since this date, the majority of renal transplant patients received sequential quadruple induction therapy based on antithymocyte globulin, azathioprine and steroids, followed by delayed ciclosporine introduction. Maintenance immunosuppression consisted of cyclosporine plus azathioprine. Acute rejection episodes were treated with IV steroid pulses for 5 consecutive days. An antithymocyte globulin cure was only given in case of steroid-resistance.

Results

Table 1 shows the total number of malignancies encountered among our transplant patient population.

Table 2 shows the outcome of malignancies encountered among the pancreas/renal transplant patients.

Table 2. Outcome of malignancies among pancreas/renal transplant patients

	Onset	Immunos	Therapy	Outcome
PTLD	M4	reduced	no	favourable
Myeloma	M18	stopped	yes	death
Pancreas	M60	unchanged	no	death
Graft	M48	unchanged	surgery	death
Testis	M9	reduced	surg/yes	favourable
Skin	M29	unchanged	surgery	no recurrence
Skin	M24	unchanged	surgery	no recurrence

Onset: time (months after transplantation) of cancer diagnosis; Immunos: maintenance immunosuppression; Therapy: specific anti-tumoral treatment; Surg: cancer's surgery.

Table 3. Age: years at transplantation time. Immunos.: induction immunosuppression; ATG, antithymocyte globulin; quad, quadruple immunosuppression including ATG or 33B3.1 (an anti-IL2-R MoAb), CsA, steroids and azathioprine. Rejection: presence or absence of an acute episode of rejection and its therapy. R/P funct.: denotes renal and pancreas graft function (yes or no) at the time of cancer diagnosis

PTLD	28	ATG/quad	yes/ATG	yes/yes
Myeloma	50 (2 TX)	ATG/quad	no	yes/yes
Pancreas	54	ATG/quad	no	yes/yes
Graft	33	33B31/quad	yes/OKT3	yes/no
Testis	43	ATG/quad	no	yes/yes
Skin	56	ATG/quad	no	yes/yes
Skin	49	33B31/quad	yes/OKT3	yes/yes

Onset: time (months after transplantation) of cancer diagnosis; Immunos: maintenance immunosuppression; Therapy: specific anti-tumoral treatment; Surg: cancer's surgery.

Table 3 shows characteristics of the immunosuppressive regimens given to the 7 pancreas/renal transplant patients developing cancer.

Discussion

We found a similar incidence of malignancies among diabetics who received combined pancreas/renal transplants and recipients of renal transplant alone (almost all non-diabetics). However, the small number of diabetic patients analyzed as well as the shorter follow-up after transplantation impede final conclusions.

One of the main differences among pancreas/renal and renal transplant patients was the immunosuppressive therapy given following transplantation. As previously described, pancreas/renal transplant patients received heavier prophylactic immunosuppression as compared to renal transplant patients. In addition, acute rejection episodes occuring among diabetics were treated with monoclonal or polyclonal anti-lymphocyte sera, both agents well known to be potent immunosuppressants. Fortunately, only one PTLD was encountered among our diabetic transplant population. This patient in doing well with normal pancreatic and renal functions seven years after PTLD's diagnosis, although immunosuppression was continued.

Whether the risk of pancreatic cancer is increased among pancreas/renal transplant patients is unknown. Two out of 107 pancreas/renal transplant patients developed pancreatic cancer. One was located to the graft and the other to the native pancreas. This last patient had history of insulin-dependent diabetes secondary to chronic pancreatitis. In spite of an uncomplicated post-transplant course, suggesting the absence of a pre-transplant occult cancer, the patient died 66 months after transplantation because of generalized metastasis of the pancreatic cancer. Concerning the pancreatic graft cancer, the diagnosis was done 1 year after the graft stopped functioning because of a probable artery thrombosis. At that time, no sign of tumoral mass was observed at the angiogram or the CT scan. One year later, when diagnosis of cancer was done, multiple extra-pancreatic metastasis were present, in addition to the extensive infiltration of the graft. Death occured 6 months later. These two observations are unfrequent when the transplant literature is examinated. By comparison, no pancreatic cancer was yet observed among our recipients of renal transplant alone.

Diabetes seems to be a risk factor for skin cancer, principally melanoma, clear cell syringomata (with increased numbers of clear cells within the eccrine glands), and APUDomas. None of these types of cancer were observed in our pancreatic transplant population. Two patients developed squamous cell carcinoma of the skin, a well known skin cancer following renal transplantation.

So far, malignancies (including skin ones) do not seem more frequent after pancreas/renal than renal transplantation. Multicentre cancer data from diabetic patients undergoing pancreas transplantation is necessary to better understand the occurrence and type of malignancies encountered among this particular patient population.

References

1. Marble A. Diabetes and cancer. N Engl J Med, 1934; 211: 339.
2. Bell ET. Carcinoma of the pancreas. I. A clinical and pathologic study of 609 necropsied cases. II. The relation of carcinoma of the pancreas to diabetes mellitus. Am J Pathol, 1957; 33: 449.
3. Green RC. Diabetes mellitus in association with primary carcinoma of tha pancreas. Diabetes, 1958; 7: 308.
4. Clark CG. Diabetes mellitus and primary carcinoma of the pancreas. BMJ, 1961; 2: 1259.
5. Karmody AJ. The association between carcinoma of the pancreas and diabetes mellitus. Br J Surg, 1969; 56: 362.
6. Kessler II. Cancer and diabets mellitus. A review of the literature. J Chron Dis, 1971; 23: 579.
7. Ragozzino M. Subsequent cancer risk in the incidence cohort of Rochester, Minnesota, residents with diabetes mellitus. J Chron Dis, 1982; 35: 13.
8. Ariela N. Diabets and pancreatic cancer: clues to the early diagnosis of pancreatic malignancy. JCE&M, 1994; 79: 1223.
9. Gullo L. Diabetes and the risk of pancreatic cancer. N Engl J Med, 1974, 331: 81.
10. Albrecht M. Occurrence of oral leukoplakia and lichen planus in diabets mellitus. J Oral Pathol Med, 1992; 21: 364.
11. Saitoh A. Clear cells of eccrine glands in a patient with clear cell syringoma associated with diabetes mellitus. Amm J Dermatopathol, 1993; 15: 166.
12. Buchanan KD. APUDomas and diabetes mellitus. Baillieres Clin Endocrinol Metab, 1992; 6: 899.
13. Kessler II. A genetic relationship between diabetes and cancer. Lancet, 1970; 1: 218.
14. Gruber SA. De novo cancer in cyclosporine-treated and non-cyclosporine-treated adult primary renal allograft recipients. Clin Transplant, 1994; 8: 388.

PART FOUR

Immunosuppression and cancer

14. Cancer risk factors in transplantation

ERIC ALAMARTINE, NABIL DIAB, JEAN-PIERRE DE FILIPPIS &
FRANÇOIS BERTHOUX

Introduction

It is now without doubt that organ transplant recipients are prone to develop malignancies. A major role seems to be played by oncogenic viruses in these cancers. Different clinical risk factors have been sought after, mainly the type and the amount of immunosuppression. Azathioprine has been suspected to have its own oncogenic effect. More recently, reports pointed out the excessive immunosuppression achieved with long lasting use of anti-CD3 monoclonal antibodies. The actual influence of the induction protocols is still controversial and we cannot identify the patients who are at risk to eventually develop a tumour.

In order to find out possible clinical risk factors, we conducted a retrospective analysis of de novo tumours among the 611 renal transplant recipients in our center. Most of the usual items of transplant data were collected to compare cancer patients with noncancer patients, and the various malignancies within themselves.

Patients and methods

Between 1979 and 1995, we performed 692 renal transplantations in 611 patients. Virus-related tumours such as skin cancers, cancers of the cervix, lymphomas and Kaposi's sarcomas were identified as specific tumours, whereas other cancers were named common tumours. The mean age of the recipients was 42 ± 12 years at the time of grafting. The ethnical and/or geographical origin of the patients was France in 66%, Italy in 25%, Africa in 9%, and Asia in less than 1%. The first 108 transplantations were achieved before cyclosporine A was available. The prophylactic immunosuppressive regimens changed throughout these years.

J.L. Touraine et al. (eds.), Cancer in Transplantation. Prevention and Treatment, 123–129.

For all these patients, we gathered the following clinical and biological data: patient's characteristics (sex, age, ethnic and/or geographical origin, primary renal disease), immunological status (HLA-A, B, DR phenotype, number or transfusions, PRA, number of grafts), graft's characteristics (HLA match and mismatch, cold and warm ischemia, graft and patient's survival), complications (number of rejections, CMV, EBV and HCV infections), and immunosuppression (prophylactic regimen, treatments of acute rejection episodes). For the patients transplanted during the cyclosporine era, a "cumulative amount of immunosuppression" was defined: we added up every treatment steroids, anti-lymphocyte or anti-thymocyte globulins, and OKT3, whether in induction protocols or anti-rejection treatments.

Univariate analysis of risk factors for de novo malignancies

We observed 63 solid tumours in 53 patients, thus the cancer prevalence in these recipients was 8.6%. These tumours were common malignancies for 41% of them (17 adenocarcinomas, 6 epitheliomas, 1 leiomyosarcoma, 1 malignant multiple plastocytoma, and 1 fibrohistiocytoma), and transplant-related cancers for 59% of them (1 immunoblastic B lymphoma, 6 Kaposi's sarcomas, 14 basal cell carcinomas and 14 squamous cell carcinomas of the skin, and 2 uterine cervix carcinomas).

We compared all the available data between cancer patients and noncancer patients. We did not find any difference between cancer and noncancer patients in regard to sex (66 v 68% males), primary renal disease, number of transfusions (8 ± 4 v 9 ± 8), PRA (19 ± 29 v 16 ± 26%), but the cancer patients were older at the time of the transplantation than the others (49 ± 10 v 42 ± 12 years, $p = 0.0004$).

As for graft characteristics, we respectively found the same number of second grafts (12 v 11%), total HLA match (3.07 ± 0.93 v 2.88 ± 0.69) and mismatch (2.48 ± 1.2 v 2.71 ± 1.0). Six of the tumours occurred under immunosuppression without cyclosporine (5.5% out of 108) and 57 occurred since the cyclosporine era (11.3% out of 503). We included ALG, ATG, or OKT3 in the prophylactic regimen of 49% of the cancer patients and 37% of the noncancer patients ($p = 0.17$). The number of acute rejection episodes was not different in cancer and noncancer patients (0.91 ± 0.90 v 0.89 ± 0.86). Therefore, the cumulative immunosuppression above the cyclosporine scheme was similar in cancer patients and noncancer patients, with respectively 0 treatment in 14 v 22%, 1 or 2 treatments in 77 v 67%, 3 or 4 treatments in 9 v 11% ($p = 0.55$). On the other hand, the graft survival was longer in cancer patients (5.8 ± 2.9 years) than in noncancer patients (3.8 ± 3.1 years, $p < 10^{-4}$). To visualize how the duration of graft survival influences the occurrence of tumours, we calculated an actuarial survival rate using the duration of graft survival for lifetime and the occurrence of a tumour for censoring. The cumulative rate of cancer-free patients was 98.3% at 1 year, 96.9% at 2 years, 92.2% at 5 years, and 84.2% at 10 years. This calculation was also done to compare patients under conventional immunosuppression and patients treated with cylosporine. The cumulative rate of cancer-free patients was lower in patients under cyclosporine (91% at 5 years, 79% at 10 years) than in patients with no cyclosporine (97% at 5 years, 87% at 10 years, $p = 0.10$).

Multivariate analysis of risk factors for de novo malignancies

The occurrence of a tumour was analysed as the dependent variable of a multivariate logistic regression, in which were included as independent variables: sex, recipient's and donor's ages, HLA-A, B, DR match and mismatch, ordinal number of graft, number of transfusions, PRA, cold ischemia, CMV and HCV infections, prophylactic use of ALG, ATG, OKT3, number of acute rejections, the cumulative amount of immunosuppression, and duration of graft survival. Among these 15 parameters, only 2 were selected as risk factors: the recipient age (β/SE = 3.35, $p = 0.001$) and the duration of graft survival (β/SE = 2.91, $p = 0.004$).

Stratification on recipient age

As the age of the patients is the most relevant factor to the occurrence of a cancer, as well as in the general population, we sorted out the data in patients over forty-five years old. In these older patients it was not possible to identify new risk factors. We only noticed that a heavier immunosuppression favoured the earlier appearance of cancers: On the basis of the cumulative amount of immunosuppression, the cumulative rate of cancer-free patients at 5 years was 88% in patients who received up to one treatment and 80% in patients who received two or more treatments. Nevertheless, the two curves joined together at 10 years (Figure 1).

Comparison of the various kinds of tumours

We compared the 26 common tumours to the 30 tumours of the skin and the cervix, and to the 6 Kaposi's sarcomas.

At the time of diagnosis, patients with a Kaposi's sarcoma were younger (37 ± 9 years) than the other cancer patients (common tumours: 55 ± 6 years, skin and cervix tumours: 56 ± 7 years). The outset of these tumours spread over a large period after grafting for common tumours (43 ± 31 months) and for skin and cervix tumours (52 ± 35), but remained in a narrow interval

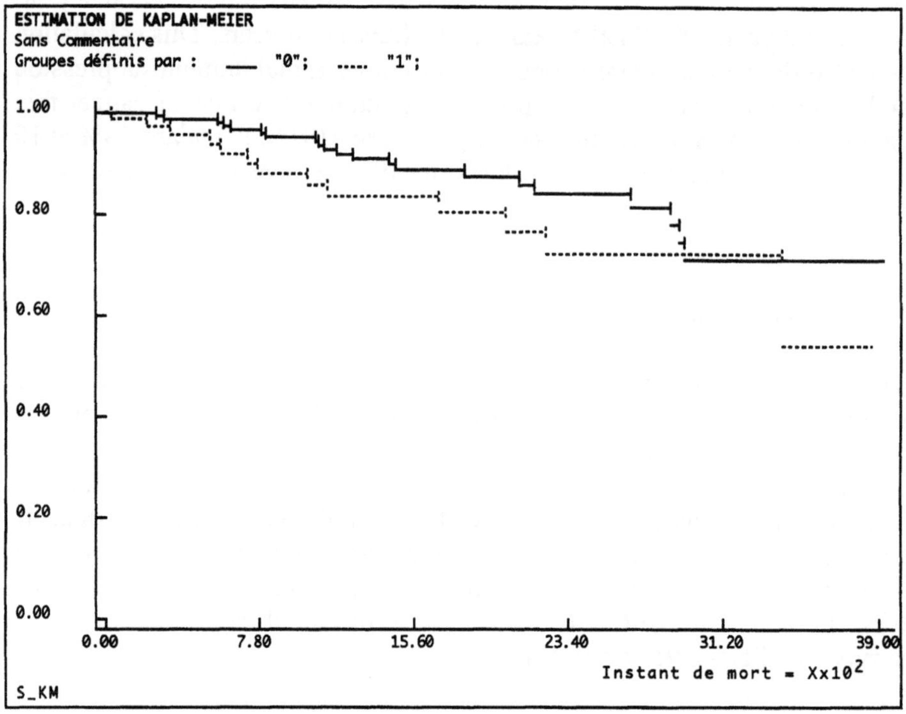

Fig. 1. Kaplan–Meier estimate of cancer-free patients in over forty-five recipients. The comparison was done in 262 recipients over forty-five years old at time of grafting according to the cumulative amount of immunosuppression (full line is up to one treatment, dotted line is more than one treatment). Breslow: $p = 0.05$; Mantel: $p = 0.13$.

for Kaposi's sarcomas (8 ± 4 months). The distribution of the ethnic and/or geographical origins only differed in Kaposi's sarcomas: these were noticed in 5 Italian people and 1 African from Nigeria. We also looked into a possible association with the various HLA-A, B, or DR antigens. We did not find any association in skin cancers, but 4 out of the 6 patients with a Kaposi's sarcoma were HLA-DR5 positive (67%). The frequency of HLA-DR5 in the Italian people we transplanted was only 35% (74/209, p = ns).

The mean number of rejection was 0.6 ± 0.7 in common tumours, 0.7 ± 0.8 in skin and cervix tumours, and 1.8 ± 1.1 in Kaposi's sarcomas ($p < 0.05$). We sorted out the therapeutic immunosuppression used in these patients: 55% of the common cancers received ALG and 20% OKT3, 60% of the skin and cervix cancers received ALG and 28% OKT3, 100% of the Kaposi's sarcomas received ALG and 50% OKT3. The immunosuppression could have been considered as excessive in 50% of the Kaposi's sarcomas, 25% of the skin cancers and only 10% of the common cancers.

On the whole, the rate of CMV infection in our centre is 38%. The occurrence of a CMV infection was 61% in skin and cervix tumours, 50% in Kaposi's sarcomas and only 25% in common cancer patients ($p < 0.05$). An obvious EBV infection was more frequent in Kaposi's sarcomas (17%) than in the other cancer patients (< 5% of skin cancers and common cancers, $p < 0.05$).

Discussion

When the de novo tumours were considered together, we found that cancer patients differed from noncancer patients for age at grafting and duration of graft survival. These two variables were significant in both univariate and multivariate analyses. Increased age at the time of transplantation was the strongest risk factor in our study. Age has already been reported as a risk factor for squamous cell carcinoma in kidney recipients [1]. Duration of graft survival was the second risk factor we found out. In a previous report we wrote out 4 years ago [2], the prevalence of solid tumours was only 4.9% in 389 kidney recipients. The difference with our present data is striking [3], suggesting the hypothesis that the frequency of tumours in transplanted patients will increase in the forthcoming years.

The introduction of cyclosporine was mainly believed to shift the distribution of cancers from skin cancers towards lymphomas [4]. Nevertheless, this change is likely to be due to the introduction of heavy immunosuppressive protocols, as in nonrenal recipients [5]. We noticed an increased risk for all cancers in patients treated with cyclosporine when compared to patients treated in the pre-cyclosporine era. More precisely, we found a higher yearly cumulative percentage of cancer patient. A similar result has recently been reported [6]. Once again, age and graft survival are more likely to explain this finding than any oncogenic effect of cyclosporine.

Taking into account the age of the patients is important to obtain reliable figures regarding the incidence of malignancies [7]. We have stratified our patients on the basis of age at grafting.This procedure did not allow us to find more clinical risk factors, excepted for the cumulative amount of immunosuppression. In patients over forty-five, a heavy immunosuppression seemed to increase cancer incidence, especially in the short term.

Overimmunosuppression is assumed to play a major role in the occurrence of malignancies. The introduction of OKT3 could have increased post-transplant lymphoproliferative disorders, but controversy is not closed [8, 9]. It may be noteworthy that in our experience, we encountered a very low number of lymphoma. This finding is consistent with the absence of significant overimmunosuppression in our cancer patients. Nevertheless, when we carefully looked at the different types of malignancies, we found important differences. Patients with common cancers received less immunosuppression, whereas patients with Kaposi's sarcomas received the strongest immunosuppression. In between were the patients with skin and cervix cancers. An oversuppression in the genesis of Kaposi's sarcoma has already been emphasized, mainly because of the early outset of this disease [10].

Kaposi's sarcoma remains a badly understood malignancy in organ recipients [11]. In our experience, they appeared to be particular tumours among transplant-related malignancies. Despite the few six of them, we noticed that they occurred in younger people, appearing within the first year of transplantation, in patients having more acute rejection episodes and therefore more immunosuppressive treatments. The higher risk for Kaposi's sarcoma in Mediterranean people has been known for long, and the weak association we noticed with HLA-DR5 strengthens the idea of a genetic background lying behind this disease. A genetically programmed susceptibility to corticosteroid-related Kaposi's sarcoma has recently been described [12].

A particular immunogenetic background should lay in organ recipients who develop a cancer. We expected some possible associations of skin cancers with HLA antigens, due to such description in transplanted patients, as in the general population [13–15], but we failed to find such a linkage in our patients.

Conclusions

In this one-center study on de novo malignancies in kidney recipients, age at grafting and duration of graft survival were the two main clinical risk factors, isolated by univariate and multivariate analyses. It remained difficult to establish the actual influence of overimmunosuppression. Virus-related transplant-specific cancers, especially Kaposi's sarcomas, seemed to be linked to more immunosuppression than common cancers. Heavy immunosuppression was also associated with an accelerated incidence of tumours in the over forty-five patients. Common cancers and skin carcinomas are more likely to be related to the length of follow-up.

References

1. Roeger RS, Sheil AGR, Disney APS, Mathew TH, Amiss N: Risk factors associated with the development of squamous cell carcinomas in immunosuppressed renal transplant recipients. Clin Transplantation 1992; 6: 202–211.
2. Alamartine E, Berthoux F: Oncological complications after renal transplantation. Press Med 1991; 20: 891–895.
3. Alamartine E, Berthoux F: Tumours in kidney transplanted patients: A comprehensive one-centre study. Transplant Proc 1995; 27: 1761–1763.
4. Penn I: Cancers following cyclosporine therapy. Transplantation 1987; 43: 32–35.
5. Penn I: Malignancy. Surg Clin North Am 1994; 74: 1247–1257.

6. Hiesse C, Kriaa F, Rieu P et al: Incidence and type of malignancies occuring after renal transplantation in conventionally and Cyclosporine-treated recipients: Analysis of a 20-year period in 1600 patients. Transplant Proc 1995; 27: 972–974.
7. Brunner FP, Landlais P, Selwood NH: Malignancies after renal transplantation: the EDTA-ERA registry. Nephrol Dial transplant 1995; S10: 74–80.
8. Swinnen LJ, Costanzo-Nordin MR, Fischer SG et al: Increased incidence of lymphoproliferative disorder after immunosuppression with the monoclonal antibody OKT3 in cardiac transplant recipients. N Engl J Med 1990; 323: 1723–1728.
9. Emery RW, Lake KD: Post-transplantation lymphoproliferative disorder and OKT3. N Engl J Med 1990; 324: 1437.
10. Montagnino G, Bencini PL, Tarantino A, Caputo R, Ponticelli C: Clinical features and course of Kaposi's Sarcoma in kidney transplant recipients: report of 13 cases. Am J Nephrol 1994; 14: 121–126.
11. Farge D: Kaposi's sarcoma in organ transplant recipients. Eur J Med 1993; 2: 339–343.
12. Trattner A, Hodack E, David M, Sandrack M: The appearance of Kaposi sarcoma during corticosteroid therapy. Cancer 1993; 72: 1179.
13. Bouwes-Bavinck JN, Gissman L, Glaas FHJ: Relation between skin cancer, humoral responses to human Papillomavirus, and HLA class II molecules in renal transplant recipients. J Immunol 1993; 151: 1579–1586.
14. Bouwes-Bavinck JN, Koote AMM, van der Woude FJ, Vanderbrouke JP, Vermeer BJ, Claas FHJ: HLA-A11-associated resistance to skin cancer in renal-transplant recipients. N Engl J Med 1990; 323: 1350.
15. Czarnecki D, Zalcberg J, Nicholson I, Tait B: Skin cancer and HLA antigens. N Engl J Med 1992; 326: 765.

15. Risk of cancer in transplant patients treated with recombinant growth hormone

PIERRE COCHAT, MARIE-HÉLÈNE SAÏD, CATHERINE LESAGE, CÉCILE GOUFFRANT & PASCALE BERLIER

Introduction

Growth hormone (GH) is a potent stimulator of insulin-like growth factor-1 (IGF-1), which in its turn has been proven to stimulate both cell proliferation and protein synthesis in various systems. Thus, the question may be raised whether the therapeutic use of GH, particularly in transplant patients, may increase the risk of developing malignant tumors or causing recurrence of a previous tumor that is thought to be under control [1].

In vitro data suggest that GH and IGF-1 may promote blast cell proliferation [2]. In rat experiments, malignant tumors have been induced following administration of supraphysiological doses of GH, whilst in other studies in hypophysectomized animals a lower than normal incidence of carcinogen-induced neoplasms was reported [3]. Moreover, in acromegaly in which there is a sustained high GH level, there is a significantly increased incidence of cancer in general and specifically of colonic neoplasia [3]. Studies in patients with GH deficiency (GHD) treated with human recombinant GH (rhGH) have shown that there is no compelling evidence that tumor recurrence or *de novo* neoplasia is a practical concern.

Is cancer a possible adverse event following GH treatment?

As of January 1st 1993, 12039 patients were followed in the Kabi International Growth Study (KIGS); 1495 adverse events were reported in 1371 patients (11.4%); 65 neoplasms were diagnosed in 61 patients (0.5%) (Table 1) [4]. The duration of GH treatment at the time of diagnosis of the tumor ranged from a few months up to 9 years and the cancer sometimes occurred after discontinuation of rhGH. However, in children who were treated because of

J.L. Touraine et al. (eds.), Cancer in Transplantation. Prevention and Treatment, 131–133.

Table 1. Five years' experience in the KIGS: cancer following rhGH treatment [4]

Brain tumour (n = 45)	Duration of GH treatment at time of diagnosis: 0.1 to 8.7 years
recurrence of craniopharyngioma (n = 23)	
other CNS tumour recurrences (n = 22)	
Secondary tumours (n = 5)	Duration of GH treatment at time of diagnosis: 0.9 to 4.5 years
3 in children with GHD after treatment for leukaemia	
1 in a child with primary medulloblastoma	
1 in a child with optic glioma	
De novo tumours (n = 2)	Duration of GH treatment at time of diagnosis: 2 to 4 years
reported in 2 patients with idiopathic GHD	
1 renal papillary carcinoma, 1 chondrocarcinoma	
Leukaemia (n = 4)	Duration of GH treatment at time of diagnosis: 0.3 to 2 years
de novo leukaemia (n = 1) in a child with IUGR	
recurrence of leukaemia (n = 3)	

rhGH, recombinant human growth hormone
KIGS, Kabi International Growth Study
CNS, Central Nervous System
GHD, growth hormone deficiency
IUGR, intrauterine growth retardation

GHD secondary to neoplasms (craniopharyngioma, medulloblastoma, astrocytoma, ependymoma), the relapse rate was not significantly different from patients who did not receive GH and the risk of developing leukemia in GH-treated children without risk factors – i.e. Fanconi anemia, myelodysplastic syndrome, Bloom syndrome, radiation, chemotherapy [3, 5, 8] – is comparable to the normal population, but seems to be higher in Japanese [4, 7]. It is hard to know whether the risk of Wilms tumor is increased since the number of cases is very small [8].

Recently, a significant but reversible increased growth rate of pigmented naevi has been shown in a longitudinal study and an increased activity of naevocytes was also demonstrated by immunohistochemistry [9]; however, no malignant melanoma has been reported in the literature.

Is the risk of cancer increased in transplant patients treated with rhGH?

The administration of rhGH has a selective effect on lymphocyte immune function and its role in the initiation or regulation of antigen-mediated immune responses has been suggested [10].

However, a great number of growth-retarded renal transplant children are currently under rhGH treatment and the potential risk of neoplasm in these patients must be assessed [6, 11]. Theoretically, the risk of cancer is mainly increased by the associated immunosuppression, the duration on therapy and the relatively high dose of rhGH (0.6 to 1.2 U/kg/week *versus* 0.4 to 0.8 U/kg/week in GHD patients) [1, 5]. However, despite such a potential risk, no case of neoplasm has been reported to-date in pediatric transplant patients.

Conclusion

Because of the well-known long-term risk of cancer in adult transplant recipients, children with short stature should be successfully treated with growth hormone under certain conditions. Patients with previous cancer, leukemia or Fanconi should be excluded. In those children who are elected for growth hormone treatment, skin lesions should be carefully screened. Transplant patients who are – or have been – under growth hormone treatment should remain under long term surveillance.

References

1. Ritzén EM. Does growth hormone increase the risk of malignancies? Horm Res 1993; 39: 99–101.
2. Zadik Z, Estrov Z, Karov Y, Hahn T, Barak Y. The effect of growth hormone and IGF-1 on clonogenic growth of hematopoietic cells in leukemic patients during active disease and durning remission – A preliminary report. J Pediatr Endocrinol 1993; 6: 79–83.
3. Ogilvy-Stuart AL, Shalet SM. Tumour occurrence and recurrence. Horm Res 1992; 38 (suppl 1): 50–55.
4. Wilton P. Adverse effect during growth hormone treatment: 5 years' experience in the Kabi International Growth Study. In: Ranke MB, Gunnarsson R, editors. Progress in Growth Hormone Therapy – 5 years of the KIGS. Mannheim, Germany: J & J Verlag, 1994: 291–307.
5. Stahnke N. Leukemia in growth-hormone-treated patients: an update, 1992. Horm Res 1992; 38 (suppl 1): 56–62.
6. Butturini A, Bernasconi S, Izzi G, Gertner JM, Gale RP. Short stature, Fanconi's anemia, and risk of leukaemia after growth hormone therapy. Lancet 1994; 343: 1576.
7. Watanabe S, Mizuno S, Oshima LH, Tsunematsu Y, Fujimoto J, Komiyama A. Leukemia and other malignancies among GH users. J Pediatr Endocrinol 1993; 6: 99–108.
8. Momoi T, Yamanaka C, Yorifuji T et al. Wilms tumour in a patient with growth hormone replacement therapy. Eur J Pediatr 1989; 149: 159–161.
9. Bourguignon JP, Pierard E, Ernould C et al. Effects of human growth hormone therapy on melanocytic naevi. Lancet 1993; 341: 1505–1506.
10. Petersen BH, Rapaport R, Henry DP, Huseman C, Moore WV. Effect of treatment with biosynthetic human growth hormone on peripheral blood lymphocyte populations and function in growth hormone-deficient children. J Clin Endocrinol Metab 1990; 70: 1756–1760.
11. Tönshoff B, Haffner D, Mehls O et al. Efficacy and safety of growth hormone treatment in short children with renal allografts: three year experience. Kidney Int 1993; 44: 199–207.

16. Malignancies in transplant patients under cyclosporine treatment for more than 10 years

ULRICH FREI, VOLKER KLIEHM, MARTIN KOLDITZ, MATTHIAS BEHREND & REINHARD BRUNKHORST

Introduction

Long-term immunosuppressive therapy after renal transplantation with different kinds of drugs carries an increased risk of development of malignant disease [1–4]. Except for preexisting or undetected cases most of the malignancies in graft recipients are de-novo malignancies developing at various times after transplantation. Due to the growing number of patients exposed to the risk a careful follow-up observation with documentation of developing malignancies is mandatory. This is in particular important for newer drugs such as cyclosporine A (CsA). The number of reports concerning the risk of developing de-novo malignancies under use of CsA has increased during the last years [5–8]. However in most of them only short observation times were covered. To evaluate if there is a excess risk in the long-term a suitable number of patients observed for 10 ore more years is necessary. In other reports the numbers of patients without malignancy were not reported. Furthermore they consisted of heterogeneous populations with different therapeutic regimens and different ethnic and geographic background. A comparison to a nontransplantated control population was often not made. The purpose of the present study was to give an update of our previous reports [5, 9] and to analyze the risk for development of malignant disease in a homogenous population in respect to immunosuppressive treatment and ethnic and geographic background. A regional cancer registry was used for comparison.

J.L. Touraine et al. (eds.), Cancer in Transplantation. Prevention and Treatment, 135–139.

Patients and methods

Patients: Between 1981 (when CsA was introduced in the Medizinische Hochschule Hannover) and the end of 1994 a total of 2054 kidney transplants were performed at our institution, 1875 of them were first transplants. Last date of follow up was 31 of December 1994. 1198 transplants were performed in male, 856 in female recipients. Total observation time was 9060 observation years (5292 in male and 3768 in female patients). Patient characteristics did not differ significantly from our previous reports. Mean age of the recipients at time of transplant was 39.5 years (Median 41.9, range 1–73 years; mean of male patients was 40.2, of female 38.4 years). The majority received cadaver grafts, 11% received grafts from living related donors. Grafts were allocated according to EUROTRANSPLANT exchange criteria. More than 60% of the grafts were shipped from elsewhere for optimal HLA-matches. Mean HLA-mismatches achieved were: mean MM-HLA A: 0.7, Mean MM-HLA B: 0.8, Mean MM-HLA DR: 0.4.

The data for comparison with a control population were taken from the cancer registry of Saarland (German federal state of 1 mill. inhabitants). Patient follow up: All patients were seen at the outpatient clinic in close cooperation with the referring nephrologists. A screening program for detection of tumors and skin malignancies was carried out in regular intervals. Major efforts were made to collect all available information in particular for skin cancers from general practitioners, dermatologists and nephrologists who are in care of our population.

Immunosuppression: Prophylactic immunosuppression consisted of prednisolone 1 mg/kg body weight(BW)/day initially which was tapered down to 0.1 mg/kg BW/day after three months to a final maintenance dose of 7.5 mg/day. CsA was administered at 10 mg/kg BW per day postoperatively and subsequently adjusted to RIA whole blood trough levels. Until 1984 the initial dose was 14 mg/kg BW/day. Levels of 400–800 ng/ml until 1984 and 300–600 ng/ml until 1988 measured by the polyclonal RIA were tolerated. Thereafter the therapeutic range was 100–150 ng/ml measured by the specific monoclonal assay (RIA). In addition 20% of the patients received azathioprine (2 mg/kg BW/day) for some periods because of initial nonfunction or cyclosporine toxicity. Rejection treatment consisted of 3–5 times methylprednisolone boluses (500 mg) intravenously, in steroid resistant rejections poly-or monoclonal antilymphocytic sera were given in 7% of the patients.

Results

Incidence of de-novo malignancies: Development of a de-novo malignant disorder was observed in 123 patients (in 74 males and 49 females). A total of 155 de-novo malignancies were counted in the population. Mean age of the

Table 1. Percentage of patients developing per posttransplant year a de-novo malignancy

Postop. years	Pat. at risk	n (neoplasms)	% per year
1	1875	19	1.01
2	1560	16	1.02
3	1350	13	0.96
4	1166	11	0.94
5	996	15	1.51
6	816	13	1.59
7	658	9	1.38
8	523	7	1.34
9	379	3	0.79
10	262	9	3.44
11	188	0	0.00
12	128	2	1.56
13	88	5	5.68

recipients developing a malignancy was 49.4 years (range 11–69 years) at the time of transplant. Mean age at the time when the malignancy was diagnosed was 53.8 years (male 54.8, female 53.2 years).

The incidence for development of a malignant disease per posttransplant year is given in Table 1. The table shows that the incidence was around 1/100 patient years until year four after transplant. In the following years the incidence rose to numbers between 1.3 and 5.7 cases per 100 patient years.

Sites of malignancies: 76 out of 155 malignancies detected after kidney transplantation were skin cancers, three of them malignant melanomas. 7 lymphomas were observed, one of them Hodgkin's lymphoma. None of these patients ever received poly- or monoclonal antibodies. Time of development ranged between 8 and 128 months after transplant. The remaining malignancies consisted of solid tumors of different sites resembling the distribution in a nontransplanted population except for urotheliomas which were found in 8 cases. Original disease in 7 of them was analgesic nephropathy. 13 lung cancers, 15 tumors of the gastrointestinal tract (8× colorectal, 2× oropharynx, 1× oesophagus, 3× pancreas, 1× hepatocellular carcinoma; 6× breast carcinoma, 11× of the female genital tract, 6× of the male genital tract, 6× kidney and 7 others). 188 patients had a follow-up longer than 10 years. 5 malignancies were diagnosed in this population. The sites did not differ from the other population.

Risk estimation: The ratio between expected and observed de-novo malignancies was calculated for all age groups in five year intervals comparing the study population with a cancer registry a described previously [5]. For 3768 observed patient years in the female population the expected number of malignancies was 11 compared to 24 in our population resembling a 2.2 fold increase if nonmelanotic skin cancers were excluded and 5.7 when included; in 5292 patient years observed in males the expected number was 20, we found 58 resembling a 2.4 fold increase if nonmelanotic skin cancers were excluded and a 4.6 fold increase when included.. This difference was significant ($p < 0.01$, x-square). When the cumulative risk to develop a de-novo malignancy (including skin cancers) was calculated by life table analysis, the risk after 10 years was 14%.

Survival: The development of a malignant disorder after kidney transplantation affected highly significant the patient survival, when the patient survival curve for affected and nonaffected patients was compared by life table analysis. The patient survival after 10 years was in the affected population 40% less than in the unaffected population.

Discussion

During the last years the risk of malignant disease in immunosuppressed population was well recognized. Serious problems were reported for Australia [10] and North America [11] at least concerning skin cancer. Lymphoproliferative disorders were observed in kidney as well as in heart transplanted patients [12–13]. Unfortunately most studies only gave the percentage of affected patients out of the total population irrespective of time of exposure to risk. Furthermore mode of immunosuppression and racial and geographic background were reported inadequately. No attempts were made to address the question if there is an excessive risk with increasing posttransplant years. The present study analyzed a population homogenous with respect to selection criteria, mode of immunosuppression and ethnic and geographic background. Compared to a regional cancer registry the risk to develop de-novo malignancy was 2.2–2.4 fold for males and females, and markedly greater if skin cancers were included. The limited sun expose in Northern Europe did not exclude the development of skin cancers, as also reported by Dutch investigators [14, 15]. This is in agreement with the report of Walz et al from a different German region [6]. In contrast to other reports we found under our conditions of limited immunosuppression with steroids and CsA and cautious use of poly- and monoclonal antibodies no excess numbers of lymphomas nor a higher incidence of tumors in the first posttransplant period. However our data suggest an increasing incidence of malignancies with time of exposure irrespective of age. Therefore the cumulative risk to develop a malignancy within a 10 years interval is 14%. Development of malignancy after kidney transplantation worsened markedly survival in affected patients. Therefore at least under our conditions of cautious immunosuppression development of malignancy is a serious problem which has to be considered more intensively in the next years. In particular this should be considered in populations using in a higher proportion of patients antilymphocytic preparations, azathioprine or newer developed drugs.

References

1. Rao KV, Andersen RC. Long-term results and complications in renal transplant recipients. Observations in the second decade. Transplantation 1988; 45: 45–52.
2. Birkeland SA. Malignant tumors in renal transplant patients. The Scandia transplant material. Cancer 1983; 51: 1571–1575.
3. Sheil AG, May J, Mahoney JF et al. Incidence of cancer in renal transplant recipients. Proc Eur Dial Transplant Assoc 1980; 17: 502–506.
4. Birkeland SA, Kemp E, Hauge M. Renal transplantation and cancer in the Scandiatransplant material. Scand J Urol Nephrol Suppl 1980; 54: 11–15.
5. Vogt P, Frei U, Repp H, Bunzendahl H, Oldhafer K, Pichlmayr R. Malignant tumours in renal transplant recipients receiving cyclosporin: survey of 598 first-kidney transplantations. Nephrol Dial Transplant 1990; 5: 282–288.
6. Walz MK, Albrecht KH, Niebel W, Eigler FW. De novo malignant tumors during drug immunosuppression. The findings following 1245 cadaveric kidney transplants in 1080 patients. Dtsch Med Wochenschr 1992; 117: 927–934.
7. Penn I, First MR. Development and incidence of cancer following cyclosporine therapy. Transplant Proc 1986; 18: 210–215.
8. Cockburn IT, Krupp P. The risk of neoplasms in patients treated with cyclosporine A. J Autoimmun 1989; 2: 723–731.
9. Frei U, Bode U, Repp H et al. Malignancies under cyclosporine after kidney transplantation: analysis of a 10-year period. Transplant Proc 1993; 25: 1394–1396.
10. Sheil AG, Disney AP, Mathew TH, Amiss N. De novo malignancy emerges as a major cause of morbidity and late failure in renal transplantation. Transplant Proc 1993; 25: 1383–1384.
11. Gruber SA, Gillingham K, Sothern RB, Stephanian E, Matas AJ, Dunn DL. De novo cancer in cyclosporine-treated and non-cyclosporine-treated adult primary renal allograft recipients. Clin Transplant 1994; 8: 388–395.
12. Swinnen LJ, Costanzo-Nordin MR, Fisher SG et al. Increased incidence of lymphoproliferative disorder after immunosuppression with the monoclonal antibody OKT3 in cardiac-transplant recipients [see comments]. N Engl J Med 1990; 323: 1723–1728.
13. Cockfield SM, Preiksaitis J, Harvey E et al. Is sequential use of ALG and OKT3 in renal transplants associated with an increased incidence of fulminant posttransplant lymphoproliferative disorder? Transplant Proc 1991; 23: 1106–1107.
14. Bourke JF, Mellott GJ, Young M, Donohoe J, Carmody M, Keogh JA. Skin cancer in an Irish renal transplant population. Ir J Med Sci 1992; 161: 116–117.
15. Bouwes Bavinck JN, Vermeer BJ, van der Woude FJ et al. Relation between skin cancer and HLA antigens in renal-transplant recipients [see comments]. N Engl J Med 1991; 325: 843–848.

17. Risk of malignancies in patients treated with Sandimmun® for autoimmune diseases

V. LAMARQUE, C. MONKA, M.C. COMMARE & P. KRUPP

Introduction

Cyclosporine A was first isolated in 1970 from the fungal species Tolypocladium inflatum gams.

It was found to have potent immunosuppressive effects. During clinical studies in 1978 beneficial effects of Sandimmun® have been shown in prevention of graft rejection following kidney transplantations [1]. After the first approval in renal transplantation in 1983, a large clinical programme was begun in many diseases in which immune mechanisms are suspected (autoimmune diseases). This has led to the first registration of Sandimmun® for the treatment of severe forms of endogenous uveitis in 1988. Then it was registered for severe stage of psoriasis, rheumatoid arthritis, nephrotic syndrome in 1990 and more recently in 1993 for atopic dermatitis.

However the development of immunosuppressive agents has been associated to the occurence of malignancies especially virus related such as lymphomas and squamous skin cell cancers, before the introduction of Sandimmun® .

The use of Sandimmun® in transplantation has been also related with an increased risk of malignancies due to immunosuppressive properties. But the relative risk was comparable to the data of conventional immunosuppressive therapy (azathioprine or cyclophosphamide and prednisone).

Moreover the pattern of malignancies seen with Sandimmun® (usually given with prednisone) was different. The analysis had shown the incidence of lymphomas and Kaposi's sarcoma was higher than in the patients with conventional immunosuppressive therapy and a lower incidence of skin cancers [2].

In addition the lymphomas occured earlier and were predominantly constituted by B-cells [2,3].

J.L. Touraine et al. (eds.), Cancer in Transplantation. Prevention and Treatment, 141–148.

What is the magnitude of the risk of malignancies in the patients treated with Sandimmun® in autoimmune diseases? It can be estimated from animal studies, clinical studies, epidemiological studies, spontaneous reports and published cases.

In experimental studies Sandimmun® is neither mutagenic nor carcinogenic [4,5].

With respect to clinical data in autoimmune diseases, the information in psoriasis and in rheumatoid arthritis will be discussed because we have at disposal, for these two indications, an estimate of the treated patients from the sales tracking studies.

Material and methods

Information on the malignancies in autoimmune diseases was collected from clinical trials, spontaneous reports, published cases and from the long term safety survey in the psoriasis. The data for renal transplantation result only from a study prospective multicentre, non controlled, non randomised long term survey with 56 centres in 17 countries including 4595 patients. A patient was enrolled for this study after being treated for at least two weeks with Sandimmun® after renal transplantation. Patients whose treatment was discontinued prior to the two-week limit were not included in the survey. Follow-up examinations were conducted regularly at 3, 6 and 12 months and at one year for up to seven years.

The following data were analysed for the 3 groups.

(1) the total number of malignancies reported
(2) the type and incidence of malignancies
(3) the average age of patients
(4) the relative risk of malignancies

The analysis (1) and (3) included all patients, who represent about 50 000 patients in psoriasis indication and about 24 000 patients in rheumatoid arthritis indication. In contrast the analysis (2) and (4) were evaluated for the 1657 patients who were treated with Sandimmun® in psoriasis clinical trials and for the 2800 patients in rheumatoid arthritis clinical trials. The malignancies described in spontaneous reports had to be excluded in the last estimates because the denominator is not known with enough precision.

The 95% confidence interval was calculated using a "Poisson distribution".

Results

The calculations were made for all malignancies irrespective of the causality assessment including preexisting lesions in order to counterbalance the underreporting. The total number of malignancies, in about 50 000 psoriatic patients, was 109 (0.22%) and, in about 24 000 Sandimmun® treated rheumatoid arthritis patients, was 47 (0.20%). During the long term safety survey in

Table 1.

Sandimmun® -type and incidence of malignancies						
	Renal transplantation LTSS[a] n = 4 595		Psoriasis Clinical studies n = 1 657		Rheumatoid arthritis Clinical studies n = 2 800	
Malignancies	n	incidence %	n	incidence %	n	incidence %
Skin	44	0.97	17	1.02	12	0.43
Solid tumors	59	1.28	16	0.97	23	0.82
Lymphoproliferative disorders	12	0.26	2	0.12	4	0.15
Kaposi sarcoma	6	0.13	1	0.06	–	–
Total	121	2.63	36	2.17	39	1.39

[a] Long term safety survey.

renal transplantation, the total number of malignancies was 121 (2.63%). It should be noted that the patients in renal transplantation received higher doses of Sandimmun® and other immunosuppressive agents. Only 1.2% of the patients were treated by Sandimmun® as monotherapy. The incidence of all malignancies estimated from the clinical studies in psoriasis indication was 2.17% and in rheumatoid arthritis 1.39%. The different types of malignancies are summarized in Table 1. The analysis in the psoriatic patients showed a high incidence of skin malignancies. Most Sandimmun® -treated patients who presented malignancies had a long history of psoriasis with previous treatments. All the patients with skin cancers recovered after appropriate treatment.

Skin malignancies were reported in 17 psoriatic patients (1.02%) in 12 rheumatoid arthritis patients (0.43%) and in 44 renal transplant recipients (0.97%).

With the respect to the skin malignancies, the incidence of squamous cell carcinomas was the highest in the psoriasis patients "Table 2".

Malignant lymphoproliferative disorders were reported in 2 psoriatic patients (0.12%), 4 rheumatoid arthritis patients (0.15%) and 12 renal transplant recipients (0.26%) "Table 3".

In the psoriasis indication, the relationship to Sandimmun® treatment is questionable for the 2 cases.

Regarding the solid tumors, the analysis was performed on all solid tumors and does not result in a definite conclusion.

Table 2.

Sandimmun® -type and incidence of skin cancers

	Renal transplantation LTSS[a] n = 4 595		Psoriasis Clinical studies n = 1 657		Rheumatoid arthritis Clinical studies n = 2 800	
Skin malignancies	n	incidence %	n	incidence %	n	incidence %
BBC[b]	22	0.48	6	0.36	9	0.32
SCC[c]	15	0.33	10	0.60	1	0.04
Others	7	0.16	1	0.06	2	0.07

[a] Long term safety survey.
[b] Basal cell carcinoma.
[c] Squamous cell carcinoma.

Table 3.

Sandimmun® -type and incidence of lymphoproliferative disorders

	Renal transplantation LTSS[a] n = 4 595		Psoriasis Clinical studies n = 1 657		Rheumatoid arthritis Clinical studies n = 2 800	
Lymphoproliferative disorders	n %	incidence	n %	incidence	n %	incidence
Lymphoma	12	0.26	2	0.12	3	0.11
Myeloma	–	–	–	–	1	0.04

[a] Long term safety survey.

Table 4 shows the average age of patients in the 3 indications comparable in the three groups.

The results of the relative risk (RR) estimated for skin cancers and malignant lymphoproliferative disorders are provided (Table 5).

Sandimmun® treatment is associated with a 7.5 fold increase of RR for skin cancers in the psoriatic patients. There was no definite change related to the malignant lymphoproliferative disorders.

In contrast in the rheumatoid arthritis patients, the RR for lymphomas is increased by a factor of 10.7. The relative risk of skin cancers was only increased 2.6 fold.

Table 4.

Sandimmun® -average age of patients developing malignancies						
	Renal transplantation LTSS[a] n = 4 595		Psoriasis All sources n = 50 000		Rheumatoid arthritis All sources n = 24 000	
Malignancies	mean age (years)	range (years)	mean age (years)	range (years)	mean age (years)	range (years)
Skin	52.9	25–72	53.3	33–82	62.9	54–75
Solid tumors	53.0	23–74	53.4	24–73	59.7	36–35
Lymphoproliferative disorders	46.7	22–64	62.3	44–75	57.0	50–62

[a] Long term safety survey.

Table 5.

Sandimmun® -relative risk of malignancies						
	Renal transplantation LTSS[a] n = 4 040		Psoriasis Clinical studies n = 1 657		Rheumatoid arthritis Clinical studies n = 2 800	
Malignancies	RR[b]	CI[c]	RR	CI	RR	CI
Skin	6.8		7.52	4.37–11.52	2.61	1.35–4.56
Lymphoproliferative disorders	27.5		1.52	0.14–4.31	10.7	2.21–31.31

[a] Long term safety survey.
[b] Relative risk.
[c] 95% Confidence interval.

Discussion

In *psoriasis* the analysis of 1 657 patients included in the clinical studies showed an incidence of 1.02% skin malignancies, 0.97% solid tumors and 0.12% lymphomas. These studies enrolled patients with severe psoriasis resistant to other treatments.

The estimates of relative risk is in favour that the use of Sandimmun® was associated with a 7.5 fold increased risk of skin malignancies. Most skin cancers were squamous cell carcinomas.

The patients with severe psoriasis are exposed to other forms of therapies known to be carcinogenic and/or immunosuppressive, i.e. arsenic, tar, ionizing radiation and PUVA. Arsenic induces skin carcinoma in a dose-dependent manner in up to 8% of the patients treated [6]. The previous exposure to ionizing radiation has been associated to a significant increase in cutaneous cancers [7].

But the most important contributing factor is represented by the pretreatment with PUVA. PUVA therapy has been associated with an increased risk of skin tumors development, particularly of squamous cell carcinoma (SCC) with a relative risk of 2.6 to 16.2 [8–10]. Usually the risk of SCC is related significantly with the doses and the duration of PUVA treatment. There was also a small dose dependent increase in the risk of basal cell carcinomas 11].

The relative risk for psoriatic patients treated with Sandimmun® to develop malignant lymphoproliferative disorders was 1.52 including an inferior limit below 1 and does not allow a definite conclusion about a strong association between the exposition of Sandimmun® and the occurrence of lymphomas.

In *rheumatoid arthritis* the analysis of 2800 rheumatoid arthritis patients exposed to Sandimmun® during clinical trials showed a crude incidence of 0.43% skin malignancies, less than in psoriasis ($p<0.02$). The most frequent skin tumors were represented by basal cell carcinomas. The other incidences for solid tumors and malignant lymphoproliferative disorders, respectively 0.82% and 0.15%, were comparable to those estimated in psoriatic patients. The average of the exposure time during clinical studies was about 6 months.

Considering the relative risk, it appears that its of malignant lymphoproliferative disorders is increased by a factor of 10.7 in the rheumatoid arthritis patients treated with Sandimmun® . The patients exposed to Sandimmun® had the most advanced and severe form of the disease.

However, several studies suggested an increase of lymphomas and hematological malignancies among patients with rheumatoid arthritis without any treatment. From different epidemiological studies, the estimates of lymphoma relative risk varied from 3 to 24.1 [12–14]. It was postulated as a possible predisposing factor, a combination of defective T cell function and persistent Epstein-Barr virus infection [15].

The risk for the development of non-Hodgkin's lymphoma in rheumatoid arthritis patients treated with azathioprine or cyclophosphamide was increased 10 fold [16]. Some cases have been also described in associated with methotrexate [17,18].

To conclude it appears that the incidence of malignancies is a little higher in renal transplantation than in autoimmune diseases. But the total number of patients exposed is higher and the duration of the surveillance longer in renal transplantation long term survey, compared to the data in clinical trials for autoimmune diseases. Consequently these results should be considered with care and only as a tendency.

The type of tumors more frequently observed is represented by the skin cancers in the psoriasis patients and malignant lymphoproliferative disorders in rheumatoid arthritis patients treated with Sandimmun® .

However the risk of skin tumors is in the range of that described in psoriatic patients treated with previous carcinogenic and/or immunosuppressive agents. The present clinical experience in rheumatoid arthritis suggests that the use of Sandimmun® increases the risk of lymphoma by approximately the same magnitude as other rheumatoid arthritis treatments [16,19].

In addition, in rheumatoid arthritis, the disease per se is associated with an increased risk of lymphoproliferative disorders.

An important point is that the relative risk does not allow to evaluate the respective contribution of different factors, the disease itself, the age of the patients, the role of the different previous and concomitant drugs...

In order to perform this analysis, a long term safety survey of Sandimmun® in psoriasis started in 1992 and the same survey will be initiated in the first quarter of 1996 in rheumatoid arthritis, coordinated by SANDOZ Pharma Ltd.

These long term surveillances with prospective data will supply with the accurate information on the incidence and risk factors in psoriasis and rheumatoid patients treated with Sandimmun® .

References

1. Gupta AK, Ellis CN, Goldfarb MT, et al. Cyclosporine A. Clin Dermatol 1989; 73: 98–110.
2. Penn I. The changing pattern of posttransplant malignancies. Transplant Proc 1991; 23: 1101–3.
3. Cockburn ITR, Krupp P. The risk of neoplasms in patients treated with cyclosporine A. J Autoimmun 1989; 2: 723–31.
4. Zwanenburg TSB, Suter W, Matter BE. Absence of genotoxic potential for Sandimmun® in experimental systems. Transplant Proc 1988; 20(suppl 3): 931–3.
5. Ryffel B. Experimental toxociological studies with cyclosporine A. In "Cyclosporine A", Proc Internat Conference on Cyclosporin A, Cambridge (UK), September 1981. Publ. DJG White (Cambridge). Elsevier, Amsterdam, New York, Oxford; 1982: 45–75.
6. Tanew A. Hönigsmann H, Ortel B et al. Nonmelanoma skin tumors in long-term photochemotherapy treatment of psoriasis. J Am Acad Dermatol 1986; 15: 960–5.
7. Stern RS, Zierler S, Parrish JA. Skin carcinoma in patients with psoriasis treated with topical tar and artificial ultraviolet radiation. Lancet 1980; 1: 732–5.
8. Lindelöf B, Sigurgeirsson B, Tegner E, et al. PUVA and cancer: a large-scale epidemiological study. Lancet 1991; 338: 91–3.
9. Stern RS, Laird N, Melski J, et al. Cutaneous squamous-cell carcinoma in patients treated with PUVA. N Engl J Med 1984; 310: 1156–61.
10. Stern RS, Lange R. Non-melanoma skin cancer occurring in patients treated with PUVA five to ten years after first treatment. J Invest Dermatol 1988; 91: 120–4.
11. Epstein JH. Phototherapy and photochemotherapy. N Engl J Med 1990; 322: 1149–51.

12. Symmons DP. Neoplasms of the immune system in rheumatoid arthritis. Am J Med 1985; 78: 22–8.
13. Pearce N, Porta M. Association of non-Hodgkin's lymphoma with rheumatoid arthritis. Am J Med 1986; 81: 747–8.
14. Hakulinen T, Isomaki H, Knekt P. Rheumatoid arthritis and cancer studies based on linking nationwide registries in Finland. Am J Med 1985; 78: 29–32.
15. Weir AB, Herrod HG, Lester Ep. Diffuse large-cell lymphoma of B-cell origin and deficient T-cell function in a patient with rheumatoid arthritis. Arch Intern Med 1989; 149: 1688–90.
16. Kinlen LJ. Incidence of cancer in rheumatoid arthritis and other disorders after immunosuppressive treatment. Am J Med 1985; 78(suppl 1A): 44–9.
17. Cobeta-Garcia JC, Ruiz-Jimeno MT, Fontova-Garoffé R. Non-Hodgkin's lymphoma, rheumatoid arthritis and methotrexate. J Rheumatol 1993; 20: 200–2.
18. Taillan B, Garnier G, Ferrari E, et al. Lymphome malin et polyarthrite rhumatoîde traitée par méthotrexate. Rev Med Int 1992; 13: S 477.
19. Arellano F, Krupp P. Malignancies in rheumatoid arthritis patients treated with cyclosporin A. Br J Rheumatol 1993; 32(suppl 1): 72–75.

18. De novo malignancies following renal transplantation

NORIO YOSHIMURA & TAKAHIRO OKA

Introduction

As renal transplantation is being increasingly undertaken for growing numbers of patients with end-stage renal disease, there has been a trend toward offering this treatment to patients who have undergone successful treatment for malignant disease. Malignancies following immunosuppressive therapy have been observed at all transplantation centers and much material has been published on this subject in recent years [1–8].

Since 1970, 449 patients have been transplanted in our center, 31 of whom developed malignant diseases after their transplantation. These included 10 cancer of skin and lips, 4 breast cancers,5 hepatobiliary carcinoma and others. We present herein our experiences of malignancies following renal transplantation.

Patient and methods

Patients

Between April 1970 and April 1995, 433 patients received 449 renal allografts (448 renal, and 1 combined renal and pancreas grafts) at the Kyoto Prefectural University of Medicine (Kyoto, Japan). Three-hundred two transplants were performed in males, and 131 in females. Living-related and unrelated donations totaled 393, and 56 were cadaveric donations. The mean age at the time of transplantation was 31.6 years. For primary immunosuppression, 178 patients (39.6%) received azathiorine (Az), and prednisolone (Pred), while 107 patients (23.8%) received cyclosporine (CsA) and Pred (CsA-Pred group, April 1982 to December 1986), and 144 patients (36.6%) received triple (CsA-Az-Pred) therapy from January 1987 to present (Table 1). Only six patients

J.L. Touraine et al. (eds.), Cancer in Transplantation. Prevention and Treatment, 149–158.

Table 1. Kyoto prefectural university of medicine. The second department of surgery (1970. 4 ~ 1995. 4)

		No. of malignancies
Az/Pred (1970. 4 ~ 1982. 3) . . .	198	22 (71.0%)
CsA/Pred (1982. 4 ~ 1986. 12)	107	5 (16.1%)
CsA/Az/Pred (1987. 1 ~ 1995. 4)	144	4 (12.9%)
	449	31

received FK 506 and Pred. The remaining three received RS-61443, CsA, and Pred.

Immunosuppression

Az administration (3 mg/kg/d) was begun 5 days before transplantation, and the dose decreased gradually to maintenance levels of 2.0 to 2.5 mg/kg/d. Pred was started on the day of intravenous (IV) Methylprednisolone (MP) for the first 3 posttransplant days, and decreased gradually until a maintenance dose of 10 mg/kg/d was reached. In CsA-Pred group,CsA was administered orally in a dose of 10 mg/kg for 5 days prior to transplantation. Postoperatively, it was started at a dose of 14 mg/kg orally and was tapered by 2 mg/kg every 2 weeks thereafter until a daily maintenance dose of 5 to 6 mg/kg, which was subsequently adjusted to maintain serum trough levels at 100 to 200 ng/ml by radioimmunoassay (RIA), was reached.

In CsA-Az-Pred group (Figure 1), CsA was administered orally in a dose of 12 mg/kg for 2 days prior to transplantation. On the day of transplantation, 3 mg/kg of CsA was administered intravenously. Postoperatively, it was started at a dose of 12 mg/kg orally and was tapered by 2 mg/kg every week until a daily dose of 6 mg/kg, and 1.0–1.5 mg/kg of Az was added (9).

The dose of Pred given in combination with CsA was 50 mg/d initially, supplemented by 500 mg of IV MP during operation, and was gradually tapered every 10 days to a maintenance daily dose of 10 mg/d at 6 months. Rejection episodes in the Az group were treated with 1 g of MP IV, followed by a dose reduced by half every 3 days until remission was achieved. In the CsA group, MP administration was started from a daily dose of 500 mg/d and was reduced by harf every 3 days until remission.

The person-years method

The number of years from the day of transplantation to the day the malignance was diagnosed, the day of the patient's death, April 30, 1995, was calculat-

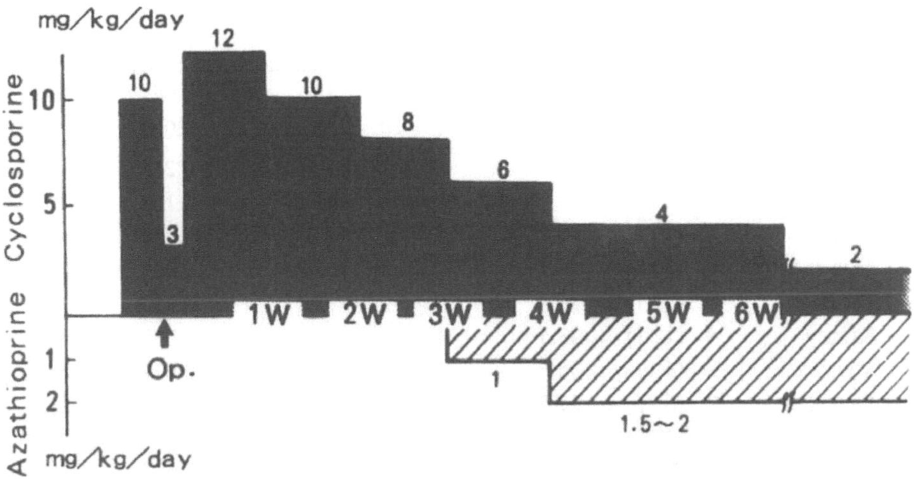

Fig. 1. Triple drug therapy with CsA/Az/Pred in living related renal transplant recipients. CsA was administered orally in a dose of 12 mg/kg for 2 days prior to transplantation. On the day of transplantation, 3 mg/kg of CsA was administered intravenously. Postoperatively, it was started at a dose of 12 mg/kg orally and was tapered by 2 mg/kg every week until a daily dose of 6 mg/kg, and 1.0–1.5 mg/kg of Az was added.

ed. Total observation time was 4011 patient-years. The expected number of cancers was calculated on the basis of sex and age-matched general population in our country (10). Risk ratios (observed/expected numbers of cancers) were calculated and subjected to standard significance tests under the Poisson assumption.

Patient and graft survival rates were calculated by the Kaplan–Meier method. Statistical significance was determined with the log-rank test.

Results

Incidence of post-transplant malignancies

In our institution, de novo malignancies developed in 30 recipients of living-related donor renal allografts and 1 of cadaveric donor grafts (Table 1). The total number of cancers was 33, with two patients exhibiting two cancers (Table 2).

Table 2. De novo malignancies following renal transplantation

Site of malignancy	No. of malignancies n	(%)	Mean age of patients (y)	Sex M	F	Time of diagnosis posttransplant (mo)	Expected no.	Risk ratio
Esophagus*	1	(3.0)	55	1[a]	0	139	0.061	16.4
Stomach	1	(3.0)	44	1	0	120	1.004	1.0
Colon†	1	(6.1)	40	0	2[b]	160	0.214	9.4
Rectum	1	(3.0)	57	0	1	151	0.168	6.0
Liver	5	(15.2)	43.2	5	1	125.2	0.259	19.2
Skin and lips	10	(30.3)	47.1	7	2	166.0	0.035	285.7
Breast	5	(15.1)	36.3	0	5	92.3	0.230	17.4
Kidney	4	(12.1)	43.5	4	0	73.5	0.050	40.0
Thyroid	2	(6.1)	35.5	1	1	135.5	0.077	26.0
Leukemia	2	(6.1)	27.5	2	0	80.5	0.126	15.8
Total	33		40.1	21	12	128.4	2.224	14.8

[a] This patient had both esophageal cancer and leukemia.
[b] One patient had both colon and rectal carcinomas.

Age and sex of patients

The mean age at the time of transplantation was 31.6 years. The mean age at the time of the diagnosis of malignancy was 40.9 years (range, 12 to 57 years). Eleven (35.5%) patients developed malignancies thirties, and 9 (29.0%) patients developed it fourties (Figure 2). Nineteen of 31 recipients were male (61.2%) and others were female (38.8%).

Interval between transplantation and cancer

The average interval from transplantation to the time of diagnosis was 128.4 months (range, 18 to 255 months). Malignancies developed in 5 (16.1%) of 31 patients within 5 years posttransplantation, 5 patients developed malignancies between 5 year and 10 years posttransplantation (Figure 3). Moreover, malignancies occurred in 21 (67.8%) patients who survived over 10 years with a functioning grafts. Twenty one of one hundred forty three patients who showed over 10 years graft survival developed malignancies. Therefore, 14.6% of patients whose graft functions over 10 years developed malignancies.

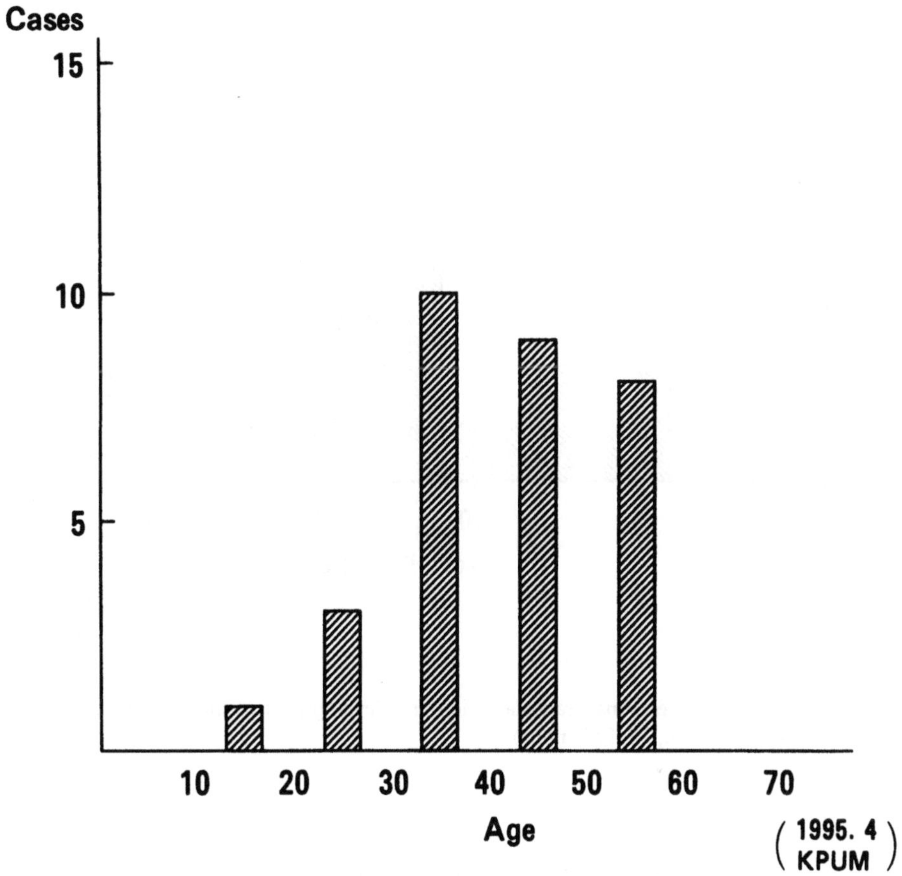

Fig. 2. Age at the development of malignancies in renal transplant recipients. Mean age was 40.9 years old.

Immunosuppression of patients with cancer

Since nephrotoxicity is a major side effect, some patients were changed CsA to Az at some time after transplantation. Therefore, twenty six patients received Az-Pred, three received CsA-Pred and two patient received CsA-Az-Pred at the development of malignancies.

Sites of cancer

Although cancer occurred in 10 sites, 11 tumors (33.3%) involved the digestive system (Table 2). No malignant lymphomas, which occur frequently in

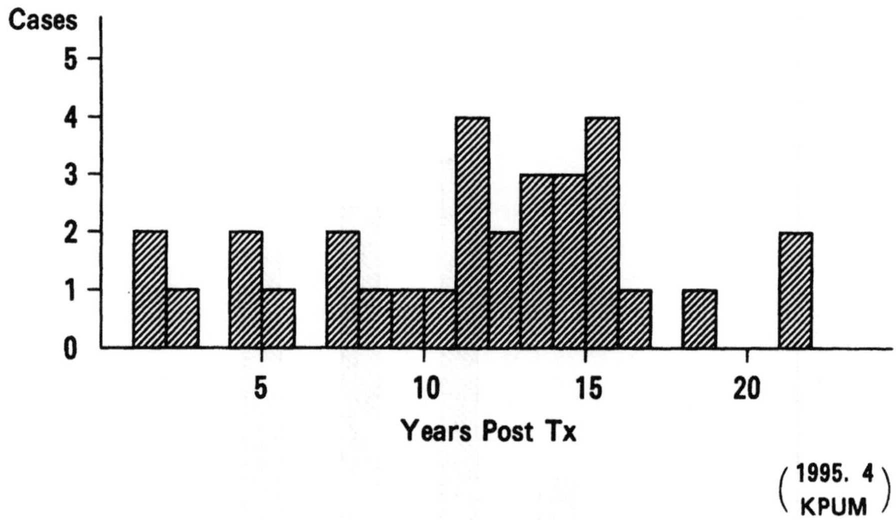

Fig. 3. Intervals between renal transplantation and development of malignancies. Average was 128.4 months (range, 18–255 months).

Table 3. Observed and expected number of de novo malignancies in renal transplant recipients

	Observed no.	Expected no.	Risk ratio
Male	20	2.487	8.1[a]
Female	11	0.934	11.8[a]
Overall	31	3.421	9.1[a]

[a]$P < 0.01$.

renal transplant recipients in Western countries, were identified. Nine patients (29.0%) developed cancers at skin and lips, which was lower rate compared with that of Western countries.

Table 4. Risk of acquiring de novo malignancies following renal transplantation

Years posttransplant	Observed no.	Expected no.	Risk ratio
0 to 5	5	0.152	33.1[a]
5 to 10	8	0.607	13.2[a]
10 to 15	13	1.285	10.1[a]

[a]$P < 0.01$.

The risk of malignancy

The risk of developing a malignance was increased following renal transplantation (Table 3). Compared with sex- and age-matched Japanese control, the incidence of cancer was 8.1 times greater for males, 11.8 times greater for females, and 9.1 times greater overall ($p < 0.01$). Of note was the fact that the risk was increased at all sites except the stomach (Table 2). The risk of acquiring a malignancy at 5-year intervals following transplantation was 33.1 times greater from 0 to 5 years ($p < 0.05$), 13.2 times greater from 5 to 10 years ($p < 0.01$), and 10.1 times greater from 10 to 15 years ($p < 0.01$; Table 4).

Patient and graft survival rates with cancer

Patient and graft survival rates after transplantation were compared among patients with and without cancer (Figure 4). The patient survival rate was lower in the cancer group over 10 years posttransplantation ($p < 0.05$). The graft survival rate was not significantly different in either group. Up to 10 years after transplantation, patient and graft survival in the cancer group was better than in the noncancer group. However, beyond 10 years after transplantation, patient survival was worse in the cancer group, mainly because of deaths due to cancer.

Treatment of patients

Twenty four patients were able to have surgical treatment (67.8%), and 5 patients were not able to have operation due to dissemination. Nineteen patients are alive.

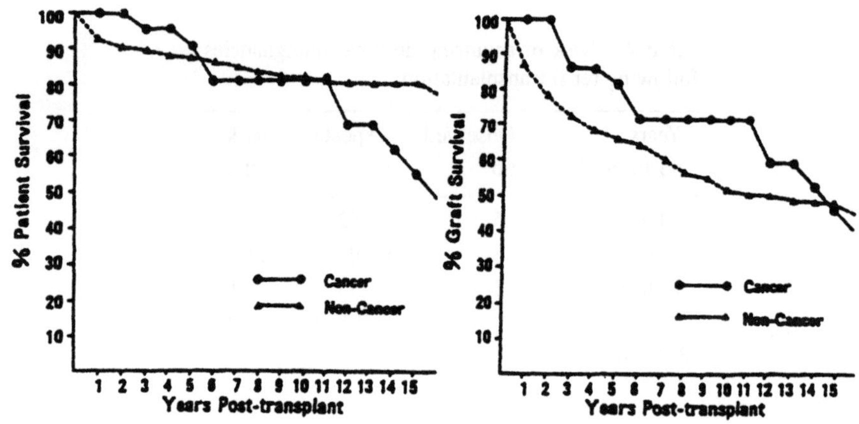

Fig. 4. Patient and graft survival in living related renal transplantation.

Discussion

Organ-allograft recipients have an increased incidence of cancers that arise de novo after transplantation. The prevalence in several large series ranges from 4 to 18%, with an average of 6%. However, this figure underestimates the true incidence because patients with short survival times or short lengths of follow-up are included. Since the number of patients gradually increased in japan and the number of patients with long-term graft survival increased, the risk of malignant disease in the immunosuppressed population has been well recognized recently.

Serious problems were reported for Australia [11] and North America [12], at least concerning skin cancer. Increased numbers of lymphoproliferative disorders were observed in heart transplanted patients [13] as well as in some kidney-grafted populations [14].

In our series, the incidence of cancer was 6.8%, which is similar to that found in Western countries. The risk of developing a malignancy in renal transplant recipients was 9.1 times greater when compared with agematched Japanese controls. The cancer risk in renal transplant recipients in Western countries has been calculated to be 3- to 10-fold.

Eleven of 33 tumors (33.3%) involved the digestive system. No malignant lymphomas occurred in this series. The distribution of cancers was similar to that in the Japanese general population. The risk was increased at all sites except the stomach (Table 2). Sheil et al [6] also reported an increased risk for all de novo malignancies.

Although 21 of 31 patients (67.8%) developed malignancies 10 years after transplantation, the risk of acquiring malignancies at 5-year intervals of transplantation increased at every interval over 15 years after transplantation. Frei et al [7] reported that the incidence of malignancy increases after 5 years posttransplantation. Although patient and graft survival for the cancer group was better in the early posttransplant years, survival worsened in the cancer group because of cancer related deaths 10 years after transplantation in our experiences (Figure 4).

The exact mechanism of carcinogenesis due to immunosuppression, in man, cannot be explained at the present time. Several suggested explanations have been proposed [1–5], such as impaired immunosurveillance, increased susceptibility to oncogenic viruses, chronic antigenic stimulation from the graft and carcinoneogenic effects of immunosuppresive agents. The occurrence of malignant disease in patients with transplants is presumably due to an interplay of these factors. In our laboratory, chromosomal abnormalities of peripheral blood leukocytes have been observed in patients receiving prolonged immunosuppressive therapy [15]. Chromatid gaps were observed in 22 of 60 kidney transplant recipients and several aberrations of chromosomes, such as breaks, translocations or extra fragments were found in 8 of the 60 patients. No such chromosomal abnormality, however, was found in the patient reported here.

The incidence of malignant disease, an important complication in the late period of post transplantation, should be borne in mind during the management of long-term survivors.

Development of malignancy after kidney transplantation worsened the survival of affected patients markedly. Therefore, at least under our conditions of cautious immunosuppression, development of malignancy is a serious problem that has to be considered more intensively over the next several years.

References

1. Penn I. Cancers of the anogenical region in renal transplant recipients. Analysis of 65 cases. Cancer 1986; 58: 611–616.
2. Penn I. Why do immunosuppressed patients develop cancer?, in Pimentel E (ed): CRC Critical reviews in oncogenesis. Boca Raton, FL, CRC, 1989; 27–52 .
3. Penn I. Post-transplant kidney cancers and skin cancers (including Kaposi's sarcoma), in Schmahl D, Penn I (eds): Cancer in organ transplant recipients. New York, NY, Springer-Verlag, 1991; 46–53.
4. Penn I. Immunosuppression-A contributory factor in lymphoma formation. Clin Transplant 1992; 6: 214–219.
5. Penn I. Immunosuppression and opportunistic tumors: Do viruses play a role?, in Dammacco F (ed): Advances in tumor immunology and allergic disorders. Immuno Incontri, Milan, Italy, Edi Ermes, 1992; 139–162.
6. Sheil AJR. De novo malignancy emerges as a major cause of morbidity and late failure in renal transplantation. Transplant Proc, 1993; 25: 1383.
7. Frei U, Bode U, Repp H et al. Malignancies under cyclosporine after kidney transplantation: Analysis of a 10-year period. Transplant Proc, 1993; 25: 1394.

8. Shel AJR. Development of malignancy following renal Transplantation in Australia and New Zealand. Transplant Proc, 1992; 24: 1275.
9. Oka T, Ohmori Y, Aikawa I et al. Early conversion of CsA to Az in living related renal transplantation. Transplant Proc, 1989; 21: 1645–1648.
10. Tokoro Y, Asano T, Nakagouri T et al. A Statistical Study of Cancer Incidence in Renal Transplant Patients. Transplant Proc, 1992; 24: 1588–1590.
11. Sheil AGR, Disney APS, Mathew TH et al. Cancer development in cadaveric donor renal allograft recipients treated with azathioprine (AZA) or cyclosporine (CyA) or AZA/CyA. Transplant Proc, 1991; 23: 1111–1112.
12. Gruber SA, Skjei KL, Sothern RB et al. Cancer development in renal allograft recipients treated with conventional and cyclosporine immunosuppression. Transplant Proc, 1991; 23: 1104–1105.
13. Swinnen LJ, Constanzo-Nordin MR, Fisher SG et al. Increased incidence of lymphoproliferative disorder after immunosuppression with the monoclonal antibody OKT3 in cardiac-transplant recipients. N Engl J Med 1990; 323: 1723–1728.
14. Cockfield SM, Preiksaints J, Harvey E et al. Is sequential use of ALG and OKT3 in renal transplants associated with an increased incidence of fulminant posttransplant lymphoproliferative disorder? Transplant Proc 1991; 23: 1106–1107.
15. Fukuda M, Aikawa I, Ohmori Y et al. Chromosome aberration in kidney transplant recipients. Transplant Proc 1987; 19: 2245–2247.

PART FIVE

Epstein-Barr virus related malignancies

19. Virus induced cancer: The lesson of Epstein–Barr virus

MARIA G. MASUCCI, VICTOR LEVITSKY, TERESA FRISAN, JELENA LEVISTKAYA & PEDRO O. DE CAMPOS-LIMA

Virally induced tumors provide the strongest case of host surveillance against neoplastic cells and their precursors. There is now substantial evidence that Epstein–Barr virus (EBV), hepatitis-B and C viruses (HBV and HCV), several types of papilloma viruses (HPV), Human Herpesvirus type 8 (HHV8) and human T-cell leukemia-lymphoma virus type I (HTLV I) and type II are responsible for approximately 15–20% of the total cancer incidence in the world. These viruses are widespread in populations where the associated diseases are seen at the highest incidence. In the vast majority of cases primary infection is either asymptomatic or is accompanied by benign proliferations of virus infected cells that often appear in concomitance with disturbances of the host immune responses and tend to regress spontaneously once full immunocompetence is restored. This, together with the observation that progression to malignancy occurs after long latency periods, and that the tumors are usually monoclonal, indicates that none of these viruses is by itself tumorigenic. An important aspect of viral oncogenesis is, therefore, the establishment of persistent asymptomatic infection where the transforming potential of the virus is controlled by a combination of cellular control mechanisms that regulate the expression of viral genes, and by strong immune responses that prevent the proliferation of virus infected cells.

The complexity of the interaction between oncogenic viruses and their hosts is clearly illustrated by Epstein–Barr virus (EBV), a gamma-herpesvirus with double tropism for lymphoid and epithelial cells. EBV causes a benign lymphoproliferative disease, infectious mononucleosis (IM) [1] and has been implicated in the pathogenesis of an increasing number of human malignancies. The best characterized are the immunoblastic lymphomas (IL) arising in immunosuppressed patients [2], endemic Burkitt's lymphoma (BL) [3] and undifferentiated nasopharyngeal carcinoma (NPC) [4], where the virus is found in virtually all tumors. Well established is the association of EBV with up to 40% of Hodgkin's lymphomas [5], anaplastic large cell lymphomas of both B- and T-cell origin [6, 7], a proportion of peripheral T-cell lym-

J.L. Touraine et al. (eds.), Cancer in Transplantation. Prevention and Treatment, 161–175.

phomas [8] and in nasal T-cell lymphoma of the midline granuloma type [9]. In addition, the virus has been implicated in the pathogenesis of thymic lymphoepithelioma-like carcinomas [10], some gastric carcinomas [11] and leiomyosarcomas arising in organ transplant children [12] and HIV patients [13]. The association of EBV with such broad spectrum of malignancies stands in sharp contrast to its spread in all human populations and its capacity to persist asymptomatically as a life-long infection of healthy hosts. When blood lymphocytes from EBV carriers are cultured *in vitro*, EBV transformed lymphoblastoid cell lines (LCLs) arise spontaneously provided that immune T cells are removed or inhibited by cyclosporin-A [14]. This phenomenon highlights the importance of EBV-specific T cells in restricting the potentially harmful consequences of virus infection. Here, we shall summarize the most recent advances in our understanding of the immune controls that regulate the persistence of EBV infected cells in healthy virus carriers and the escape mechanisms that are likely to operate in the pathogenesis of EBV associated malignancies.

Latent EBV infection in normal and malignant cells

EBV infects B lymphocytes via binding to the CR2 receptor [15], and induce their immortalization *in vitro* [16]. EBV carrying LCL cells constitutively express the viral genes encoding for six nuclear antigens (EBNA 1, 2, 3, 4, 5 and 6) and three membrane proteins (LMP1, 2A and 2B) (reviewed in [17]. mRNAs encoding the individual EBNAs are generated by alternative splicing of long rightward transcripts initiated at one of two promoters in the BamHI C and BamHI W regions of the genome (Cp and Wp). The LMPs transcripts are expressed from separate promoters in BamHI N (Np) which run in opposite orientation but apparently share the same bidirectional control region. The mechanism of action of these viral products and their role in B cell transformation are still largely unknown. Studies on natural or *in vitro* generated EBV deletion mutants clearly indicates that immortalization of B cells involves the coordinate action of several viral gene functions. LCLs express high levels of the B cell activation markers CD23, CD30, CD39 and CD70 and the adhesion molecules LFA1, LFA3 and ICAM1 resembling, in this respect, mitogen or antigen-induced B blasts [18, 19]. This suggests that EBV induced immortalization my be achieved through the constitutive triggering of physiological pathways of B cell activation.

EBV transformed lymphoblasts are detected in the blood of patients with infectious mononucleosis [20]. They may represent as much as 15–20% of the circulating B lymphocytes during the acute phase of the disease but promptly disappear following activation of T cell responses. The infected cells are not eradicated, however. Using highly sensitive PCR methods the virus has been demonstrated in one in 10^5–10^6 resting blood B lymphocytes [21]. mRNAs encoding the nuclear antigen EBNA1 and the membrane protein LMP2A have been demonstrated by RT-PCR [22, 23] while messages for EBNA2-6 and LMP1 have not been detected. These cells are likely to represent the latent reservoir from which lytic infection is periodically reactivated leading to reinfection of epithelia and spread to new hosts. The EBV positive immunoblastic B cell lymphomas arising in immunocompromised patients, such as allograft recipients receiving long term immunosuppressive therapy, AIDS patients and patients with primary immunodeficiencies, are the *in vivo* counterpart of *in vitro* immortalized LCLs [reviewed in 24]. The surface marker phenotype of the lymphoma cells resemble that of LCLs with high expression of activation and adhesion molecules. A different type of EBV latency in B cells has been revealed by studies of biopsies from endemic BLs and early passage BL lines. Only EBNA1 is selectively expressed in the tumor cells while the remaining EBNAs and LMPs are down-regulated [25, 26]. EBNA1 specific mRNAs are transcribed from an alternative promoter which was initially localized in the BamHI F region of the viral genome [27]. However, recent data suggest that the latent transcript is initiated from an adjacent promoter in the BamHI Q fragment while the Fp promoter is active during the lytic cycle [28]. The silencing of Cp, Wp and Np in BL cells correlates with methylation of critical sites within the control regions [29–31]. BL cells display a distinct cell surface phenotype characterised by expression of CD10 (CALLA) and CD77 (BLA) but no or low expression of the activation markers and adhesion molecules that are expressed in LCLs [32].

In recent years, evidence has accumulated which implicates EBV in the aetiology of other malignancies of the hemopoietic system including Hodgkin's disease (HD), midline granuloma and peripheral T cell lymphoma. One unusual feature of HD is that the malignant population of Hodgkin and Reed–Sternberg cells (HRS) constitutes only a minority of the tumor mass. The HRS cells themselves are of uncertain lineage since many of the conventional markers which distinguish T- from B-cells and monocytes are either absent or expressed in atypical combinations [33]. EBV genomes have been detected in HRS cells of about 40% of HD cases by in situ hybridization [34]. Immunohystochemical analysis has shown that the EBV positive HRS cells express LMP1 in the absence of EBNA2. This is supported by transcription studies which have also revealed expression of both LMP2A and 2B [35]. A similar pattern of viral gene expression has been regularly detected in EBV positive T cell malignancies [36] suggesting that expression of EBNA2-6 and usage of Wp and Cp may be restricted to the B cell lineage.

The tropism of EBV for epithelial cells is reflected by the association of the virus with numerous epithelial tumors. These tumors regularly express EBNA1 which is transcribed from Fp. LMP1, LMP2A and LMP2B specific transcripts have been detected in virtually all NPCs by sensitive PCR and *in situ* hybridization techniques [37, 38] while LMP1 has been detected in

Table 1. Patterns of viral gene expression in EBV associated malignancies

Cell type	Tumor	EBV gene expression		
		EBNA1	EBNA2-6	LMP1-2
B lymphocyte	Immunoblastic B-lymphoma	+	+	+
B lymphocyte	Burkitt's lymphoma	+	–	–
HRS cells	Hodgkin's Disease	+*°	–**	+*°
T lymphocyte	Immunoblastic T-lymphoma	+*°	–**	+*°
T lymphocyte	Midline granuloma	+°	–**	+*°
Nasal epithelium	Nasopharyngeal carcinoma	+	–	+ (60%)
Thymic epithelium	Thymic lymphoepithelioma	+	–	+
Gastric epithelium	Gastric lymphoepithelioma	+	–	–
Smooth muscle	Lejomiosarcoma	+	+**	–°

*Detected by RT-PCR.
°Detected by immunohistochemistry.
**Only EBNA2 has been tested.

approximately 60% of the cases by immunoblotting with specific monoclonal reagents [39]. Undifferentiated carcinomas located at other anatomical sites and morphologically resembling NPC are frequently EBV positive. Best documented are the association of the virus with undifferentiated gastric and thymic carcinomas [40]. These tumors are also described as lymphoepitheliomas due to the extensive lymphoid infiltrate. Thymic carcinoma appears to be always EBV positive and express an NPC-like pattern of viral gene expression (EBNA1 and LMPs) while gastric carcinomas resemble BL cells and express EBNA1 only.

Perhaps most surprising is the presence of EBV in smooth-muscle tumors of severely immunocompromised patients suffering from advanced AIDS or receiving immunosuppressive therapy after organ transplantation. Two independent studies have demonstrated the expression of EBNA1 and EBNA2 but not LMP1 in EBV carrying leiomyomas and leiomyosarcomas cells [12, 13], suggesting the existence of a novel, previously uncharacterized form of EBV latency. A still unresolved question is the route of viral entry in smooth-muscle since these cells do not express classical CR2 receptors.

In Table 1 is a summary of the different pattern of viral antigen expression identified in EBV associated malignancies. The diversity of these patterns is likely to mirror the complex balance between the influence of the virus on the cells and the effects of cellular factors on the control of EBV gene expression. While EBV driven proliferation may be the primary oncogenic event in IL, other EBV associated malignancies probably represent more complex entities in which malignant transformation is brought about by the concerted action of EBV and other genetic events.

T cell control of viral latency in immunocompetent host

The capacity of EBV to infect and transform B lymphocytes *in vitro* has provided an accessible cell culture system with which to search for evidence of virus specific T cell mediated immunity. Thus, the outgrowth of EBV transformed B cells frequently regresses in *in vitro* infected cultures of blood lymphocytes from EBV immune but not from EBV seronegative donors [41]. The regression is predominantly mediated through reactivation of memory cytotoxic T cell responses [42]. Expansion and subsequent cloning of the reactive T cells demonstrated that the effector cells are EBV specific, recognizing LCLs but not mitogen induced B-blasts, and restricted through HLA class I and occasionally through HLA class II [43, 44]. Analysis of CTL responses within this complex viral system has been made possible by the construction of a set of vaccinia recombinants expressing individual viral genes derived from the B95.8 EBV strain [45–48]. A systematic survey of MHC:viral antigen combinations yielding CTL target epitopes in donors of different HLA class I type had led to several important observations. In any one individual EBV specific CTL responses were shown to be a composite of reactivities against different viral antigens the identity of which is determined by the HLA class I type of the responder. Thus, HLA-A2 molecules present epitopes from LMP2; HLA-B8 presents epitopes from EBNA3; HLA-A11 presents epitopes from EBNA4 and EBNA6; HLA-B7, B27 and B44 present epitopes from EBNA6 [46–49]. Interestingly, certain alleles appear to act as preferred restriction elements as clearly illustrated by the dominance of HLA-A11 restricted responses in polyclonal CTL cultures reactivated from HLA-A11 positive individuals.

The molecular basis of this phenomenon were investigated by comparing the response to two HLA A11 restricted epitopes localized in residues 399–408 and 416–424 of the EBNA4 protein [45, 50]. Clonal analysis performed in four HLA A11 positive EBV positive individuals revealed a strong predominance of clones specific for the 416–424 epitopes with the 399–408 specific clones being about 10 fold less frequent. This correlated with a different efficiency of lysis of HLA A11 positive LCLs. Thus, while targets prepulsed with optimal concentrations of the relevant peptide were killed equally well by effectors of both specificities confirming that the clones had identical lytic capacity, untreated LCL cells were lysed more efficiently by the 416–424 specific effectors over a wide range of effector:target ratios (Table 2). EBNA4 399–408 specific lysis could be increased several fold by preincubation with the corresponding synthetic peptide or by over expression of the protein following recombinant vaccinia virus infection while no or very small increase of 416–424 specific lysis could be achieved under the same conditions (Table 2). It seems therefore that the strength of CTL responses to a given epitope may be determined by the efficiently of presentation at the surface of EBV infected cells. In this particular setting, differences in

Table 2. Induction of IVT and AVF specific lysis by preincubation of HLA A11 positive B95.8 virus transformed LCLs with synthetic peptides

	% Specific lysis[a]					
	IVT			AVF		
Cell line	−pep.	+pep.	*ratio*[b]	−pep.	+pep.	*ratio*[b]
QJZ-B2	51	64	*1.3*	13	73	*5.6*
BK-B4	37	59	*1.6*	13	74	*5.7*
SI-B1	26	44	*1.7*	15	81	*5.4*
GD-B1	24	57	*2.3*	10	69	*6.9*
JAC-B2	54	82	*1.5*	18	89	*5.0*
Mean ± SD			*1.68 ± 0.33*			*5.72 ± 0.63*

[a]Untreated and peptide pulsed LCLs (10^{-9}M for 1 hr) were tested for sensitivity to lysis by CTL clones specific for the EBNA4 416–424 (IVT) and EBNA4 399–408 (AVF) epitopes. Mean % specific lysis at 10:1 effector:target ratio in three experiments.
[b]Calculated by the formula:% specific lysis of peptide pulsed LCL/% specific lysis of untreated LCL.

immunogenicity could be accounted for by the structure of the epitopes, their different processing and/or the interaction of the relevant peptides with the presenting MHC allele. The stability of MHC:peptide complexes is likely to play an important role since HLA A11 molecules induced at the surface of the peptide transporter defective mutant T2 cell line by incubation with the 416–424 peptide had a significantly longer half life at 37°C compared to molecules containing the 399–408 peptide (Figure 1).

The importance of immunodominant epitopes in the control of EBV infection is underscored by the demonstration that the two EBNA4 epitopes are selectively mutated in EBV strains from South East Asia where the HLA A11 allele is expressed in over 50% of the population [50, 51]. All 33 Chinese and Papuan isolates that were sequenced carried mutations within the immunodominant 416–424 epitope. The mutations selectively affected residues 2 and 9 of the peptide, which are critical for binding to the groove of A11 molecules. Moreover, about half of the Chinese isolates and all the Papuan isolates had additional mutations in the 399–408 epitope, which again selectively affected amino acids 1 and 2. Memory CTL responses specific for the variant epitopes were not detected in HLA A11 positive Chinese donors infected with the mutated viruses [50]. Thus, elimination of reactivities to these CTL epitopes seems to have conferred a selective advantage to the mutated EBV strains in human populations where the relevant restriction element is over-represented. The exclusive expression of EBNA4 in EBV transformed immunoblasts suggests that strain selection may occur at the time of primary infection. A delay of effective rejection may allow the estab-

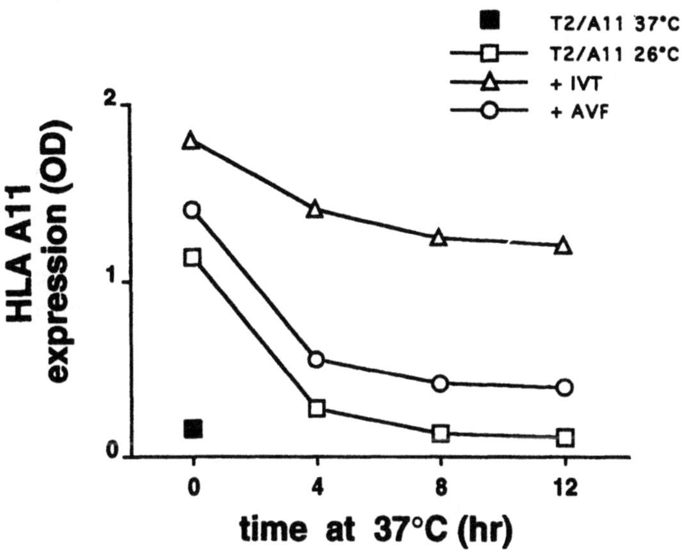

Fig. 1. Surface HLA A11 expression was induced by incubation of metabolically labelled T2/A11 cells over night at 26°C either alone □ or in the presence of 100 μM IVT △ or AVF ○ peptides. After extensive washing to remove the excess peptide the cells were incubated at 37°C for the indicated time and surface HLA A11 molecules were then immunoprecipitated using the W6/32 mouse monoclonal antibody that reacts with a monomorphic determinant on class I molecules. HLA A11 was detected by isoelectrofocusing and the level of expression was measured by densitometry scanning of the autoradiograms.

lishment of a larger pool of latently EBV infected cells increasing the chance of viral reactivation later in life, and of transmission to new hosts.

A puzzling feature of EBV specific CTL responses has been the consistent failure to demonstrate EBNA1 specific CTLs in individuals of different HLA class I backgrounds. EBNA1 is the only viral antigen regularly expressed in all EBV infected cells. This observation and the finding that EBNA1 expression cannot induce rejection of non-immunogenic mouse mammary carcinoma lines in syngeneic hosts [52], have been taken to suggest that this viral antigen may not be recognized as efficiently as other viral gene products. Recent evidence has confirmed this assumption and unravelled a previously unknown mechanism of escape from CTL surveillance. EBNA1 is a phosphoprotein composed of unique N- and C-terminal domains joined by an internal glycine-alanine repeat. Glycine-alanine repeats of different length are present in all EBV isolates and represent the major target of EBNA specific antibody responses but their function is unknown. The possibility that presence of repetitive sequences covering over one third of the molecule could influence the recognition of EBNA1 by the cellular immune system was tested using recombinant vaccinia viruses expressing chimeric genes that contained the

EBNA4 416–424 epitope inserted in frame within the intact EBNA1, or within EBNA1 deletion mutants lacking the glycine-alanine repeats [53]. Presence of the repeats abolished recognition of the EBNA1 chimeras while insertion of the glycine-alanine sequence in EBNA4 hampered presentation of both the 416–424 and 399–408 epitopes. These findings suggest that the repeats generate a cis-acting signal which either prevents processing or, alternatively, sequesters the processing products to a cellular compartment which is inaccessible to MHC class I restricted presentation. Failure to undergo processing of a constitutively expressed viral protein may afford protection independently of the class I type of the host and favour the long term persistence of virus infected cells without involving immunosuppression.

Failure of T cell surveillance in EBV associated malignancies

Immunoblastic lymphoma

The role of immunosurveillance in limiting the proliferative potential of EBV infected cells *in vivo* is clearly illustrated by the development of EBV positive immunoblastic lymphomas in immunosuppressed individuals. These tumors present as multifocal lesions within lymphoid tissues and/or in the central nervous system and are often oligoclonal with a small number of distinct clones being present either in the same lesion or at distinct anatomical sites. The phenotypic similarity between *in vitro* transformed LCLs and the lymphoma cells suggest that these tumors represent EBV-driven lesions growing out opportunistically in the absence of immune control. This is also in line with the observation that while lymphomas arising in bone marrow recipients are of donor origin, organ transplant lymphomas are usually of recipient type. Thus, the predominant B cell compartment seems to determine the origin of the lymphoma. Indeed, regression has been reported following relaxation of immunosuppressive therapy in kidney transplant recipients [54], as it would be expected if the recovering virus specific T cell surveillance could recognize and eliminate the tumor cells. The concomitant rejection of the graft precludes the use of this therapeutic regimen in heart, liver or bone marrow recipients. Recently, passive transfer of blood lymphocytes or in vitro activated EBV specific CTL cultures of donor origin has been successfully applied in bone marrow recipients developing immunoblastic lymphomas [55, 56]. A single CTL infusion lead to a complete disappearance of lymphoma in the majority of patient with no or very mild symptoms of GVHD. The success of the clinical trials combined with our rapidly increasing knowledge of CTL epitopes and their corresponding restriction elements opens the possibility to apply passive immunotherapy to other forms of EBV associated malignancies.

Table 3. Possible routes of immunoescape in EBV positive Burkitt's lymphoma

	Defect
VIRUS RELATED	• EBNA1 cannot serve as rejection target due to selective inhibition of processing by the glycine-alanine repeats
PHENOTYPE RELATED	• Low expression of MHC class I antigens • Low expression of adhesion molecules • Low expression of TAPs and proteasome subunits
TUMOR ASSOCIATED	• Transcriptional downregulation of EBNA2-6 and LMP1-2 due to methylation of regulatory sequences • Selective loss of HLA class I alleles • Selective defects of antigen processing

Table 4. Possible routes of immunoescape in LMP1 expressing malignancies

	Defect
VIRUS RELATED	• Involvement of specific EBV strains with mutations resulting in loss of antigenic epitopes or hampered antigen processing
TUMOR ASSOCIATED	• Low expression of MHC class I antigens and adhesion molecules in EBV positive HRS cells • Low expression of TAPs or proteasome subunits • Mutations of the viral antigen resulting in loss of antigenic epitopes, generation of antagonist peptides or hampered antigen processing • LMP1 induced production of TH2 lymphokines causing local T-cell energy

Burkitt's lymphoma

Burkitt's lymphoma provides one of the best know example of tumor that escape immunosurveillance (Table 3). Normal levels of EBV specific CTLs precursors can be demonstrated in BL patients [56], whereas the tumor cells are often insensitive to CTL lysis [57, 58]. In addition to the restricted expression of viral antigens and non-immunogenicity of EBNA1 discussed above, studies on BL cell lines that have retained the tumor cell phenotype *in vitro* have identified at least three consistent features which may affect recognition by the immune system: (i) a very low expression of the cell adhesion molecules LFA3 and ICAM1, which are normally involved in mediating target cell conjugation with effector T cells [59, 60], (ii) a selective down-regulation of HLA class I expression often accompanied by selective loss of certain alleles, the best example being the down-regulation of HLA-A11 (reviewed in [61, 62], and (iii) a down-regulation of various components of the antigen processing/presentation pathway, in particular the transporters associated with antigen processing (TAPs) [63]. Whilst collectively these features may facilitate the immune evasion by BL cells, their individual contributions to the overall effect is difficult to assess. Moreover, the BL cell phenotype is reminiscent of germinal center centroblasts suggesting that the poor immunogenicity of the tumor may partly reflect the characteristics of normal B cells in a particular stage of activation/differentiation. The selective downregulation of certain HLA alleles appears to be the only phenotypic characteristic unequivocally associated with tumor progression. Reconstitution of MHC class I expression along with a relevant antigenic T-cell epitope renders BL cells sensitive to CTL lysis. This together with the demonstration that selective downregulation of MHC alleles is observed in both EBV carrying and negative BL lines suggests that the putative rejection target recognized by the immune system on BL cells may be of cellular rather than viral origin.

LMP expressing tumors

Similar to BL, NPC and HD arise and develop in relatively immunocompetent individuals. It is therefore quite surprising that expression of at least two potentially highly immunogenic viral antigens, LMP1 and LMP2, does not lead to rejection. A possible clue may be found in recent experiments where LMP1 genes derived from a Chinese NPC and from the B95.8 virus were transfected in the mouse mammary carcinoma line S6C. This cell line becomes highly immunogenic when transfected with the B95.8 derived LMP1, leading to rejection of the transfected cells in virtually all previously immunized mice. In contrast, transfectants carrying the NPC derived gene remained non-immunogenic in spite of a similar level of LMP1 expression [64]. Thus, mutations within the LMP1 gene may alter the antigenicity of the protein and/or its capacity to be efficiently processed.

A characteristic feature of LMP1 expressing tumors is the presence of abundant lymphoid infiltrate. Recently, we have performed a comparative study monitoring EBV specific responses in the tumour and peripheral blood of patients with EBV positive and EBV negative HD [65]. EBV specific reactivity was detected in tumor infiltrating lymphocytes (TILs) from 3 donors with EBV negative HD but was absent in TILs isolated from 6 EBV positive tumors. EBV specific memory CTL responses were detected in blood lymphocytes suggesting that virus specific responses may be selectively suppressed in the tumor. The demonstration that LMP1 expression influences antigen processing and MHC class II restricted presentation in Burkitt's lymphoma cells [66], and the finding of multiple sequence variations in EBV isolates from HD lesions , support the possibility that EBV positive HRS cells may present altered peptides that act as competitors for EBV as well as tumor specific responses. In addition, the finding that LMP1 upregulates hIL-10 production in transfected sublines of EBV negative BLs [67] suggests that selective inhibition of IL-2 driven responses could be mediated by local production of IL-10 (Table 4).

Conclusions

Epstein–Barr virus, a herpesvirus with dual tropism for lymphoid and epithelial cells, is one of the most potent transforming agents known, yet it persists in most individuals as a lifelong asymptomatic infection. We are rapidly gaining insights on the nature and regulation of the mechanisms controlling the spread of the virus and the persistence of virus infected cells in healthy immunocompetent hosts. The failure to mount effective CTL responses to EBNA1, which is required for EBV episome maintenance and is the only viral antigen regularly expressed in all EBV carrying cells, is likely to play a key role in virus persistence and pathogenesis. Recent studies have identified the targets of EBV-specific cytotoxic T lymphocytes and mapped antigenic peptide epitopes within the primary sequences of several of the viral proteins expressed in transformed cells. These peptides may be good candidates for immune interventions aiming to activate and/or enhance CTL responses directed to immunodominant rejection targets. Passive transfer of *in vitro* reactivated EBV specific CTLs could provide an efficient means of specific intervention for immunoblastic lymphomas in immunocompromised individuals. Other EBV associated malignancies develop in relatively immunocompetent hosts. The cell phenotype associated downregulation of all highly immunogenic viral antigens, together with defects of MHC class I expression and antigen processing/presentation are likely to favour the immunoescape of Burkitt's lymphoma. Suppression of EBV specific responses may play an important role in the pathogenesis of LMP1 expressing tumors. This may be achieved by selective mutations affecting the antigenicity and/or immunogenicity of this viral antigen or by induction of TH2 lymphokines, leading to local T-cell anergy.

Acknowledgments

The work of the authors was supported by grants from the Swedish Cancer Society, the Karolinska Institute and the Magnus Bergvalls Stiftelse, Stockholm, Sweden; the Concern II Foundation, Los Angeles, CA (USA).

References

1. Henle G, Henle W, Diehl V. Relation of a Burkitt tumor associated herpes-type virus to infectious mononucleosis. Proceedings of the National Academy of Sciences USA 1968; 59: 94–101.
2. Hanto DW, Gajl-Peczalska KJ, Frizzera G et al. Epstein–Barr virus (EBV) induced polyclonal and monoclonal B-cell lymphoproliferative diseases occurring after renal transplantation. Ann. Surg. 1983; 198: 356–369.
3. Epstein MA, Achong BG, Barr YM. Virus particles in cultured lymphoblasts from Burkitt's lymphoma. Lancet 1964; i: 702–703.
4. Wolf H, zur Hausen H, Becker V. EB-viral genomes in epithelial nasopharyngeal carcinoma cells. Nature (Lond.) 1973; 244: 245–247.
5. Herbst H, Dallenbach F, Hummel M et al. Epstein–Barr virus latent membrane protein expression in Hodgkin and Reed–Sternberg cells. Proceedings of the National Academy of Sciences USA 1991; 88: 4766–4770.
6. Herbst H, Dallenbach F, Hummel M et al. Epstein–Barr virus DNA and latent antigens in Ki-1 (CD30)-positive Anaplastic Large Cell lymphoma. Blood 1991; 78: 2666–2673.
7. Anagnostopoulos I, Herbst H, Niedobetek G, Stein H. Demonstration of monoclonal EBV genomes in Hodgkin's disease and Ki-1 positive anaplastic large cell lymphoma by combined Southern blot and in situ hybridization. Blood 1989; 74: 810–816.
8. Pallesen G, Hamilton-Dutoit SJ, Zhou X. The association of Epstein–Barr virus (EBV with T cell lymhpoproliferations and Hodgkin's disease: Two new developments in the EBV field. Advances in Cancer Research 1993; 62: 180–239.
9. Harabuchi Y, Yamanaka N, Kataura A et al. Epstein–Barr virus in nasal T-cell lymphomas in patients with lethal midline granuloma. Lancet 1990; 335: 128–130.
10. Leyvraz S, Henle W, Chahinian AP et al. Association of Epstein–Barr virus with thymic carcinoma. New England Journal of Medicine 1985; 312: 1296–1299.
11. Imai S, Koizumi S, Sugiura M et al. Gastric carcinoma: monoclonal epithelial malignant cells expressing Epstein–Barr virus latent infection proteins. Proceedings of the National Academy of Sciences USA 1994; 91: 9131–9135.
12. Lee ES, Locker J, Nalesnik M et al. The association of Epstein–Barr virus with smooth-muscle tumors occurring after organ transplantation. New England Journal of Medicine 1995; 332: 19–25.
13. McClain KL, Leach CT, Jenson HB et al. Association of Epstein–Barr virus with leiomyosarcomas in young people with AIDS. New England Journal of Medicine 1995; 332: 12–18.
14. Rickinson AB, Rowe M, Hart IJ et al. T-cell-mediated regression of "spontaneous" and of Epstein–Barr virus-induced B cell transformation *in vitro*: Studies with cyclosporin A. Cell. Immunol. 1984; 87: 646–658.
15. Nemerow GR, Wolfert R, McNaughton MW, Cooper NR. Identification and characterization of the Epstein–Barr virus receptor on human B lymphocytes and its relationship to the C3d complement receptor (CR2). Journal of Virology 1985; 55: 347–351.
16. Miller G, Lipman M. Release of infectious Epstein–Barr virus by transformed marmoset leukocytes. Proceedings of the National Academy of Sciences USA 1973; 70: 190–194.

17. Kieff E, Liebowitz D. Epstein–Barr virus and its replication. In: Fields B, Knipe D, ed. Virology, 2nd Edition. New York: Raven press, 1990: 1889–1920. vol 2).
18. Ehlin-Henriksson B, Manneborg-Sandlund A, Klein G. Expression of B-cell-specific markers in different Burkitt lymphoma subgroups. Int. J. Cancer 1987; 39: 211–218.
19. Rowe M, Rooney CM, Edwards CF, Lenoir GM, Rickinson AB. Epstein–Barr virus status and tumour cell phenotype in sporadic Burkitt's lymphoma. Int. J. Cancer 1986; 37: 367–373.
20. Robinson J, Smith D, Niederman J. Mitotic EBNA-positive lymphocytes in peripheral blood during infectious mononucleosis. Nature 1980; 287: 234–235.
21. Miyashita EM, Yang B, Lam KM, Crawford DH, Thorley-Lawson DA. A novel form of Epstein–Barr virus latency in normal B cells in vivo. Cell 1995.
22. Tierney RJ, Steven N, Young LS, Rickinson AB. Epstein–Barr virus latency in blood mononuclear cells: analysis of viral gene transcription during primary infection and in the carrier state. Journal of Virology 1994; 68: 7374–7385.
23. Chen F, Zou JZ, di Rienzo L et al. A subpopulation of latently EBV infected normal B-cells resembles Burkitt lymphoma (BL) in expressing EBNA1 but not EBNA2 or LMP1. Journal of Virology 1995; 1995: 3752–3758.
24. Thomas J, Allday M, Crawford D. Epstein–Barr virus-associated lymphoproliferative disorders in immunocompromised individuals. Advances in Cancer Research 1991; 57: 329–380.
25. Rowe DT, Rowe M, Evan GI, Wallace LE, Farrell PJ, Rickinson AB. Restricted expression of EBV latent genes and T-lymphocyte-detected membrane antigen in Burkitt's lymphoma cells. EMBO J. 1986; 5: 2599–2607.
26. Rowe M, Rowe DT, Gregory CD et al. Differences in B cell growth phenotype reflect novel patterns of Epstein–Barr virus latent gene expression in Burkitt's lymphoma. European Molecular Biology Organization Journal 1987; 6: 2743–2751.
27. Sample J, Brooks L, Sample C et al. Restricted Epstein–Barr virus protein expression in Burkitt lymphoma is due to a different Epstein–Barr Nuclear Antigen-1 transcriptional initiation site. Proceedings of the National Academy of Sciences USA 1991; 88: 6343–6347.
28. Lear AL, Rowe M, Kurilla MG et al. The Epstein–Barr virus (EBV) nuclear antigen 1 BamHI F promoter is activated on entry of EBV-transformed B cells into the lytic cycle. Journal of Virology 1992; 66: 7461–7468.
29. Masucci MG, Contreras-Salazar B, Ragnar E et al. 5-Azacytidine up-regulates the expression of Epstein–Barr virus nuclear antigen 2 (EBNA-2) through EBNA-6 and latent membrane protein in the Burkitt's lymphoma line Rael. J. Virol. 1989; 63: 3135–3141.
30. Jansson A, Masucci MG, Rymo L. Methylation of discrete sites within the enhancer region regulates the activity of the EBV BamHI W promoter in Burkitt's lymphoma lines. Journal of Virology 1992; 66: 62–69.
31. Hu LF, Minarovits J, Cao SL et al. Variable Expression of Latent Membrane Protein in Nasopharyngeal Carcinoma Can Be Related to Methylation Status of the Epstein–Barr Virus BNLF-1 5'-Flanking Region. J. Virol. 1991; 65(3): 1558–1567.
32. Gregory CD, Murray RJ, Edwards CF, Rickinson AB. Down regulation of cell adhesion molecules LFA-3 and ICAM-1 in Epstein–Barr virus-positive Burkitt's lymphoma underlies tumour cell escape from virus-specific T cell surveillance. J. Exp. Med. 1988; 167: 1811–1824.
33. Herbst H, Trippelmann G, Anagnostopoulos I et al. Immunoglobulin and T cell receptor gene rearrangements in Hodgkin's disease and Ki-1 positive anaplastic large cell lymphoma: dissociation between phenotype and genotype. Leukemia Research 1989; 13: 103–116.
34. Weiss LM, Movahed LA, Warnke RA, Sklar J. Detection of Epstein–Barr virus genome in Reed–Sternberg cells of Hodgkin's Disease. New England Journal of Medicine 1989; 320: 502.

35. Deacon EM, Pallesen G, Niedobitek G et al. Epstein–Barr virus and Hodgkin's disease: transcriptional analysis of virus latency in the malignant cells. Journal of Experimental Medicine 1993; 177: 339–349.
36. Pallesen G, Hamilton-Dutoit SJ, Zhou X. The association of Epstein–Barr virus (EBV with T cell lymhpoproliferations and Hodgkin's disease: Two new developments in the EBV field. Advances in Cancer Research 1993; 62: 180–239.
37. Brooks L, Yao QY, Rickinson AB, Young LS. Epstein–Barr virus latent gene expression in nasopharyngeal carcinoma cells: coexpression of EBNA1, LMP1 and LMP2 transcripts. Journal of Virology 1992; 66: 2689–2697.
38. Busson P, McCoy R, Sadler R, Gilligan K, Tursz T, Raab-Traub N. Consistent tanscription of the Epstein–Barr virus LMP2 gene in nasopharyngeal carcinoma. Journal of Virology 1992; 66: 3257–3262.
39. Fåhraeus R, Li-Fu H, Ernberg I et al. Expression of the Epstein–Barr virus genome in nasopharyngeal carcinoma. Int. J. Cancer 1988; 42: 329–338.
40. Niedobitek G, Herbst H. Epstein–Barr virus associated carcinomas. Epstein–Barr virus report 1994; 1: 81–85.
41. Moss D, Rickinson A, Pope J. Long-term T-cell mediated immunity to Epstein–Barr virus in man: III. Activation of cytotoxic T cells in virus infected leukocyte cultures. International Journal of Cancer 1978; 23: 618–625.
42. Rickinson AB, Moss DJ, Wallace LE et al. Long-term T-cell-mediated immunity to Epstein–Barr virus. Cancer Res. 1981; 41: 4216–4221.
43. Wallace LE, Rickinson AB, Rowe M, Epstein MA. Epstein–Barr virus-specific cytotoxic T-cell clones restricted through a single HLA antigen. Nature 1982; 297: 413–415.
44. Misko I, Pope D, Hütter R, Soszynski T, Kane R. HLA-DR antigen associated restriction of EBV specific cytotoxic T-cell colonies. International Journal of Cancer 1984; 33: 239–243.
45. Gavioli R, Kurilla M, de Campos-Lima P-O et al. Multiple HLA A11 restricted CTL epitopes of different immunogenicity in the Epstein–Barr virus (EBV) encoded nuclear antigen-4 (EBNA4). Journal of Virology 1993; 67: 1572–1578.
46. Gavioli R, De Campos-Lima P-O, Kurilla MG, Kieff E, Klein G, Masucci MG. Recognition of the EBV encoded nuclear antigens EBNA-4 and EBNA-6 by HLA A11 restricted cytotoxic T-lymphocytes. Implications for the down-regulation of HLA A11 in Burkitt's lymphoma. Proceedings of the National Academy of Sciences USA 1992; 89: 5862–5866.
47. Khanna R, Borrows S, Kurilla M et al. Localisation of Epstein–Barr virus cytotoxic T cell epitopes using recombinant vaccinia: Implications for vaccine development. Journal of Experimental Medicine 1992; 176: 169–176.
48. Murray R, Kurilla M, Brooks J et al. Identification of target antigens for the human cytotoxic T cell response to Epstein–Barr virus (EBV): implications for the immune control of EBV-positive maligancies. Journal of Experimental Medicine 1992; 176: 157–168.
49. Khanna R, Jacob C, Borrows S et al. Expression of Epstein–Barr virus nuclear antigens in anti-IgM stimulated B cells following recombinant vaccinia infection and their recognition by human cytotoxic T cells. Immunology 1991; 74: 504–510.
50. de Campos-Lima PO, Levitsky V, Brooks J et al. T cell responses and virus evolution: Epstein–Barr virus isolates from highly HLA A11-positive populations carry mutations selectively involving anchor residues of A11-restricted CTL epitopes. Journal of Experimental Medicine 1994; 179: 1297–1305.
51. de Campos-Lima P-O, Gavioli R, Zhang Q-J et al. HLA-A11 epitope loss isolates of Epstein–Barr virus from a highly $A11^+$ population. Science 1993; 260: 98–100.
52. Trivedi P, Masucci M, Wimberg G, Klein G. The Epstein–Barr virus encoded membrane protein LMP but not the nuclear antigen EBNA-1 induces rejection of transfected murine mammary carcinoma lines. International Journal of Cancer 1991; 48: 794–800.

53. Levitskaya J, Coram M, Levitsky V et al. Inhibition of antigen processing by the internal repeat region of the Epstein–Barr Virus nuclear antigen-1. Nature (London) 1995; 375: 685–688.
54. Starlz TE, Nalesnik MA, Porter KA et al. Reversibility of lymphomas and lymphoproliferative lesions developing under cyclosporin-A-steroid therapy. Lancet 1984; I: 583–587.
55. Papadopulos AB, Landanyi M, Emanuel D et al. Infusion of donor leukocytes to Epstein–Barr virus associated lymphoproliferative disorders after allogeneic bone marrow transplantation. New England Journal of Medicine 1994; 330: 1185–1191.
56. Rooney C, Rickinson AB, Moss DJ, Lenoir GM, Epstein MA. Cell-mediated immunosurveillance mechanisms and the pathogenesis of Burkitt's lymphoma. In: Lenoir G, O'Conor G, Olweny C, eds. Burkitt's Lymphoma: A Human Cancer Model. Lyon: IARC Scientific Publications, 1985: 249–264. vol 60).
57. Rooney CM, Rowe M, Wallace LE, Rickinson AB. Epstein–Barr virus-positive Burkitt's lymphoma cells not recognized by virus-specific T-cell surveillance. Nature 1985; 317: 629–631.
58. Torsteinsdottir S, Masucci MG, Ehlin-Henriksson B et al. Differentiation dependent sensitivity of human B-cell derived lines to major histocompatibility complex-restricted T-cell cytotoxicity. Proceedings of the National Academy of Sciences USA 1986; 83: 5620–5624.
59. Patarroyo M, Prieto J, Ernberg I, Gahmberg C. Absence or low expression of the leukocyte adhesion molecules CD11 and CD18 on Burkitt lymphoma cells. International Journal of Cancer 1988; 41: 901–907.
60. Gregory CD, Murray RJ, Edwards CF, Rickinson AB. Down regulation of cell adhesion molecules LFA-3 and ICAM-1 in Epstein–Barr virus-positive Burkitt's lymphoma underlies tumour cell escape from virus-specific T cell surveillance. J Exp Med 1988; 167: 1811–1824.
61. Masucci MG. Cell phenotype dependent down-regulation of MHC class I antigens in Burkitt's lymphoma cells. Current Topics in Microbiology and Immunology 1990; 166: 309–316.
62. Rowe M, Masucci MG. Cellular adhesion molecules and MHC antigens in cells infected with Epstein–Barr virus: implications for immune recognition. In: Blair GE, Maudsley DJ, Pringle CR, eds. Modulation of MHC antigen expression and disease. Cambridge University Press, 1995 (in press).
63. Khanna R, Borrows SR, Agaet V, Moss DJ. Endoplasmic reticulum signal sequence facilitated transport of peptide epitopes restore immunogenicity of an antigen processing defective tumor cell line. International Immunology 1994; 6: 639–645.
64. Trivedi P, Hu L, Chen F et al. The EBV encoded membrane protein LMP1 from a nasopharyngeal carcinoma is non-immunogenic in a murine model system, in contrast to a B-cell derived homologue. European Journal of Cancer 1994; 30A: 84–88.
65. Frisan T, Sjöberg J, Dolcetti R et al. Local suppression of Epstein–Barr virus (EBV) specific cytotoxicity in biopsies of EBV positive Hodgkin's Disease. Blood 1995; 86: 1493–1501.
66. de Campos-Lima PO, Torsteinsdottir S, Klein G, Solitzeanu D, Masucci MG. Antigen processing and presentation by EBV carrying cell lines. Phenotype dependence and influence of the EBV encoded LMP1. International Journal of Cancer 1993; 53: 856–862.
67. Nakagomi H, Dolcetti R, Bejarano MT, Pisa P, Kiessling R, Masucci MG. The Epstein–Barr virus latent membrane protein-1 (LMP1) induces production of interleukin-10 in Burkitt lymphoma lines. International Journal of Cancer 1994; 57: 240–244.

20. Nonlymphoid Epstein–Barr virus induced neoplasms after organ transplantation

PAUL S. DICKMAN

Introduction

The increased incidence of neoplasms following organ transplantation is well documented [1, 2]. By far, the most common type of post-transplant neoplasm is Epstein–Barr virus (EBV) induced lymphoproliferative disease (PTLD). Non-lymphoid post-transplant tumors associated with EBV have only recently been described and are decidedly rare, even compared to PTLD. To date, descriptions of four cases have been published [3–5]; an additional five cases are known to the author [6–10]. All cases are spindle cell tumors, most having the histologic features of smooth muscle, with confirmation by immunohistochemistry and/or electron microscopy. In the eight cases in which tumor tissue has been evaluated, evidence of latent EBV infection has been found in six.

The following is a summary of the clinicopathologic features of the tumors and of the relationship of the tumors to EBV.

Clinical features

Clinical data regarding the known cases of EBV related post-transplant spindle cell tumors (PTST) is summarized in Table 1. Several clinical features are noteworthy. All but one of the patients were children. Tumors developed in patients on either cyclosporine or FK506 (tacrolimus) based immunosuppressive regimens. The interval between transplantation and tumor diagnosis ranged from 1 to $5\frac{1}{2}$ years (mean, approximately 2 yrs., 10 mos.), which is a considerably longer period than for the development of the majority of cases of PTLD. Sites have included both the allograft organ and native organs. In the seven cases in which the imaging has been studied [5, 6, 11], the findings were of masses which were often suggestive of PTLD [6].

J.L. Touraine et al. (eds.), Cancer in Transplantation. Prevention and Treatment, 177–187.

Table 1. Clinical features of post-transplant spindle-cell tumors

Pt. #	Age	Sex	Allo. organ	Immuno-suppr. regimen	Interval to tumor	Site(s)	PTLD status	Patient status	Ref.
1	$4\frac{1}{2}$ yrs	F	Liver	CYS	3 yrs	Allo. liver	None	NED	3
2	$6\frac{3}{4}$ yrs	F	Liver	CYS	$5\frac{1}{2}$ yrs	Allo. liver, lung, retroperit., GI tract	None	DWD	3
3	$2\frac{2}{3}$ yrs	F	Liver, small bowel	FK	1 yr	Large bowel	Prior to PTST	DWD	3
4	$8\frac{1}{2}$ yrs	M	Liver, small & large bowel	FK	$1\frac{1}{2}$ mos	Allo. small bowel	Immed. after PTST	DWD	6
5	9 yrs	M	Liver	CYS	2 yrs	Allo. liver	None	DWD	7, 8
6	12 yrs	F	Liver	CYS	5 yrs	Peritoneal soft tissue	None	NED	7, 8
7	10 yrs	F	Heart/DL	CYS	4 yrs	Small bowel mesentery	Prior to PTST	DWD	9
8	51 yrs	F	DL	unknown	3 yrs	Bronchus, allo. lung	unk.	AWD	10
9	11 yrs	F	Liver	CYS	2 yrs	Allo. liver	None	AWD	5, 13

Abbreviations: CYS, cyclosporine; allo., allograft; NED, no evidence of disease; GI, gastrointestinal; DWD, dead with disease; FK, tacrolimus (FK506); PTST, post-transplant spindle-cell tumor; DL, double lung; AWD, alive with disease.

In several patients, immunosuppression was withdrawn in order to induce regression of the tumors; the neoplasms responded by shrinking, but they rapidly recurred when immunosuppression was reinstituted. The tumors showed no response to antiviral therapy, interferon therapy, or immune globulin administration. In three cases, antineoplastic chemotherapy consisting of vincristine, dactinomycin, and cyclophosphamide was given, and in one case (Patient 9) cisplatin and etoposide were also used; but the tumors did not respond, or responded only minimally, to this treatment [3, 5, 7, 8, 12].

Pathologic features

Light Microscopy: All lesions had a spindle cell morphology, resembling smooth muscle cells, with little pleomorphism (Figure 1). Occasional cases have had increased numbers of mitotic figures or necrosis [7,8,13]. The lesions tended to be well circumscribed, and were either single or multiple.

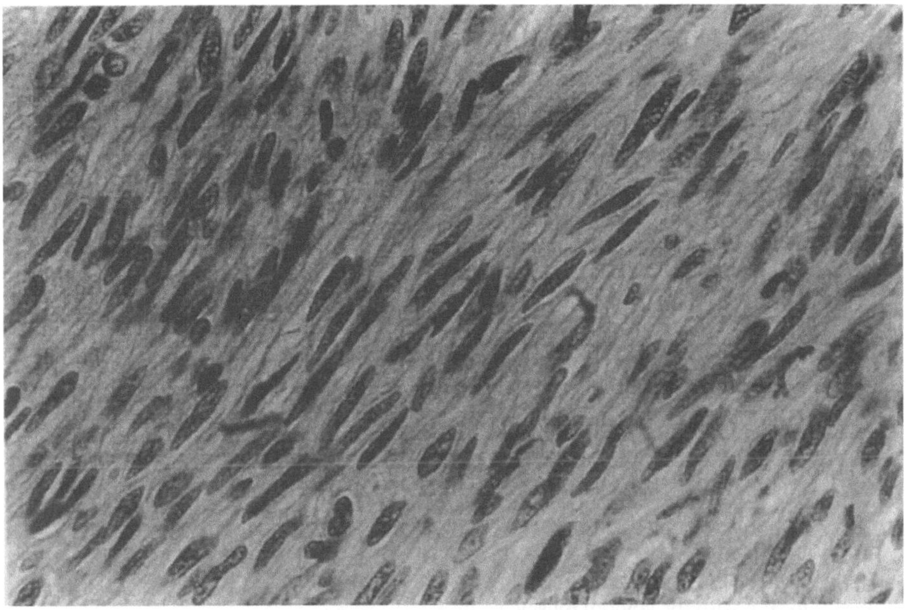

Fig. 1. Histology of post-transplant spindle cell tumor, patient #2. Tumor is composed of elongated, bland cells with blunt-ended nuclei and contains little extracellular stroma. The cells resemble smooth muscle cells. (Hematoxylin & eosin; original magnification, X400.)

Immunohistochemistry: Immunohistochemical features are summarized in Table 2. With the exception of case 4, all tumors for which immunohistochemical results were available expressed one or more markers of muscle or smooth muscle differentiation. No specific evidence of other types of differentiation has been found in the cases studied to date.

Electron microscopy: In each case in which EM has been performed, the tumor cells have consistently exhibited the ultrastructural features of smooth muscle cells, including cytoplasmic actin filaments, cytoplasmic focal densities, pinocytotic vesicles, and basal laminae [3, 7, 8].

In summary, all tumors could be characterized histologically as smooth muscle lesions, with confirmation by other methods in all but one patient. The pathobiology is still insufficiently characterized to determine whether these lesions should best be designated "leiomyoma" or "leiomyosarcoma", but most have behaved in a benign fashion.

Epstein–Barr virus studies

Serologic studies of EBV in these patients is incomplete. Prior to transplantation, Patients 1 and 3 had EBV serology indicative of past infection (elevated IgG directed against viral capsid antigen); Patient 2 had negative pretransplant EBV serology; and the results in Patient 4 were consistent with remote

Table 2. Immunohistochemistry of spindle-cell tumors. +, positive staining; 0, unstained; ND, not done; –, unknown

Patient	Vimentin	Muscle-specific	Desmin	S-100	Factor VIII:RAg	EBV LMP	EBNA-2	CD21
1	+	+	+	0	0	0	+	0
2	+	+	+[a]	0	0	0[b]	+	0
3	+	+	+	0	0	0	ND	ND
4	ND	0	ND	ND	ND	ND	ND	ND
5	+	+[c]	0	0	–	–	–	–
6	–	+[d]	–	–	–	–	–	–
7	–	–	–	–	–	–	–	–
8	–	–	–	–	–	–	–	–
9	+	+	+	0	ND	0	ND	ND

[a]Positive in liver only.
[b]Rare positive cell in retroperitoneal tumor only.
[c]Weak, focal positivity, smooth muscle actin.
[d]Smooth muscle actin.

infection. Seven of the tumors have been studied by *in situ* hybridization using the EBER-1 probe, which is a 30 mer probe recognizing EBV mRNA transcribed in latently and lytically infected cells; in six of the cases, strong nuclear positivity was found (Figure 2).

Immunohistochemistry for EBNA-2 was positive in the two cases in which it was studied. CD21, the B-lymphocyte EBV receptor, was also examined immunohistochemically but, except for focal positivity in one lesion of Patient #2, was absent in the cases studied [3].

In four of the cases, molecular biologic studies of EBV were carried out. In three of these cases, there was evidence of clonal Epstein–Barr virus, ranging from 1 to 25 copies of EBV DNA per haploid genome [3]. The viral DNA was usually found as a circularized episome, but in one instance (Patient 2) it was integrated into the host DNA, a rare but previously reported event in latent EBV infection [14].

In the latter patient, who had widespread disease, EBV DNA from two separate lesions was studied. This patient had a large retroperitoneal mass and multiple smaller masses in many organs (see Table 1). The patterns of DNA hybridization demonstrated that the retroperitoneal mass and a smaller lung lesion contained the same viral clone, most likely from the initial virus infection. This finding suggested that the two nodules represented a primary tumor and a metastasis [3].

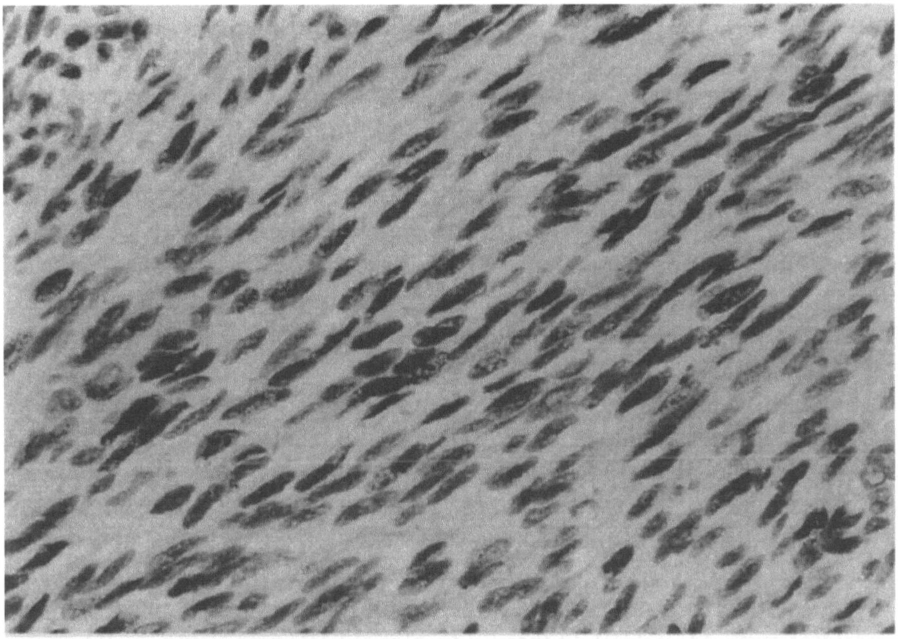

Fig. 2. *In situ* hybridization of spindle cell tumor using EBER-1 probe. Darkly stained nuclei represent positive reaction, indicating frequent presence of EBV in tumor cells. (Hematoxylin counterstain; original magnification, X400.)

Origin of tumor cells

The question of the origin of the tumor cells from donor or recipient cells was studied in four of the patients [3, 5]. In Patient 1, the only sex-mismatched transplant in the reported series, *in situ* hybridization for Y-chromosome revealed that the tumor arose from donor cells; this result was also demonstrated using microsatellite analysis for uniqueness testing [15]. In two other cases [7, 8], tumor cells were derived from donor tissue in one case and recipient (native) tissue in the other. The tumor of Patient 9 arose from donor tissue [5].

Discussion

EBV-associated PTST expressing features of smooth muscle tumors are unusual in the organ transplant population observed to date. By way of comparison, at Children's Hospital of Pittsburgh (CHP), only 4 cases of PTST were observed between 1989 and the present, a very low incidence among all transplant recipients (590 transplant recipients at CHP, excluding intestinal and multivisceral, 1988–1993). During a roughly equivalent period, the annual rate of PTLD in transplanted patients at CHP was approximately 9% [16].

Now that PTST has been described in the literature, the index of suspicion for the diagnosis of these neoplasms will undoubtedly be raised. Prior to the description of the post-transplant tumors, similar lesions had been reported in both adults and children with the acquired immune deficiency syndrome. The tumors in AIDS patients were multifocal, arose in various organ sites, and were clinically heterogeneous, as were the post-transplant tumors. For example, five pediatric patients with HIV had liver tumors which were cured surgically or were found incidentally at post-mortem examination. Deaths of these patients were due to various causes, often unrelated to the tumors [17]. Smooth muscle tumors in AIDS patients also have been found in lung, colon and ileum [18–23].

The possible association of EBV infection with smooth muscle tumors in AIDS patients was studied in a very limited fashion until recently. One patient had elevated EBNA titers [17]. *In situ* hybridization for EBV RNA (EBER) sequences was negative in one tumor in a case of AIDS [18]. In another case, EBER in situ hybridization demonstrated EBV RNA in tumor cell nuclei [17].

A recent report confirmed the significance of EBV in smooth muscle tumors in children with AIDS [19]. In that study, clonal EBV was found in all tumors in the 6 cases examined. This finding supports the possibility that EBV is an essential cofactor in the development of these tumors in AIDS patients, similar to the virus's presumed role in both lymphoid and spindle cell post-transplant tumors. The exact relationship of tumor development to immunodeficiency in both these groups of patients is unknown; patterns of expression of EBV-related proteins may provide a clue to the specific influence of the altered immune system on the development of the tumors. It will also be of interest to explore the role of immunosuppression with regimens including cyclosporine and tacrolimus, since the tumors have only been noted since the time the use of these agents for transplant immunosuppression became a regular practice.

In patients with AIDS, the non-lymphoid lesions have been characterized as leiomyomas, leiomyosarcomas, or simply "smooth-muscle tumors" [7, 8, 18–23]. In the transplanted patients, the lesions have tended to be only locally invasive, even if multifocal, except in one instance. The latter case, Patient 2, developed multiple tumors which were resistant to chemotherapy. Molecular biologic studies indicated that lesions in two different sites were derived from the same EBV infection, suggesting that the two tumors may have represented primary and metastatic disease; this patient died with numerous tumor nodules but the death was attributable to Candidal sepsis. In other patients, the tumors have behaved in a benign fashion. In the cases in which chemotherapy was used, no clinical response was observed; aggressive tumors may respond to chemotherapeutic regimens other than vincristine-dactinomycin-cyclophosphamide or cisplatin-etoposide. For the more indolent tumors, conservative therapy is indicated in the absence of involvement of vital structures.

In all cases the tumor cells had the histological features of smooth muscle cells, a finding generally confirmed by immunohistochemistry and electron microscopy, and were indistinguishable from conventional smooth muscle tumors. The bland histologic appearance of most of the lesions was comparable to leiomyomas in the non-transplanted population. Only the occasional case with pleomorphic histology (Patient 5) or widespread disease (Patient 2) might justify the designation "leiomyosarcoma". Because the biologic potential of these lesions is not yet fully characterized, perhaps the terms "smooth muscle tumor" or "spindle cell tumor" would be more accurate for diagnostic purposes. It is of interest that in one patient seen at CHP, a fibromatosis was diagnosed following transplantation; this lesion, however, was not associated with EBV infection [Dickman, unpublished data].

An entity which may cause both clinical and pathologic diagnostic confusion with these neoplasms is the mycobacterial-induced spindle cell nodule, which has been described in HIV-infected and transplant patients [24–27]. These lesions represent an inflammatory reaction to mycobacteria, containing lymphocytes, plasma cells, proliferating blood vessels, and histiocytes with numerous acid-fast bacilli in the cytoplasm. When one is aware of the clear distinctions between the two entities, the mycobacterial nodules should not present a diagnostic problem.

In patients with EBV-associated PTLD in which more than one lesion is present, it has been demonstrated that the individual tumors can be associated with different viral clones [28, 29]. In the one spindle-cell tumor patient in which this phenomenon was examined (Patient 2), only a single EBV infection could be documented. However, in children with AIDS in which multiple smooth muscle tumors were studied, clonal EBV DNA was found but with different clones in each tumor [19; Dickman, unpublished data]. Thus, it is possible that multiple post-transplant smooth-muscle tumors may also have multiclonal origins.

The latent status of EBV in the transplant-associated tumors is supported by the findings of particular EBV-associated proteins expressed by the tumor cells, including EBER and EBNA-2 [30]. In previous studies, EBV-related neoplasms have shown several different patterns of viral gene expression [31, 32]. One of the patterns includes tumors such as Burkitt's lymphoma, which express only EBNA-1, an antigen which is not targeted by cytotoxic lymphocytes. Another pattern includes post-transplant lymphoproliferative tumors, which express an array of immunogenic proteins, including EBNA-2 through EBNA-6. The immunosuppressed condition may favor the development of neoplasms such as PTLD and the spindle cell tumors which are associated with this pattern of expression of multiple EBV antigens.

The available information on EBV serology of the PTST patients is of uncertain significance. Preliminary data suggests that patients undergoing organ transplants who are EBV-seronegative prior to transplant are at an increased risk for development of PTLD [12]. Of the 4 PTST patients for whom pretransplant EBV serology results are known, only one (Patient 2) was seronegative. It is of interest that this seronegative patient had widespread, multiorgan distribution of tumors, but data on more patients with PTST will be required in order to evaluate the possible significance of EBV serology.

Several of the findings in PTST remain unexplained or contradictory. Immunohistochemical studies of PTST have failed to demonstrate expression of CD21, the EBV receptor on B-lymphocytes, T-lymphocytes and, most likely, epithelial cells [33–35]. It is possible that CD21 was expressed at levels too low to be detected by immunohistochemistry. Alternatively, an EBV receptor may be present on the smooth muscle cells which does not cross-react with antibodies directed against CD21. If CD21 or a similar receptor is truly absent from the spindle cells, however, other mechanisms for viral entry into the smooth muscle cells (or, more likely, their mesenchymal precursors) must be postulated. It has been demonstrated that EBV may enter epithelial cells, which were otherwise inaccessible to the virus, by first binding to EBV-specific IgA; transport occurred via binding to secretory component (SC), an epithelial transmembrane protein, with subsequent internalization of the virus-IgA-SC complex [36]. Similar mechanisms may govern EBV infection in PTST cells. Other possibilities include viral binding to as yet unidentified receptors, or even fusion of previously latently infected cells with the cells giving rise to the tumors [32].

Limited information is available regarding the origin of post-transplant smooth muscle tumors from donor or recipient cells. It has been shown that PTLD may, on occasion, arise from recipient B-lymphocytes which have been infected by EBV transmitted by the donor organs [37]. Spindle-cell tumors have been documented as arising from either donor or recipient tissues [3, 7, 8, 15]. The clonality of the EBV in each tumor examined indicates that the tumor progenitor cell was infected by virus, rather than that tumors were superinfected by virus.

EBV latent membrane protein (LMP) is involved in neoplastic transformation and B-cell immortalization [30], and is one of the immunogenic proteins referred to above which is coexpressed with EBNA-2 [31]; in the cases of spindle-cell tumor in which LMP expression was studied [3], the tumor cells failed to immunostain for LMP. As is the case for CD21, this negative result does not necessarily mean that LMP is not expressed by the spindle cells. The method may be insufficiently sensitive to detect the amounts of LMP produced; fixation may interfere with detection; or the properties of the antigen on smooth muscle cells may differ from those of LMP found on lymphocytes [38]. Various patterns of EBV-related protein expression have been described in lymphoproliferative disease, nasopharyngeal carcinoma, and Burkitt's lymphoma [31, 39–41], and the spindle-cell tumors may not conform to previously described patterns of antigen expression. In any case, lack of LMP expression is not unique and may still be consistent with latent EBV infection. Such limited expression of viral genes and concomitant decreased production of adhesion molecules may enhance the ability of the spindle-cell tumors to escape immune surveillance and promote tumor growth [42].

The molecular mechanisms by which EBV causes the development of mesenchymal spindle-cell tumors in both transplant patients and those with HIV infection are as yet unknown. It has been observed that smooth muscle tumors may arise as second malignant neoplasms in patients with leukemia, ataxia-telangiectasia (an immunodeficiency syndrome with which leukemia may be associated), and in a case of Poland's syndrome (which also has an increased risk of leukemia). A unique translocation, t(12;14), has been observed in smooth muscle tumors, and involves a site which is deleted in B-cell chronic lymphocytic leukemia and in non-Hodgkin's lymphomas [43]. This site is the location of the MAX gene, a regulator of the MYC oncogene, which may therefore be involved in the development of smooth-muscle tumors [44]. Another possible mechanism by which EBV may influence tumorigenesis is suggested by the relationship between EBV and bcl-2, a cellular oncogene which inhibits apoptosis, the process of programmed cell death [45, 46]. Other investigators have demonstrated an interaction between EBV and p53, the tumor suppressor gene which has been implicated in a variety of human neoplasms [47]. Exploration of the relationship of EBV to oncogene and tumor suppressor gene function represent exciting areas for future investigation in post-transplant neoplasms.

Acknowledgments

I would like to thank the following individuals for their invaluable assistance given to me in the preparation of this paper: David M.O. Becroft, Department of Obstetrics & Gynaecology, University of Auckland, New Zealand; Petrina DeFlavia, Department of Pathology, Children's Hospital of Pittsburgh; Michael Green, Division of Infectious Diseases, Children's Hospital of Pittsburgh; Ronald Jaffe, Department of Pathology, Children's Hospital of Pittsburgh; Michael Nalesnik, Division of Transplant Pathology, University of Pittsburgh Medical Center; Parmjeet S. Randawha, Division of Transplant Pathology, University of Pittsburgh Medical Center; John Wilson, University of Pittsburgh Cancer Institute; and Samuel Yousem, Department of Pathology, University of Pittsburgh Medical Center.

References

1. Mueller BU, Pizzo PA. Cancer in children with primary or secondary immunodeficiencies. J Ped 1995; 126: 1–10.
2. Penn I. Posttransplant malignancies in pediatric organ transplant recipients. Transplantation Proc 1994; 26: 2763–2765.
3. Lee ES, Locker J, Nalesnik M, et al. The association of Epstein–Barr virus with smooth-muscle tumors occurring after organ transplantation. N Engl J Med 1995; 332: 19–25.

4. Doyle H, Tzakis AG, Yunis E, Starzl TE. Smooth muscle tumor arising de novo in a liver allograft: A case report. Clin Transplantation 1991; 5: 60–62.
5. Danhaive O, Ninane J, Sokal E, et al. Hepatic localization of a fibrosarcoma in a child with a liver transplant. J Pediatr 1992; 120: 434–437.
6. Pollock AN, Newman B, Putnam PE, Dickman PS, Medina JL. Imaging of post transplant spindle cell tumors. Pediatr Radiology, in press.
7. Timmons CF, Richards S, Katz JA, Andrews WS. Hepatic leiomyosarcoma of donor genotype in a liver transplant recipient. Lab Invest 1993; 68: 9P (abstr).
8. Timmons CF, Dawson DB, Richards CS, Andrews WS, Katz JA. Epstein–Barr virus-associated leiomyosarcomas in liver transplantation recipients: Origin from either donor or recipient tissue. Cancer 1995; 76: 1481–1489.
9. Becroft DMO, Jaffe R. Personal communication.
10. Yousem S. Personal communication.
11. Ha C, Haller JO, Rollins NK. Smooth muscle tumors in immunocompromised (HIV negative) children. Pediatr Radiol 1993; 23: 413–414.
12. Green M. Personal communication.
13. Randawha PS. Personal communication.
14. Gulley M, Raphael M, Lutz C, Ross D, Raab-Traub N. Epstein–Barr virus integration in human lymphomas and lymphoid cell lines. Cancer 1992; 70: 185–191.
15. Dickman PS, Lanning R, Cooper D, Sakallah S. Microsatellite analysis (MSA) on paraffin embedded material using the polymerase chain reaction (PCR) for distinction of tissues from different individuals. Lab Invest 1995; 72: 164A (abstr).
16. Wilson J. Personal communication.
17. van Hoeven KH, Factor SM, Kress Y, Woodruff JM. Visceral myogenic tumors. A manifestation of HIV infection in children. Am J Surg Pathol 1993; 17: 1176–1181.
18. Ross JS, Del Rosario A, Bui HX, Sonbati H, Solis O. Primary hepatic leiomyosarcoma in a child with the acquired immunodeficiency syndrome. Hum Pathol 1992; 23: 69-72.
19. McClain KL, Leach CT, Jenson HB, et al. Association of Epstein–Barr virus with leiomyosarcomas in young people with AIDS. N Engl J Med 1995; 332: 12–18.
20. Mueller BU, Butler KM, Higham MC, et al. Smooth muscle tumors in children with human immunodeficiency virus infection. Pediatrics 1992; 90: 460-463.
21. Chadwick EG, Connor EJ, Hanson IC, et al. Tumors of smooth-muscle origin in HIV-infected children. JAMA 1990; 263: 3182-3184.
22. Radin D, Kiyabu M. Multiple smooth muscle tumors of the colon and adrenal gland in an adult with AIDS. AJR Am J Roentgenol 1992; 159: 545–546.
23. McLoughlin LC, Nord KS, Joshi VV, Di Carlo FJ, Kane MJ. Disseminated leiomyosarcoma in a child with acquired immunodeficiency syndrome. Cancer 1991; 67: 2618–2621.
24. Brandwein M, Choi HS, Strauchen J, Stoler M, Jagirdar J. Spindle cell reaction to nontuberculous mycobacteriosis in AIDS mimicking a spindle cell neoplasm. Evidence for dual histiocytic and fibroblast-like characteristics of spindle cells. Virchows Arch A Pathol Anat Histopathol 1990; 416: 281-286.
25. Umlas J, Federman M, Crawford C, O'Hara CJ, Fitzgibbon JS, Modeste A. Spindle cell pseudotumor due to Mycobacterium avium-intracellulare in patients with acquired immunodeficiency syndrome (AIDS). Positive staining of mycobacteria for cytoskeleton filaments. Am J Surg Pathol 1991; 15: 1181-1187.
26. Sekosan M, Cleto M, Senseng C, Garolan M, Sekosan J. Spindle cell pseudotumors in the lungs due to Mycobacterium tuberculosis in a transplant patient. Am J Surg Pathol 1994; 18: 1065–1068.
27. Chen KTK. Mycobacterial spindle cell pseudotumor of lymph nodes. Am J Surg Pathol 1992; 16: 276–281.
28. Cleary ML, Nalesnik MA, Shearer WT, Sklar J. Clonal analysis of transplant-associated lymphoproliferations based on the structure of the genomic termini of the Epstein–Barr virus. Blood 1988; 72: 349–352.

29. Raab-Traub N, Flynn K. The structure of the termini of the Epstein–Barr virus as a marker of clonal cellular proliferation. Cell 1986; 47: 883–889.
30. Middleton T, Gahn T, Martin J, Sugden B. Immortalizing genes of Epstein–Barr virus. Adv Virus Res 1991; 40: 19–55.
31. Klein G. Epstein–Barr virus strategy in normal and neoplastic B cells. Cell 1994; 77: 791–793.
32. Wolf H, Bogedain C, Schwarzmann F. Epstein–Barr virus and its interaction with the host. Intervirology 1993; 35: 26–39.
33. Bush JL, Radich PC. The Epstein–Barr virus receptor. Lab Med 1989; 20: 318–323.
34. Birkenbach M, Tong X, Bradbury LE, Tedder TF, Kieff E. Characterization of an Epstein–Barr virus receptor on human epithelial cells. J Exp Med 1992; 176: 1405–1414.
35. Paterson RLK, Kelleher CA, Streib JE, et al. Activation of human thymocytes after infection by EBV. J Immunol 1995; 154: 1440–1449.
36. Sixbey JW, Yao Q-Y. Immunoglobulin A-induced shift of Epstein–Barr virus tissue tropism. Science 1992; 255: 1578–1580.
37. Cen H, Breinig MC, Atchison RW, Ho M, McKnight JLC. Epstein–Barr virus transmission via the donor organs in solid organ transplantation: Polymerase chain reaction and restriction fragment length polymorphism analysis of IR2, IR3, and IR4. J Virol 1991; 65: 976–980.
38. Sauvageau G, Stocco R, Kasparian S, Menezes J. Epstein–Barr virus receptor expression on human CD8+ (cytotoxic/suppressor) T-lymphocytes. J Gen Virol 1990; 71: 379–386.
39. Brooks L, Yao QY, Rickinson AB, Young LS. Epstein–Barr virus latent gene transcription in nasopharyngeal carcinoma cells: Coexpression of EBNA1, LMP1, and MP2 transcripts. J Virol 1992; 66: 2689–2697.
40. Young L, Alfieri C, Hennessy K, et al. Expression of Epstein–Barr virus transformation associated genes in tissues of patients with EBV lymphoproliferative disease. N Engl J Med 1989; 321: 1080–1085.
41. Schaefer B, Woisetschlaeger M, Strominger JL, Speck S. Exclusive expression of Epstein–Barr virus nuclear antigen 1 in Burkitt lymphoma arises from a third promoter, distinct from the promoters used in latently infected lymphocytes. Proc Natl Acad Sci USA 1991; 88: 6550–6554.
42. Purtilo DT, Strobach RS, Okano M, Davis JR. Epstein–Barr virus-associated lymphoproliferative disorders. Lab Invest 1992; 67: 5-23.
43. Davies SM. EBV – in trouble again? Causes of Childhood Cancer Newsletter 1995; 6(1): 2.
44. Wagner AJ, Le Beau MM, Diaz MO, Hay N. Expression, regulation, and chromosomal localization of the Max gene. Proc Natl Acad Sci USA 1992; 89: 3111–3115.
45. Rowe M, Peng-Pilon M, Huen DS, et al. Upregulation of bcl-2 by the Epstein–Barr virus latent membrane protein LMP1: A B-cell-specific response that is delayed relative to NF-B activation and to induction of cell surface markers. J Virol 1994; 68: 5602–5612.
46. Hickish T, Robertson D, Clarke P, et al. Ultrastructural localization of BHRF1: An Epstein–Barr virus gene product which has homology with bcl-2. Cancer Res 1994; 54: 2808–2811.
47. Zhang Q, Gutsch D, Kenney S. Functional and physical interaction between p53 and BZLF1: Implications for Epstein–Barr virus latency. Mol Cell Biol 1994; 14: 1929-1938.

21. The Epstein–Barr virus latency and reactivation

ALAIN SERGEANT

Introduction

The Epstein–Barr virus (EBV) is a widely-spread human herpes virus, that persists latently for the life time of the infected host. The life-long exposure to EBV and the fact that EBV-infected B lymphocytes from the peripheral blood have the potential to proliferate continuously (immortalization), are believed to be predisposing factors for the emergence of EBV-associated human malignancies like Burkitt's Lymphoma (BL), Nasopharyngeal Carcinoma (NPC), Hodgkin's disease (HD), and B and T cell lymphomas in immunocompromised individuals [1]. Little is known about the EBV persistence *in vivo*, and the only models for EBV latency and reactivation are B-cells immortalised *in vitro* or Burkitt lymphomas cell lines. In such cells, only a minority of the viral genes are expressed and define latency. In this chapter, the molecular mechanisms of EBV-mediated immortalisation of B cells, latency and reactivation will be shortly presented.

EBV-mediated immortalisation of B cells

In *in vitro* immortalized B cells, the EBV genes expressed define a latency of type III (Figure 1), and encode the two small RNAs (EBERS), the six *E*pstein-*B*arr *N*uclear *A*ntigens (EBNA-1, 2, 3a, 3b, 3c and LP) and three *L*atency *M*embrane *P*roteins: LMP1, LMP2A and LMP2B (also called TP1 and TP2 respectively) (for a review see [1]). Six of these proteins, EBNA1, EBNA-LP, EBNA2, EBNA3a, EBNA3c and LMP1 [2–6], are essential for the sustained growth of B cells *in vitro*. The function of these proteins and their implication in B cell immortalization are summarised in the followings.

J.L. Touraine et al. (eds.), Cancer in Transplantation. Prevention and Treatment, 189–199.

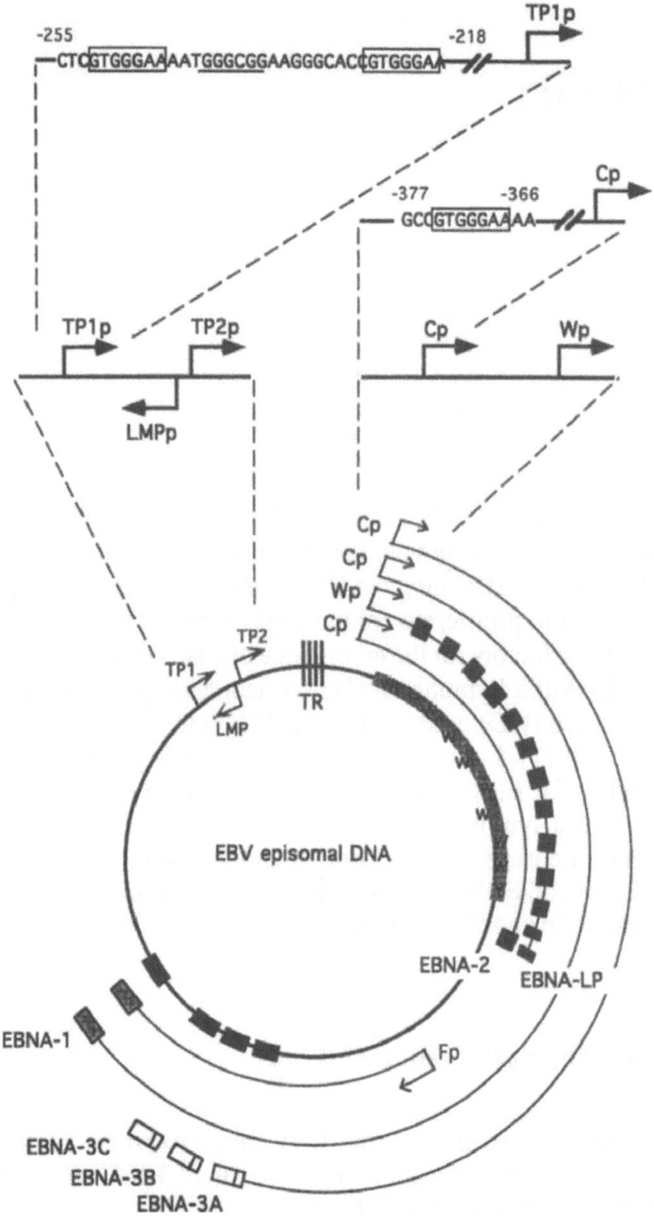

Fig. 1. EBV genes expressed during latency III. Six nuclear proteins (EBNA1, 2, 3a, 3b, 3c, and LP), translated from mRNAS generated by facultative splicing of a primary transcript initiated at promoter Cp, and three membrane proteins (LMP1, TP1 and TP2), are expressed during latency III. The EBNA2 responsive elements and the RBP-Jk binding sites in promoters Cp and TP1 are also presented. Promoter Fp from which EBNA1 transcription is initiated in Burkitt's lymphoma latency I is also presented.

EBNA1

EBNA1 is a DNA-binding protein that activates in trans the EBV origin of replication (ORIp) active during latency [7]. EBNA1 therefore ensures the equilibrated segregation and the persistence of the EBV genomes during cell mitosis. EBNA1 is also a transcription factor and as such its direct implication in B cell immortalisation has not yet been evaluated.

EBNA2

EBNA2 is a transcription factor that activates the expression of viral and cellular genes. EBNA2 activates the expression of host cell genes CD21, CD23, *c-fgr* [8–11], and activates the transcription of the three LMP genes and of all the EBNAs (Figures 1 and 2) [12–16]. Although EBNA2 does not bind directly to DNA, there are EBNA2-responsive elements in the regulatory region of EBNA2-responsive cellular and viral genes [13, 15, 17–21]. These EBNA2 responsive elements share a common DNA sequence GTGGGAA (Figure 1), to which a cellular repressor called CBF1/RBP-Jk/KBF2 binds [20–23]. Recently it has been proposed that EBNA2 is recruited to EBNA2 responsive genes through interaction with RBP-JK [24–27]. EBNA2 interaction to RBP-JK would have two consequences: masking the RBP-JK repressing domain and providing to RBP-JK a transcriptional activation domain (Figure 2C) [28].

The Drosophila homolog of RBP-Jk is Suppressor of Hairless (Su(H)), a gene whose function is important for the appropriate development of sensory organ cells in the peripheral nervous system [29, 30]. Su(H) binds to the product of the Drosophila Notch gene, a transmembrane receptor, and participates in the Notch regulated signal transduction pathway [31]. The human homolog of Notch is TAN-1, whose truncation is associated with human T lymphoblastic leukemias [32]. A pathway can be proposed for the EBNA2-induced B cell proliferation signals: EBNA2 blocks directly the RBP-JK mediated transcriptional repression of cellular genes by circumventing the TAN-1 signaling pathway.

EBNA3a, b and c

The EBNA3s are nuclear proteins whose functions are only poorly understood. EBNA3a and EBNA3c, but not EBNA3b, are essential for immortalisation of B cells [6]. Although EBNA3 proteins are identically organized and share significant amino-acids identity, their functions are different and largely unknown [6]. However, recent reports indicate that EBNA3s repress the transcriptional activation function of EBNA2 [33]. Indeed, EBNA3c, but not EBNA3a nor EBNA3b, interferes with the binding of RBP-Jk to DNA [34] and might act as a "feedback" down modulator of EBNA2-mediated tran-

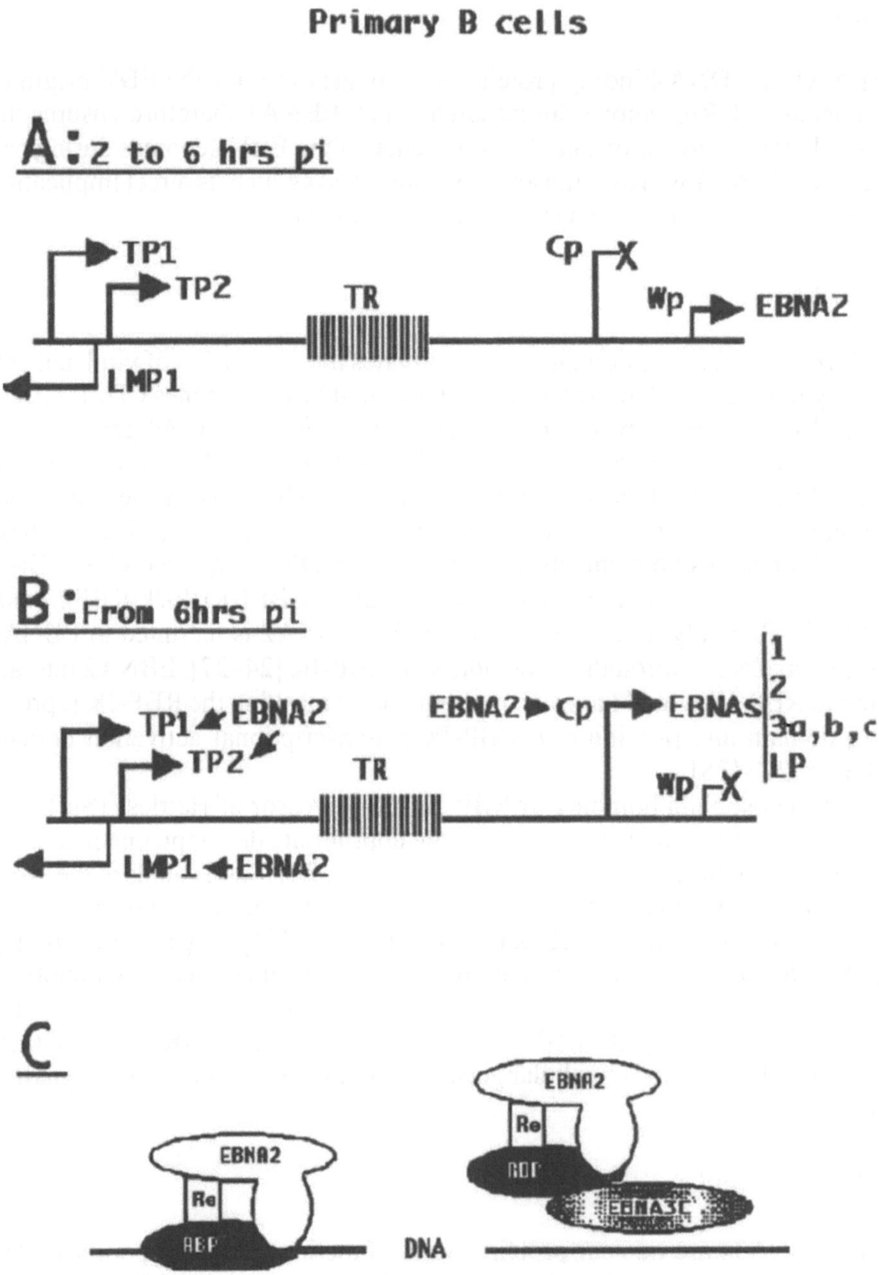

Fig. 2. Role of EBNA2 and EBNA3C in EBV infection. (A) EBV infects resting B lymphocytes. EBNA2 and EBNA-LP are the first proteins expressed from the constitutively active Wp promoter. (B) EBNA2 activates the Cp promoter and the LMP/TP promoters. The EBNAs and the membrane proteins are now made. (C) EBNA2 activates the EBV promoters (as well as cellular promoters) through contacts with the cellular protein RBP-Jk. EBNA2 interaction with RBP-Jk has two effects: 1) masking of the repressing domain in Jk (Re); and 2) providing a transcription activation domain (Act). EBNA3C binds RBP-Jk and modulates the EBNA2 activation to prevent the expression of toxic levels of LMP1 and EBNAs.

scriptional activation, principally of LMP1 whose overexpression is toxic to cells (Figure 2C).

EBNA-LP

The EBNA-LP protein is composed by a variable repetition of peptidic motifs coming from BamHIW repeats [1] (Figure 1). One report clearly demonstrated that although EBNA-LP is dispensable for the immortalisation of B cells by EBV, it is however essential for the GO to G1 transition induced by transfection of quiescent B cells by EBNA2 [35].

LMP1

LMP1 is an integral membrane protein that transform cells, possibly by constitutively activating a growth factor pathway common to many cell types [36]. In B lymphoblasts, LMP1 induces the expression of activation markers and adhesions molecules, and altered growth [37, 38]. These phenotypic effects of LMP1 are likely to be, at least in part, linked to LMP1-mediated NF-kB activation [39, 40]. There are five known members of the mammalian NF-kB/Rel family of transcription factors, that form heterodimers, and increase transcription of genes from promoter sequences that contain binding sites for NF-kB/rel proteins [41]. Recently a link has been established between LMP1 and NF-kB, by the characterisation of TRAF1 and TRAF2 (Tumor Necrosis Factor Receptor Associated Factors 1 and 2) interactions with the cytoplasmic C-terminal domain of LMP1 [42], domain required for maximal stimulation of NF-kB activity [43]. Such interactions are also a clear evidence for a central role of LMP1 as an effector of cell growth and death signalling pathways.

According to the results summarised above and in Figure 2, appropriate levels of expression of EBNAs and LMPs are essential for the infected B cell to progress through the S phase, and to proliferate continuously *in vitro*. Although, this model is quite satisfactory for *in vitro* immortalised B cells, it cannot be simply extended to the proliferating EBV positive tumor cells. Indeed, in Burkitt lymphomas biopsies, only the EBERS and EBNA1 are expressed, yet these tumor cells proliferate efficiently [44]. In NPC and Reed–Sternberg tumor cells, only EBERS, EBNA1 and LMP1 are expressed.

EBV latency and reactivation

Various chemical agents, including the tumour promoter 12-O-tetradecanoyl-phorbol-13-acetate (TPA), can cause the virus to switch from a latent to a lytic replication cycle *in vitro*. The activation seems to be linked to the expression of two EBV-encoded transcription factors: the BZLF1-encoded factor, EB1 (also

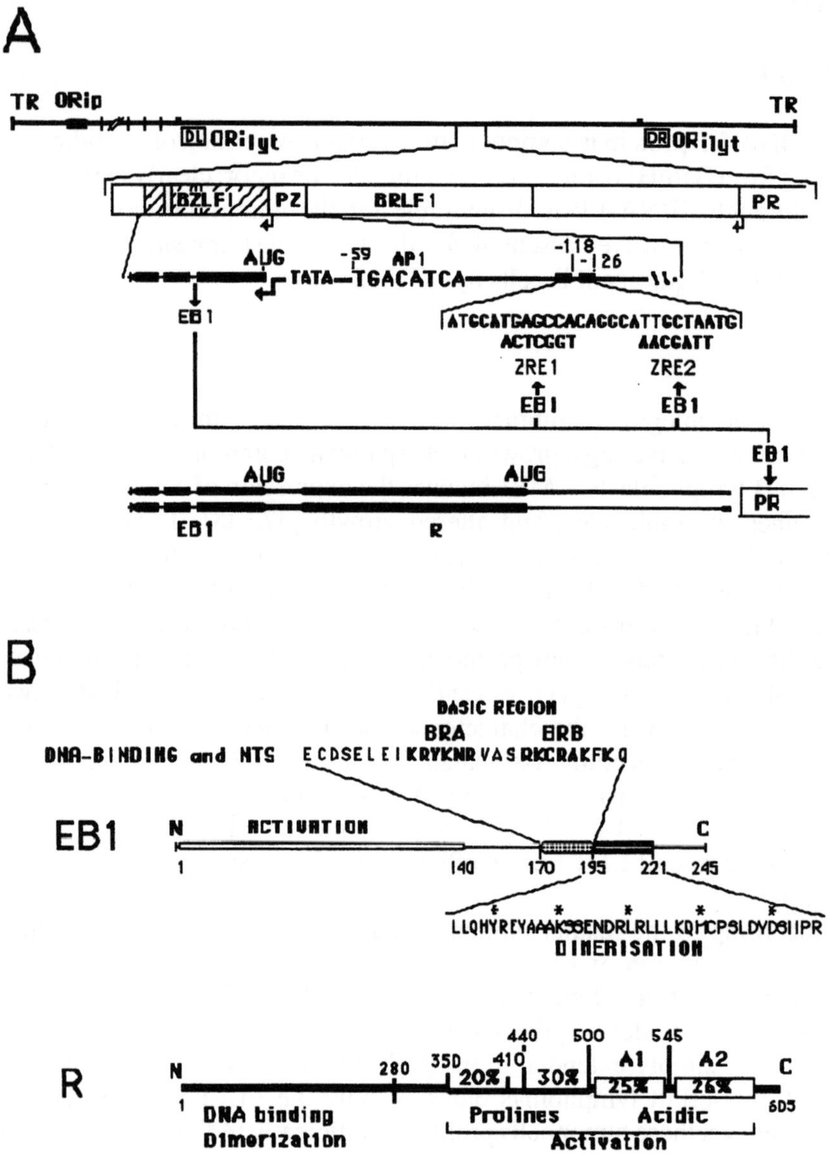

Fig. 3. Latency and reactivation of EBV. (A) Promoter PZ and PR are inactive during latency, and the EBV-encoded transcription factors EB1 and R are not detectably produced. By still unknown mechanisms, promoter PZ can be activated, leading to the expression of monocistronic mRNAs from which EB1 is translated. EB1 autoactivates his own expression and the transcription from promoter PR of bicistronic mRNAs from which both EB1 and R are translated. Once made EB1 and R activate the transcription of all the EBV early promoters, and the origin of replication active during the lytic cycle (ORIlyt). (B) Functional domains of EB1 and R.

called Z, Zta or ZEBRA) [45, 46] and the BRLF1-encoded factor, called R (or Rta) [47] (Figure 3). EB1 is a bZIP protein (basic Zipper) [48, 49] (Figure 3B) that binds as a homodimer to specific DNA sequences (ZREs) present in the promoter of many EBV early genes [50, 51]. EB1 also transactivates the origin of replication active during the lytic cycle (ORIlyt) [52], through binding to four ZREs present in a promoter overlapping the ORIlyt. R also binds directly as a homodimer to the DNA sequences: 5′-G^{T}_{G}CC-N_7-GTGGTG-3′, present in many EBV early genes promoters (Figure 3B) [53, 54].

The model which is favored for the reactivation of EBV in latently infected B cells growing in culture is the following. In such cells, the genes coding for EB1 (BZLF1) and R (BRLF1) are not detectably transcribed (Figure 3A). Upon activation of the lytic cycle, EB1 is thought to be translated either from 1 Kb monocistronic mRNAs initiated at promoter PZ, or from 3.5 Kb mRNAs initiated at promoter PR, and containing both the BZLF1 ORF and the BRLF1 ORF from which R is translated [55] (Figure 3A). However, although EB1 and R are translated upon transfection of the cDNA for the 3.5 kb mRNAs, it has not been demonstrated that EB1 and R are translated from the 3.5 kb mRNAs initiated at promoter PR from the viral genome. A weak transcriptional activation of PZ and PR promoters is seen in the absence of de novo protein synthesis, and probably requires the postranscriptional activation of pre-existing cellular factors [56]. Interestingly, promoter PZ contains a TRE (TPA Responsive Element) also called AP-1 site (TGACATCA), and this site binds dimeric AP-1 factors that are subject to post-transcriptional regulation induced by TPA (Figure 3A). However, efficient transcription from promoter PZ and PR seems to be insured by their transcriptional activation by EB1. Indeed, promoter PZ contains two EB1 binding sites called ZREZ1 and ZREZ2 (Figure 3A), and transient expression assays confirmed that EB1 autoactivates its own expression [49, 57]. Promoter PR is also activated by EB1 in transient expression assays, through two ZREs (Figure 3A) [58].

The model described above has been documented by using in transient expression assays non replicating plasmids bearing the PZ or the PR promoters and their mutated counterparts cloned upstream of a reporter gene. The model suggests that the limiting step in the activation of the lytic cycle is the translation of EB1. Once made, EB1 activates its own expression, the EBV early genes and the ORIlyt, due to unlimited accessibility of the EB1-responsive elements in the viral promoters. However, this model has not been yet evaluated in the context of the viral genome, i.e. nothing is known on the cellular factors involved in the inactivity of promoters PZ and PR, and on the mechanisms responsible for their activation.

References

1. Kieff E, Liebowitz D. Epstein–Barr virus and its replication. In: Fields B N, Knipe D M, Chanock R M, Hirsch M S, Melnick J L, Monath T P, Roizman B, editors, Virology, 2nd ed., New York: Raven Press, 1990: 1889–1920.
2. Hammerschmidt W, Sugden B. Genetic analysis of functions of Epstein–Barr virus in human B lymphocytes. Nature 1989; 340: 393–397.
3. Cohen J F, Wang F, Mannick J, Kieff E. Epstein–Barr virus nuclear protein 2is a key determinant of lymphocyte transformation. Proc Natl Acad Sci USA 1989; 86: 9558–9562.
4. Mannick J B, Cohen J I, Birkenbach M, Marchini A, Kieff E. The Epstein–Barr virus nuclear protein encoded by the leader of the EBNA RNAs is important in B cell transformation. J Virol 1991; 65: 6826–6837.
5. Kaye K, Izumi K M, Kieff E. Epstein–Barr virus latent membrane protein 1 is essential for B-lymphocyte growth transformation. Proc Natl Acad Sci USA 1993; 90: 9150–9154.
6. Tomkinson B, Robertson E, Kieff E. Epstein–Barr virus nuclear proteins EBNA3A and EBNA3C are essential for B lymphocyte growth transformation. J Virol 1993; 67: 2014–2025.
7. Yates J, Warren N, Reisman D, Sugden B. A cis acting element from the Epstein–Barr virus genome that permits stable replication of recombinant plasmids in latently infected cells. Proc Natl Acad Sci USA 1984; 81: 3806–3810.
8. Calender A, Billaud M, Aubry J-P, Banchereau J, Vuillaume M, Lenoir G M. Epstein–Barr virus induces expression of B cell activation markers on *in vitro* infection of EBV negative lymphoma cells. Proc Natl Acad Sci USA 1987; 84: 8060–8064.
9. Cordier M, Calender A, Billaud M, Zimber U, Rousselet G, Pavlish O, Banchereau J, Tursz T, Bornkamm G, Lenoir G M. Stable transfection of EBV nuclear antigen 2 in lymphoma cells containing the EBV P3HR1 genome induces expression of B-cell activation molecules. J Virol 1990; 64: 1002–1013.
10. Wang F, Gregory C D, Rowe M, Rickinson A B, Wang D, Birkenbach M, Kikutani H, Kishimoto T, Kieff E. Epstein–Barr virus nuclear protein 2 specifically induces expression of the B cell antigen CD23. Proc Natl Acad Sci USA 1987; 84: 3452–3456.
11. Knuston J C. The level of c-fgr RNA is increased by EBNA2, an EBV gene required for B-cell immortalisation. J Virol 1990; 64: 2530–2536.
12. Abbot S D, Rowe M, Cadwallader K, Ricksten A, Gordon J, Wang F, Rymo L, Rickinson A B. Epstein–Barr virus 2 induces expression of the virus-encoded latent membrane protein. J Virol 1990; 64: 2126–2134.
13. Fahraeus R, Jansson A, Ricksten A, Sjöblom A, Rymo L. Epstein–Barr virus nuclear antigen 2 activates the latent membrane protein promoter by modulating the activity of a negative regulatory element. Proc Natl Acad Sci USA 1990; 87: 7390–7394.
14. Zimber-Strobl U, Suentzenich K-O, Laux G, Eick D, Cordier M, Calender A, Billaud M, Lenoir G M, Bornkamm G W. Epstein–Barr virus nuclear antigen 2 activates transcription of the terminal protein gene. J Virol 1991; 65: 415–423.
15. Sung N S, Kenney S, Gutsch D, Pagano J S. EBNA2 transactivates a lymphoid-specific enhancer in the BamHI C promoter of Epstein–Barr virus. J Virol 1991; 65: 2164–2169.
16. Rooney C M, Brimmell M, Buschle M, Allan G, Farrell P J, Kolman J L. Host cell and EBNA2 regulation of EBV latent cycle promoter activity in B lymphocytes. J Virol 1992; 66: 496–504.
17. Tsang S-F, Wang F, Izumi K M, Kieff E. Delineation of the cis-acting element mediating EBNA2 transactivation from latent infection membrane protein expression. J Virol 1991; 65: 6765–6771.
18. Wang F, Kikutani H, Tsang S-F, Kishimoto T, Kieff E. Epstein–Barr virus nuclear antigen 2 transactivates a cis-acting CD23 DNA element. J Virol 1991; 65: 4101–4106.

19. Jin X W, Speck S. Identification of critical cis elements involved in mediating Epstein–Barr virus nuclear antigen 2-dependent activity of an enhancer located upstream of the viral BamHI C promoter. J Virol 1992; 66: 2846–2852.
20. Ling P D, Rawlins D R, Hayward S D. The Epstein–Barr virus immortalising protein EBNA2 is targeted to DNA by cellular enhance binding protein. Proc Natl Acad Sci USA 1993; 90: 9237–9241.
21. Zimber-Strobl U, Kremmer E, Grässer F, Marschall G, Laux G, Bornkamm G W. The Epstein–Barr virus nuclear antigen 2 interacts with an EBNA2-responsive cis-element of the terminal protein 1 gene promoter. EMBO J 1993; 12: 167–175.
22. Tun T, Hamaguchi Y, Matsunami N, Furukawa T, Honjo T, Kawaichi M. Recognition sequence of a highly conserved DNA binding protein RBP-J kappa. Nucleic Acids Res 1994; 22: 965–971.
23. Israel, A, Yano, O, Logeat, F, Kieran, M. and Kourilsky, P. Nucleic Acids Res 1989; 17, 5245–5257.
24. Grossman S R, Johannsen E, Tong X, Yalamanchini R, Kieff E. The EBV nuclear antigen 2 transactivator is directed to response elements by the Jk recombination signal binding protein. Proc Natl Acad Sci USA 1994; 91: 7568–7572.
25. Henkel T, Ling P D, Hayward S D, Peterson M G. Mediation of EBV EBNA2 transactivation by recombination signal binding protein Jk. Science 1994; 26: 92–95.
26. Zimber-Strobl U, Strobl L, Meitinger C, Hinrichs R, Sakai T, Honjo T, Bornkamm G. EBV nuclear antigen 2 exerts its transactivating function through interaction with recombination signal binding protein RBP-Jk, the homologue of Drosophila suppressor of Hairless. EMBO J 1994; 13: 4973–4982.
27. Waltzer L, Logeat F, Brou C, Israel A, Sergeant A, Manet E. The human Jk recombination signal sequence binding protein (RBP-JK) targets the Epstein–Barr virus EBNA2 protein to its DNA responsive elements. EMBO J 1994; 13: 5633–5638.
28. Hsieh JJ-D, Hayward SD. Masking of the CBF1/RBP-JK transcriptional repression domain by EBV EBNA2. Science 1995; 268:560–563.
29. Furukawa T, Kawaichi M, Matsunami N, Ryo H, Nishida Y, Honjo T. The drosophila RBP-J kappa gene encodes the binding protein for the immunoglobulin Jk recombination signal sequence. J Biol Chem 1991; 266: 23334–23340.
30. Schweisguth F, Posakony J W. Suppressor of Hairless, the drosophila homolog of the mouse recombination signal-binding protein gene, controls sensory organ cell fate. Cell 1992; 69: 1199–1212.
31. Fortini ME, Artavanis-Tsakonas S. The suppressor of Hairless protein participates in Notch receptor signalling. Cell 1994; 79: 273–282.
32. Ellisen LW, Bird J, West D, Soreng AL, Reynolds TC, Smith S, Sklar J. TAN-1, the human homolog of the drosophila Notch gene, is broken by chromosomal translocations in T lymphoblastic neoplasms. Cell 1991; 66: 649–661.
33. Le Roux A, Kerdiles B, Walls D, Dedieu JF, Perricaudet M. The EBV determined nuclear antigens EBNA3A, B and C repress EBNA2 mediated transactivation of the viral TP1 gene promoter. Virol 1994; 205: 596–602.
34. Robertson ES, Grossman S, Johannsen E, Miller C, Lin J, Tomkinson B, Kieff E. Epstein–Barr virus nuclear protein 3C modulates transcription through interaction with the sequence specific DNA-binding protein Jk. J Virol 1995; 69: 3108–3116.
35. Sinclair A, Palmero I, Peters G, Farrell P. EBNA2 and EBNA-LP cooperate to cause G0 to G1 transition during immortalisation of resting human B lymphocytes by EBV. EMBO J 1994; 13: 3321–3328.
36. Wang D, Liebowitz D, Kieff E. An EBV membrane protein expressed in immortalized lymphocytes transforms established rodent cells. Cell 1985; 43: 831–840.
37. Wang D, Liebowitz D, Wang F, Gregory C, Rickinson A, Larson R, Springer T, Kieff E. Epstein–Barr virus latent infection membrane protein alters the human B-lymphocyte

phenotype: deletion of the amino-terminus abolishes activity. J Virol 1988b; 62: 4173–4184.
38. Peng M, Lundgren E. Transient expression of the Epstein–Barr virus LMP1 gene in B-cell chronic lymphocytic leukaemia cells, T cells, and hematopoietic cell lines: cell-type-independent-induction of CD23, CD21 and ICAM-1. Leukemia 1993; 7: 104–112.
39. Hamarskjold M L, Simurda M C. Epstein–Barr virus latent membrane protein transactivates the human immunodeficiency virus type 1 long terminal repeat through induction of NF-KB activity. J Virol 1992; 66: 6496–6501.
40. Rowe M, Peng-Pilon M, Huen D S, Hardy R, Croom-Carter D, Lundgren E, Rickinson A B. Up regulation of Bcl-2 by the Epstein–Barr virus latent membrane protein LMP1: a B-cell specific response that is delayed relative to NF-kB activation and to induction of cell surface markers. J Virol 1994; 68: 5602–5612.
41. Liou H C, Baltimore D. Regulation of the NF-kB/rel transcription factor and IkB inhibitor system. Curr Opin Cell Biol 1993; 5: 477–487.
42. Mosialos G, Birkenbach M, Yalamanchili R, VanArsdale T, Ware C, Kieff E. The Epstein–Barr virus transforming protein LMP1 engages signalling proteins for the tumor necrosis factor receptor family. Cell 1995; 80: 389–399.
43. Mitchell T, Sugden B. Stimulation of NF-kB-mediated transcription by mutant derivates of the latent membrane protein of Epstein–Barr virus. J Virol 1995; 69: 2968–2976.
44. Rowe M, Rowe D T, Gregory C D, Young L S, Farrell P J, Rupani H, Rickinson A B. Differences in B-cell growth phenotype reflect novel patterns of Epstein–Barr virus latent gene expression in Burkitt's lymphoma cells. EMBO J 1987; 6: 2743–2751.
45. Countryman J, Miller G. Activation of expression of latent Epstein–Barr herpesvirus after gene transfer with a small cloned fragment of heterogeneous viral DNA. Proc Natl Acad Sci USA 1985; 82: 4085–4089.
46. Chevallier-Greco A, Manet E, Chavrier P, Mosnier C, Daillie J, Sergeant A. Both Epstein–Barr virus encoded trans-acting factors, EB1 and EB2, are required to activate transcription from an EBV early promoter. EMBO J 1986; 5: 3243–3249.
47. Hardwick J M, Lieberman P, Hayward S D. A new Epstein–Barr virus transactivator R, induces expression of a cytoplasmic early antigen. J Virol 1988; 62: 2274–2284.
48. Farrell P J, Rowe D T, Rooney C M, Kouzarides T. Epstein–Barr virus BZLF1 trans-activator specifically binds to a consensus AP-1 site and is related to c-fos. EMBO J 1989; 8: 127–132.
49. Urier G, Buisson M, Chambard P, A. Sergeant. The Epstein–Barr early protein EB1 activates transcription from different responsive elements including AP-1 binding sites. EMBO J 1989; 8: 1447–1453.
50. Lieberman P, Berk A J. *In vitro* transcriptional activation, dimerisation, and DNA-binding specificity of the Epstein–Barr virus Zta protein. J Virol 1990; 64: 2560–2568.
51. Kouzarides T, Packham G, Cook A, Farrell P J. The BZLF1 protein of EBV has a coiled coil dimerisation domain without a heptad leucine repeat but with homology to the CEB/P leucine zipper. Oncogene 1991; 6: 195–204.
52. Hammerschmidt W, Sugden B. Identification and characterisation of orilyt, a lytic origin of DNA replication of Epstein–Barr virus. Cell 1988; 55: 427–433.
53. Gruffat H, Manet E, Rigolet A, A.Sergeant. The EBV enhancer factor R is a sequence-specific DNA-binding protein. Nucleic Acids Res 1990; 18: 6835–6843.
54. Gruffat H, A. Sergeant. Characterisation of the DNA-binding site repertoire for the EBV transcription factor R. Nucleic Acids Res 1994; 22: 1172–1178.
55. Manet E, Gruffat H, Trescol-Biemont M C, Moreno N, Chambard P, Giot J F, Sergeant A. Epstein–Barr Virus bicistronic mRNAs generated by facultative splicing code for two transcriptional activators. EMBO J 1989; 8: 1819–1826.
56. Flemington E, Goldfeld A E, Speck S. Efficient transcription of the Epstein–Barr virus immediate-early BZLF1 and BRLF1 genes requires protein synthesis. J Virol 1991; 65: 7073–7077.

57. Flemington E, Speck S H. Autoregulation of Epstein–Barr virus BZLF1 putative lytic switch gene. J Virol 1990; 64: 1227–1232.
58. Sinclair A J, Brimmel M, Shanahan F, Farrell P J. Pathways of activation of the Epstein–Barr virus productive cycle. J Virol 1991; 65: 2237–2244.

22. Early detection of EBV infection and meaning in transplant patients

E.B. DROUET, C. CHAPUIS-CELLIER, J.L. GARNIER & J.L. TOURAINE

Epstein–Barr virus (EBV) is a human B-lymphotropic herpes virus that causes infectious mononucleosis. It has also been associated with a number of primary and reactivated diseases, such as Burkitt lymphoma (BL), nasopharyngeal carcinoma (NPC), posttransplant lymphoproliferative disease and X-linked lymphoproliferative disease.

EBV is difficult to recover from clinical samples, and that hampered the understanding of the relationship between viral excretion and possibly related diseases. The cumbersome cord blood lymphocyte immortalization bioassay, which has been used to detect the presence of the virus in clinical specimens (blood and saliva) requires 4–8 weeks of tissue culture and may favour detection of some strains of EBV over others. Usually, laboratory diagnosis of primary or reactivated EBV infections depends on a battery of serologic tests, the interpretation of which is rather difficult. This is particularly true for immunocompromised patients, in whom EBV serologic patterns are frequently modified, due to a T-cell deficiency to control the viral activity. A variety of EBV-coded antigens have previously been identified in EBV-infected cells, mainly through the use of immunofluorescence (IF) procedures. These antigens include viral capsid antigens (VCA), membrane antigens (MA), early antigens (EA) and nuclear antigens (EBNA). Initiation of the infectious productive cycle depends on the early expression of *trans*-acting factors (immediate-early or IE proteins), which include the protein ZEBRA (also known as EB1 or Zta, or BZLF1). This protein controls the switching of the viral cycle from latency to a productive cycle [1, 2] (for a review see [3]). EBV replication may be measured by the titration of anti-ZEBRA antibodies by different methods (i.e. ELISA test) [4]. Nevertheless, virological diagnosis of EBV infection needs for sensitive, specific and rapid techniques, readily applicable to a broad range of clinical specimens: The polymerase chain reaction (PCR) has been proposed to detect the presence of EBV DNA in blood [5–7], cerebrospinal fluid [8], and biopsy specimens [9].

J.L. Touraine et al. (eds.), Cancer in Transplantation. Prevention and Treatment, 201–207.

In order to find early markers for diagnosis of EBV-related diseases, we designed two tests: 1) The detection of circulating viral load by PCR after EBV DNA extraction from serum and 2) the quantification of anti-ZEBRA antibodies in serum, and we evaluate the diagnostic value in renal transplant recipients in a prospective study.

Patients and methods

288 sera from 84 patients (including 26 patients followed-up during > 100 days) after renal transplantation were screened for monoclonal Immunoglobulin (mIg) (C. Chapuis-Cellier, Lyon), serological markers of EBV infection (including anti-ZEBRA antibodies – see below) and EBV DNA. All patients were transplanted between from january 1993 and december 1993 at the Transplantation Unit, Hôpital E. Herriot, Lyon.

Standard laboratory diagnosis

Serologic diagnosis of EBV infection was performed by the standard methods: IgG antibodies to VCA and EA were determined by indirect immunofluorescence (IF) on antigen-producing P3HR-1 cells and TPA/butyrate-induced Raji cells, respectively. Antibodies against EBNA were determined by anticomplement IF (ACIF) on Raji cells. Reactivation of EBV infection is defined by the existence of elevated antibody titers to VCA IgG (> 1:320), EA (> 1:80), and the preexistence of anti-EBNA IgG antibodies (> 1:10).

Enzyme-linked immunoassay

Three antigen preparations were used for testing human sera in the ELISA test [10]: 1) Recombinant protein: rZEBRA recombinant protein (GST-ZEBRA from pGEXZ25 plasmid kindly supplied by Alain Sergeant, Lyon); 2) Two Synthetic peptides, named ZEBRAp125 (Aminoterminal region of the ZEBRA protein) and ZEBRAp130 (Carboxyterminal region of ZEBRA protein), were synthesized by Dr F. Troalen (Unité de Microchimie, Institut Gustave-Roussy, Villejuif, France).

ELISA test: One hundred μl (0.1 μg) of each peptide in coating buffer (50 mM carbonate buffer pH 9.6) was added to each well of a microtiter plate (MaxiSorp U16, Nunc, Denmark) and left to adsorb overnight at 37°C. After three washings in phosphate buffer saline pH 7.4, 0,1% Tween-20 (PBST), wells were incubated with 100 μl of serum samples diluted 1:100 in PBST with 5% fetal calf serum (PBSST) for 1 h at 37°C, followed by 3 vigorous washings in PBST. One hundred μl of peroxidase conjugated secondary antibodies at a dilution of 1:26;000 in PBST was added to each well, incubated for 30 min at 37°C, and then washed as described above.

After rinsing in water, the plate was developed in peroxidase substrate (0.5% tetramethylbenzidin, 0.05% hydrogen peroxide in citrate buffer pH 4) with 100 μl per well for 10 min at room temperature. The results were read by optical absorbance at 450 nm (A_{450}).

Detection of EBV DNA in serum samples

A quick alkaline lysis technique for extraction of DNA from serum sample was used [7]. 20 μl serum was mixed with 2 μl 1M NaOH and incubated at 37°C in a waterbath for 60 min, then neutralized with 2 μl 1M HCl. Flotation dialysis was then performed using 0.05 μm filters (Millipore, Bedford MA, USA) to eliminate salts. 10 μl of the preparation was used in a total volume of 100 μl in the PCR. Lysate aliquots (10 μl) from of each sample were subjected to DNA amplification in 100 μl reaction buffer, consisting of 50 mM KCl, 10 mM Tris HCl (pH 8.4), 1.5 mM MgCl2, 100 μg/ml gelatin, 200 μM of each deoxynucleotide triphoshate, 1 μM of each primer and 2.5 units of Taq DNA polymerase (Boehringer-Mannheim, Mannheim, Mannheim, Germany). A 186 bp DNA fragment located in the *Bam*HIW region was amplified, by using primers PER1 and PER2 framing the DNA sequence 5′ TTT GTC CCC ACG CGC GCA TA 3′ and 5′ AGG TGG CGT AGC AAC GCG AA 3′, respectively. PCR protocols and analysis of the PCR protocols were previously described in detail [7].

Results and discussion

Monoclonal immunoglobulins were found in 17/84 (20%) patients after allografting (Table 1) and no patient developed lymphoproliferative disease two years later. The positivity rate of Anti-rZEBRA IgG and IgM, Anti-ZEBRAp125 and Anti ZEBRAp130 IgGs and anti-ZEBRAp130 IgM were shown in Table 2: A high positivity rate of anti-rZEBRA IgG (77.4% and 70.6% in overall patients and in individuals with mIgs, respectively) must be noted. Interestingly, EBV viral load was detected by PCR in 27.4% and 23.5% of patients, respectively. Anti-ZEBRAp125 and Anti-ZEBRAp130 IgM were detected in 6/17 and 5/17 of patients with mIgs (35.3% and 29.5%), respectively. This positivity rate was higher than in non mIg-patients (12% and 19.4%, respectively). 26 transplanted patients (11 patients with mIgs and 15 without mIgs) were followed-up during a period of 100 days and more: 100% and 80% of patients had replication markers (anti-ZEBRA IgG and IgM), respectively. High anti-EA IgG titers were strongly correlated with high anti-ZEBRA absorbances ($A_{450} > 1.5$), and when an anti-EA increase was detected, anti-rZEBRA IgG and anti-ZEBRAp130 IgM were detectable 44 days and 60 days before increase of anti-EA IgG titers, respectively.

In the majority of cases (55.8%) and anti-rZEBRA IgG were detected just after transplantation (onset of follow-up) and this phenomenon

Table 1. Monoclonal immunoglobulins, anti-ZEBRA antibodies and EBV DNA in the sera from 17 patients with monoclonal gammapathy

Patient	Immunoglobulins (sera)	Time after transplantation	anti rZEBRA IgG	anti rZEBRA IgM	anti ZEBRA p125 IgG	anti ZEBRA p125 IgM	anti ZEBRA p130 IgG	anti ZEBRA p130 IgM	EBV ADN
1 (pM)	IgG κ	7 months	–	++	–	–	–	–	NT[a]
2 (zL)	IgG λ	3 months	–	–	–	–	–	–	+
3 (jlC)	IgG κ + IgG λ	4 months	+++	–	+++	–	–	–	–
4 (pC)	IgG κ + IgG λ	4 months	+++	–	+++	+	–	–	+ d28[b]
5 (lB)	IgG κ	1 month	–	–	–	–	–	++	+ d12
6 (cO)	IgM κ	6 weeks	+++	–	+	–	–	–	+
	IgG λ	9 weeks	+++						+
7 (aL)	–	3 weeks	++	–	++	–	–	–	0
	IgM κ	6 weeks	NT	NT	NT	NT	NT	NT	NT
8 (gA)	IgM	4 days	+++	–	–	+++	–	–	0
	IgG κ + IgG λ	2 months	NT	NT	NT	NT	NT	NT	NT
9 (gH)	IgM λ	3 weeks	++	–	–	++	–	++	0
	IgM + IgG λ	6 weeks	+++	–	+	++	–	+++	0
10 (lM)	IgG λ	1 month	–	–	–	++	–	–	+
11 (gV)	IgM (hmw[c])	8 weeks	++	–	–	+	–	++	0
	IgM hmw + IgG κ + IgG λ	11 weeks	NT	NT	NT	NT	NT	NT	NT
	IgM hmw	13 weeks	–	–	–	–	–	–	–
12 (mC)	IgG κ	11 weeks	+++	–	++	–	–	–	0
	IgG κ	17 weeks	NT	NT	NT	NT	NT	NT	NT
13 (jP)	IgM + IgG κ + IgG λ	17 days	++	–	++	–	–	–	0
14 (aPB)	–	5 weeks	++	–	+	–	–	–	0
	IgG κ + IgG λ	19 weeks	+++	++	++	–	–	–	0
15 (cZ)	–	5 weeks	+++	–	+++	–	–	–	0
	IgG κ + IgG λ	16 weeks	++	–	–	–	–	–	0
16 (mB)	–	6 weeks	–	–	–	–	–	++	0
	IgM κ + IgM λ	8 weeks	–	–	–	–	–	–	0
17 (cG)	IgG κ + IgGλ	11 weeks →	++	+	++	+++	–	+	0
		7 months	(6 weeks)	(6 weeks)	(6 weeks)	(6 weeks)	(6 weeks)	(6 weeks)	(6w)

+++ High antibody titers ($A_{450} > 1.5$); [a] NT = not tested; [b] d28 = day 28 post transplantation; [c] 5 w or 3 w = 5 weeks or 3 weeks; [d] hmw = high molecular weight.

Table 2. Positivity rate of anti-ZEBRA antibodies and EBV DNA in sera from the 84 transplant recipients, including the 17 patients with mIgs

	anti-rZEBRA IgG	anti-rZEBRA IgM	anti-ZEBRA p125 IgG	anti-ZEBRA p130 IgG	anti-ZEBRA p130 IgG	anti-ZEBRA p125 IgM	EBV DNA
Transplanted patients (n = 84)	65/84 (77.4%)	6/84 (7%)	44/84 (52.4%)	6/84 (7%)	25/84 (29.8%)	11184 (13%)	20/73 (27.4%)
Patients with monoclonal immuno-globulins (n = 17)	12/17 (70.6%)	3/17 (17.6%)	10/17 (58.8%)	1/17 (5.9%)	5/17 (29%)	6/17 (35.3%)	4/17 (23.5%)

Table 3. Precocity of anti-ZEBRA IgG and IgM in the follow-up of transplant recipients

	Detection after transplantation	Positivity rate at the onset of follow-up (day 0 posttransplantation)
anti-ZEBRAp125 IgG	4.52 days	44% of cases
anti-ZEBRAp125 IgM	13.2 days	30% of cases
anti-ZEBRAp130 IgM	15.4 days	30.4% of cases
anti-rZEBRA IgG	3.63 days	55.8% of cases
EBV DNA	27.85 days	5% of cases

Table 4. Correlation between the EBV replication activity and the appearance of monoclonal gammapathy

	Patients without monoclonal gammapathy	Patients with monoclonal gammapathy
High EBV replication activity[a]	7	11
Low or moderate EBV replication activity	6	3[b]

[a]Anti-ZEBRA IgG $A_{450} > 1.5$ (or presence of anti-ZEBRA IgM).
[b]2 serum samples EBV DNA+.

was also observed for anti-ZEBRAp130 IgM (30.4% positivity rate at the onset of follow-up). EBV DNA was detected on average 27.8 days post-transplantation (Table 3). When results were dichotomized in high replication activity (high titers of anti-ZEBRA antibodies with $A_{450} > 1.5$ and/or anti-ZEBRA IgM) and low/intermediate replication activity ($A_{450} < 1.5$ and/or without IgM), 61% of patients with mIg exhibited a high EBV replication activity, whereas a low/moderate EBV replication activity was present in 66.6% of patients without mIg (Table 4). EBV DNA was detected in two patients (with high hybridization score) with mIg and without high replication activity.

It was demonstrated that 40–50% of grafted patients exhibited restriction of immunoglobulin heterogeneity or monoclonal peak of serum immunoglobulin [11, 12], but the role of EBV was questionable. So we tried to find a correlation of replicating EBV (measured by the anti-ZEBRA antibodies), eventually the presence of EBV DNA, and the appearance of monoclonal gammapathy. In a previous report [7], we found that EBV DNA was detected in 73% and 68% of patients with AIDS-related non Hodgkin's lymphoma (ARNHL) and infectious mononucleosis, respectively, and that high EBV DNA levels in blood stream (> 20,000 EBV genome equivalents/10^4 leukocytes) were associated with the occurrence of ARNHL. The present study exhibits the high frequency of EBV replication after renal transplantation, as demonstrated the high positivity rate of anti-ZEBRA antibodies. When present, anti-ZEBRA antibodies (particularly anti ZEBRAp125 IgM or anti ZEBRAp130 IgM) are early markers of EBV reactivation. After transplantation, high replication activity (high anti-ZEBRA antibody titers, or anti-ZEBRA IgM) and in some cases EBV DNA, may select patients at risk for monoclonal gammapathy. In the future, quantitation of EBV DNA in blood (leukocyte or serum) might be a relevant marker of lymphoproliferative disorders in such patients [13]. The presence of homogeneous immunoglobulin in the serum may reflect the expansion of a B cell clone, which after proliferation and differentiation, produces monoclonal immunoglobulin. EBV (replicating) and probably other pathogens (Cytomegalovirus) might play a key role for mIg development. If so, is mIg a model of subversion of the immune system by pathogens?

References

1. Chevallier-Greco A, Manet E, Chavrier P, Mosnier C, Daillie J, Sergeant A. Both Epstein–Barr virus (EBV)-encoded transacting factors EB1 and EB2, are required to activate transcription from an EBV early promoter. EMBO J 1986; 5: 3243–3249.
2. Countryman J, Jenson H, Seibl R, Wolf H, Miller G. Polymorphic proteins encoded within BZLF1 of defective and standard Epstein–Barr viruses disrupt latency. J Virol 1987; 61: 3672–3679.
3. Miller G. The switch between latency and replication of Epstein–Barr virus. J Infect Dis 1990; 161: 833- 844.

4. Joab I, Triki H, De Saint-Martin J, Perricaudet M, Nicolas JC. Detection of anti Epstein–Barr virus trans-activator (ZEBRA) antibodies in sera from patients with human immunodeficiency virus. J Infect Dis 1991; 163: 53–56.
5. Savoie A, Perpête C, Carpentier L, Joncas J, Alfieri C. Direct correlation between the load of Epstein–Barr virus-infected lymphocytes in the peripheral blood of pediatric transplant patients and risk of lymphoproliferative disease. Blood 1994; 83: 2715–2722.
6. Crompton, CH, Cheung RK, Donjon C, Miyazaki I, Feinmesser R, Hébert D, Dosch HM.: Epstein–Barr virus surveillance after renal transplantation. Transplantation 1994; 57: 1182–1189.
7. Laroche C, Drouet E, Brousset P, Pain C, Boibieux A, Biron F, Icart J, Denoyel G, Niveleau A. Measurement by polymerase chain reaction of the Epstein–Barr virus load in infectious mononucleosis and AIDS-related non Hodgkin's lymphomas. J Med Virol 1995; 46: 66–74.
8. Cinque P, Brytting M, Vago L, Castagna A, Paravicini C, Zanchetta N, d'Arminio Monforte A, Wahren B, Lazzarin A, Linde A. Epstein–Barr virus DNA in cerebrospinal fluid from patients with AIDS-related primary lymphoma of the central nervous system. Lancet 1993; 342: 398–401.
9. Shibata D, Weiss LM, Nathwani BN, Brynes RK, Levine AM Epstein–Barr virus in benign lymph node biopsies from individuals infected with the human immunodeficiency virus is associated with concurrent or subsequent development of non-Hodgkin's lymphoma. Blood 1991; 77: 1527–1533.
10. Brousset P, Drouet E, Schlaifer D, Icart J, Payen C, Meggetto F, Marchou B, Massip B, Delsol G. Epstein–Barr virus (EBV) replicative gene expression in tumor cells of AIDS-related non Hodgkin's lymphoma in relation to CD4 cell number and antibody titers to EBV. AIDS 1994; 8: 583–590
11. Peest D, Schaper B, Nashan B, Wonigeit K, Raude E, Pichlmayr R, Haverich A, Deicher H. High incidence of monoclonal immunoglobulins in patients after liver or heart transplantation. Transplantation 1988; 389–393
12. Garnier JL, Berger F, Betuel H, Vuillaume M, Chapuis-Cellier C, Blanc N, Faure JL, Dubernard JM, Lenoir G, Touraine JL. Epstein–Barr virus associated lymphoproliferative diseases (B cell lymphoma) after transplantation. Nephrol Dial Transplant 1989; 4: 818–823.
13. Niveleau A, Drouet E, Reynaud C, Fares F, Bruno C, Pain C. Polymerase Chain Reaction products containing 5-methyldeoxycytidine: A microplate immunoquantitation method. Nucleic Acids Res 1994; 22: 5508–5509.

23. Lymphomas in the Scid/Hu mice: Effect of EBV on human B-cells in vivo

J.L. GARNIER, N. BLANC-BRUNAT, D. LAURIN, G. VIVIER, J.L. TOURAINE, A. SERGEANT, E. DROUET, M.J. GLENNIE & G.T. STEVENSON

Post-transplant Epstein–Barr Virus (EBV)-associated B-cell lymphomas still remain a serious complication that endangered the survival of the patient and the graft.

Human EBV-positive B-cell lymphomas that develop in the scid/Hu mice resemble the post-transplant lymphomas [1–4] and represent a suitable model to understand the pathogenesis of post-transplant lymphomas and to set up new non-immunosuppressive therapeutic strategies.

Material and methods

PBLs and EBV-B-cell lines: Human blood was obtained from healthy adult EBV-seronegative individuals or EBV-seropositive kidney transplant patients. Peripheral blood mononuclear leucocytes (PBLs) were separated over Ficoll-Hypaque gradients. EBV-immortalized B-cell lines (lymphoblastoid cell lines: LCL) were obtained by *in-vitro* infection of PBLs with B95-8 virus in the presence of cyclosporin 1 μg/ml. Cultures were maintained in RPMI containing antibiotics, glutamine, and 10% foetal calf serum.

Scid/hu chimeric mice: C.B.-17/scid mice were purchased from Iffa-Credo (Laboratoire des Oncins, L'Arbresle, France). They were tested for the absence of mouse immunoglobulins in the serum, and used when 6–8 weeks old. In two experiments, they received an intraperitoneal injection of 2×10^7 human PBLs from adult-EBV seronegative individuals followed by 400 μl of EBV B95-8 supernatant 7 days later. In two experiments, they received an intraperitoneal injection of 5×10^6 *in-vitro* EBV B95-8-immortalized B-cell lines.

Cell cultures: Lymphoblastoid cell lines were stimulated *in vitro* with cyclosporin (10 μg/ml) or the phorbol ester TPA (20 ng/ml) for 3 days. Akata

J.L. Touraine et al. (eds.), Cancer in Transplantation. Prevention and Treatment, 209–213.

cell lines were treated with anti-human IgG (Fab specific, Sigma Chemical Co.) 0.1 mg/ml for 16 h.

Treatment of mice with monoclonal antibodies: Anti-CD38 monoclonal antibodies were injected in the mice within five days after the injection of human cells. Mice received a sub-cutaneous or an intraperitoneal injection of 1 mg of mouse or human chimeric (human Fc_2, mouse Fab') monoclonal antibody.

Monoclonal antibodies and flow cytometry analysis: Cell suspension was taken from cultures or from collagenase-dispersed tumors. The following FITC-coupled monoclonal antibodies from Tenovus Laboratory were used: CD19 (clone RFB9), CD37 (clone WR17), CD38 (clone AT 13/5). Propidium iodide was added in the last incubation to gate out the dead cells.

Western Blot analysis for EBV-LMP expression: After extraction from cell cultures or tumors, proteins were separated by SDS-PAGE electrophoresis on 7.5% acrylamide Laemmli gels. After transfer, the nitrocellulose membrane was incubated with anti-LMP monoclonal antibody (Dako, Copenhagen, Denmark), and a secondary anti-mouse peroxydase labelled antibody (Sigma Chemical Co.). Detection was performed with the ECL method (Amersham International, Buckinghamshire, England).

Immunohistochemistry for EBV replication: Cytopsins of cultured cells or sections of frozen tissue from tumors were stained with monoclonal antibody to BZLF1 (Z125 recognizing aa 59-93), BRLF1 (5A recognizing aa 278–356) or to VCA (Viral Capsid Antigen, Virotech International, Rockville, MD, USA). Biotinylated anti mouse (Biosys, Vector, Burlingame, CA, USA), then streptavidin biotinylated horse radish peroxydase complex (Dako, Copenhagen, Denmark) were used to detect the fixation of antibody, which was revealed by the HRP substrate amino-ethyl carbazole (Dako, Copenhagen, Denmark).

Results

Scid/hu mice injected with the *in-vitro* derived LCL from PBLs of 3 kidney transplant patients developed intra-abdominal tumors within 40 days.

Phenotype analysis showed that LCL expressed CD19, CD37, and weakly CD38: tumor cells expressed CD19, had decreased CD37 and high CD38 expression.

LMP expression was strongly decreased in tumors.

Replication of EBV in the tumors was shown by the expression of BZLF1 (Zebra protein), and BCRF1 although VCA expression was weaker. LCL treated with cyclosporin or TPA displayed increased expression of Zebra and VCA, as did the control cells Akata treated with anti-immunoglobulins. Table 1.

Table 1. Immunohistochemistry analysis of EBV replication in tumors and LCL obtained from PBLs of transplanted patients (RT, GM, Bag)

Name	BZLF1	BRLF1	VCA
RT-LCL	±	–	–
RT-LCL (TPA)	+	–	–
RT-Tumor	+	–	–
GM-LCL	–	++	+
GM-LCL (TPA)	+	+++	++
GM-LCL (Cyclosporin)	++	+++	–
GM-Tumor	+	+	–
Bag-LCL	+	++	±
Bag-LCl (TPA)	++	++	++
Bag-LCL (Cyclosporin)	++	+++	++
Bag-Tumor	++	++	±
Akata	–	–	±
Akata (anti-immunoglobulins)	++	++	++

Anti-CD38 monoclonal antibodies were able to prevent the development of tumors in the Scid/Hu either reconstituted with normal human PBL (exp #1 and #2) or LCL (exp #3) (Table 2).

Discussion

Scid/Hu mice represent a good model to study the pathogenesis of post-transplant B-cell lymphomas [1–4].

By using lymphoblastoid cell lines from transplanted patients, we were able to get tumors in the mice. Those tumors present the same phenotype as the tumors that develop after the injection of PBLs from non-immunosuppressed patients [5, 6]: B-cell markers present a shift towards the late stages of B-cell differentiation, and EBV genome is closer to the type I of EBV latent gene expression observed in Burkitt's lymphomas than to the type III of EBV latent gene expression of LCLs. Early stages of EBV replication, assessed by the expression of Zebra protein (BZLF1), is demonstrated in tumors, whereas expression of the VCA late replicative protein is weak. *In vitro* induced replication of EBV in LCL from transplanted patients that have been treated with cyclosporin or TPA displays both early and late replicative protein expression in a full cycle of replication.

Table 2. Anti-CD 38 monoclonal antibody treatment in Scid/hu mice. In exp #2, 2 mice injected with the chimerized form of the antibody developed skin necrosis at the site of the injection

		Group 1 No antibody	Group 2 Chimeric MAb	Group 3 Mouse MAb
Number of mice		3	3	3
EXP #1 (PBL ip, MAb subcut.)	Tumor	2	2 (skin necrosis)	0
	Time (days)	32	43	
EXP #2 (PBL ip, MAb ip)	Tumor	3	0	1
	Time (days)	39		43
EXP #3 (LCL ip, MAb ip)	Tumor	3	0	0
	Time (days)	28		

Expression of CD38 seems to be critical in the expansion or transformation of tumor cells in vivo, since the treatment with anti-CD38 monoclonal antibodies is able to prevent the development of the lymphomas.

Acknowledgements

We acknowledge the help of G Panaye for flow cytometry with Facscan from Becton-Dickinson, San Jose, CA, USA.

This work was supported by grants from the Association pour la Recherche sur le Cancer, Villejuif, and the Région-Rhône Alpes, Lyon, France.

References

1. Mosier DE, Gulizia RJ, Baird SM, Wilson DB. Transfer of a functional human immune system to mice with severe combined immunodeficiency. Nature 1988; 335: 246–259.
2. Cannon MJ, Pisa P, Fox RI, Cooper NR. Epstein–Barr virus induces aggressive lymphoproliferative disorders of human B cell origin in SCID/hu mice. J Clin Invest 1990; 85: 1333-1337.

3. Mosier DE, Baird SM, Kirven MB, Gulizia RJ, Wilson DB, Kubayashi R, Picchio G, Garnier JL, Sullivan JL, Kipps TJ. EBV-associated B-cell lymphomas following transfer of human peripheral blood lymphocytes to mice with severe combined immunodeficiency. Curr Top Microbiol Immunol 1990; 166: 317–323.
4. Rowe M, Young LS, Crocker J, Stokes S, Henderson S, Rickinson AB. Epstein-Barr virus (EBV)-associated lymphoproliferative disease in the SCID mouse model: implications for the pathogenesis of EBV-positive lymphomas in man. J Exp Med 1991; 173: 147–158.
5. Rochford R, Hobbs MV, Garnier JL, Cooper NR, Cannon MJ. Plasmacytoid differentiation of Epstein-Barr Virus-transformed B cells in vivo is associated with reduced expression of viral latent genes. Proc Natl Acad Sci, USA 1993; 90: 352–356.
6. Garnier JL, Cooper NR, Cannon MJ. Low expression of CD20 and CD23 in Epstein-Barr Virus-induced B cell tumors cells in Scid/hu mice. Am J Pathol 1993; 142: 353–358.

PART SIX

Lymphoproliferative syndromes after transplantation

24. Types of lymphomas in transplant and other immunosuppressed patients

MARTINE RAPHAEL, SOPHIE CAMILLERI-BROET,
FRÉDERIC DAVI, ANTOINE MARTIN, SOPHIE PREVOT &
JEAN FEUILLARD

Lymphoproliferative disorders are the major neoplastic complications in acquired immunosuppressed patients after organ transplantation or HIV infection. Post transplantation lymphoproliferative disorders (PTLDs) affect approximately 2% of all organ recipients [1]. Non Hodgkin's lymphomas (NHL) arise at the time of the onset of acquired immunodeficiency syndrome (AIDS) in 3% of HIV infected patients and 10% of AIDS patients will develop a NHL [2].

PTLDs are generally Epstein–Barr virus (EBV)-driven lymphoid proliferations. In AIDS, different types of lymphomas are recognized and, their association with EBV varies according to the immune status of the patient, the site and the histology of the tumor [3].

The major characteristic of these tumors is their heterogeneity at different levels: clinical presentation, histology, immunophenotype, molecular alterations and EBV expression.

Diversity of post-transplantation lymphoproliferative disorders

The occurrence of PTLDs and the mode of presentation is different according to the nature of transplanted organ, the immunosuppressive regimen used and the age of the patient [1, 4, 5]. The interval between transplantation and the presentation of PTLPs varies widely from less than one month to several years. Post-transplant patients receiving cyclosporin A (CsA) or anti T-lymphocyte monoclonal antibodies could develop early PTLDs within one month of transplantation while in patients having immunosuppressed regimens with neither CsA nor anti-T-lymphocyte monoclonal antibodies PTLDs may occur months or even years after transplantation. The unusual anatomic distribution, especially in central nervous system, is one of the characteristics, however, the introduction of CsA and anti-T-lymphocyte monoclonal anti-

J.L. Touraine et al. (eds.), Cancer in Transplantation. Prevention and Treatment, 217–222.

body has changed not only the time of onset of PTLDs but also the clinical presentation [1] with the following differences: decrease in CNS localization, more frequent intestinal and lymph node involvement, more widespread disease with mononucleosis-like illness and frequent regression. Thus the wide spectrum of clinical presentations ranges from asymptomatic lymphadenopathy, infectious mononuclosis-like illness to one or more nodal or extra nodal tumors. Actually the nodal localization occur in half of cases, and the extra nodal localizations include the gastrointestinal tract, lung, kidney, genital tract and engrafted organ, and the central nervous system involvement occurs in patients with disseminated PTLDs [4, 5].

The wide spectrum of morphologic appearance is one of the main characteristics of PTLDs ranging from benign polymorphic aspect to monomorphic immunoblastic lymphoma. Lymph nodes involvement demonstrate a diffuse growth pattern with complete or partial architectural effacement. The cytologic features are polymorphic or monomorphic. The lesions are composed of small lymphocytes, large non-cleaved cells and a large proportion of immunoblasts showing plasmacytic differentiation. Atypical immunoblasts resembling Reed–Sternberg cells can be observed like in infectious mononucleosis lymph node lesions. Extensive areas of necrosis are common [4–6]. The principal morphologic classifications proposed to recognize polymorphic diffuse B-cell hyperplasia, polymorphic diffuse B-cell lymphoma and monomorphic proliferation aspects need additional analysis such as immunophenotypical, molecular and virological studies to characterize PTLDs and to predict clinical behavior [6, 7].

Immunophenotypic studies have shown that the vast majority of PTLDs are B-cells proliferations with variable expression of B-cell differentiation antigens. However, some T-cells CD4 or CD8 positive T-cell PTLDs have also been described [8]. Activation markers (CD23, CD30, CDw70 and CD39) are variously expressed on tumors cells as well as adhesion molecules (CD11a/CD18, CD54, CD58). The EBV is detected in nearly all cases of PTLDs, and proteins of EBV latency are expressed mostly in polymorphic cases where their expression is correlated with that of adhesion molecules. In about half cases immediate early replicative protein was detected but without any complete replicative cycle [9–11].

Some cases arising several years after transplantation are not associated with EBV and fitting the criteria of large cell/immunoblastic lymphomas of immunocompetent population [8].

The analysis of clonality with genetic studies using Southern blot technique for the immunoglobulin heavy and light chains genes and fused EBV genomic termini, demonstrate several patterns identifying various categories such as: nonclonal polymorphic, clonal polymorphic and clonal monomorphic tumors [6]. After reduced immunosuppression, nonclonal polymorphic tumors and some clonal polymorphic tumors have regressed. In some cases, these genotypic studies have demonstrated two or more distinct monoclonal populations or monoclonal and polyclonal proliferations at different tumors sites. The detection of structural alterations in proto-oncogenes and tumor suppressor genes compared with the clonality, the morphology and the clinical presentation allows the identification of three categories. The first one concerns a polyclonal plasmacytic hyperplasia arising in the oropharynx or lymph node containing multiple EBV infection events, lacking genes alterations and regressing after reduction of immunosuppression. The second one is found to be polymorphic hyperplasia or lymphoma arising in lymph node or extra nodal sites especially in lung and gastro-intestinal sites. These tumors are usually monoclonal without genetic alterations, and can regress following a reduction in immunosuppression or other therapeutical strategy such as monoclonal antibodies or chemotherapy. The third one corresponds to the morphologic criteria of immunoblastic lymphoma with plasmacytic features, with monoclonal genotypic pattern and presence of structural alterations of the c-myc, N-ras or p53 genes. Widely disseminated at the clinical presentation, these proliferations are refractory to reduction of immunosuppression, monoclonal antibodies treatment and chemotherapy [12].

All the studies highlight the polymorphism of these lymphoid proliferations, thus, the identification of different categories having clinical behaviour signification needs the comparison of clinical, morphologic and genotypic analysis.

Diversity of AIDS-related non Hodgkin's lymphomas

One of the most remarkable features of AIDS is the greatly increased incidence of NHL being 60 times more frequent than in the general population. Extra-nodal involvement and high grade of malignancy histologic subtype are the major characteristics. Some histological subtypes such as Burkitt's lymphoma (BL) or localizations such as central nervous system (CNS) are at least respectively 1000 times and 500 times more frequent than in the general population [2].

Nearly all cases are of the B-cell type belonging to high grade malignancy groups of lymphomas [13].

The most frequent extra-nodal initial sites of tumor are gastro-intestinal tract, CNS, bone marrow and oral cavity, but any site can be involved by NHL and multiple sites at presentation are also observed [14, 15].

In the large series of cases from the French Study Group of AIDS-related lymphoma, 5 histologic categories were identified [15]:

1. Small noncleaved-cell lymphoma (38% of cases) including two morphologic aspects, typical Burkitt's lymphoma and atypical Burkitt's lymphoma with plasmacytic features belonging to the provisional group so called "Burkitt like lymphoma" in the REAL classification of lymphomas.
2. Large noncleaved-cell lymphoma having the criteria of centroblastic lymphoma described in the Kiel classification (28% of cases).

3. Immunoblastic lymphoma with plasmacytic features (23% of cases).
4. Polymorphic lymphoproliferation showing the same morphologic features than in the PTLDs (6% of cases).
5. Anaplastic large cell lymphoma (4% of cases) reaching the same morphologic and immunophenotypic criteria than in the general population.

The comparison with localisations showed that in primary CNS nearly all cases are immunoblastic with plasmacytic differentiation. While in bone marrow most cases are typical Burkitt's lymphomas, Burkitt's like lymphomas are frequently observed in lymph nodes as well as in gastro-intestinal tract [14, 15].

Each of these NHL categories has different characteristics reflecting the complexity of these NHL developed in AIDS-patients.

Burkitt's and Burkitt's like lymphomas are defined by their morphologic criteria, the monoclonality, the classical translocation between c-myc and Immunoglobulins genes and can appear in patients without evidence of profound immunosuppression. Their association with EBV varies between 30 to 60% of cases and the genetic events involving c-myc oncogene but also the structural alterations of p53 gene are predominant in the pathogenesis of these lymphomas [16, 17].

Large cell and immunoblastic lymphomas with plasmacytic features especially in cases with CNS localisation, tend to be seen in the more profoundly immunocompromised patients. In predominantly immunoblastic lymphoma the high frequency of association with EBV is a major feature of these lymphomas, especially those of the immunoblastic type.

In CNS lymphomas, nearly all tumors are EBV positive [3]. The role of EBV in these tumors involves not only the production of cytokines but also the action of latent viral proteins and the targeting cellular genes such as bcl2. This was recently demonstrated in primary CNS lymphoma where a correlation between latent membrane protein (LMP1) and BCL2 expression was shown [18].

More recently unusual localisations of AIDS-related immunoblastic lymphomas so called body-cavity-based lymphoma from cavity effusion were characterized by their association with the novel Kaposi's sarcoma-associated, herpesvirus-like DNA sequences, suggesting additional factors in the complexity of the AIDS-related lymphomagenesis [19].

Cases of Hodgkin's disease which are rarely observed in post-transplant patients have been described in AIDS-patients. These cases are characterized by their clinical aggressiveness with visceral localizations such as liver and bone marrow. In a recent series of 36 cases tested for the presence of EBV, histopathological findings showed nodular sclerosis pattern in most cases (68%), mixed cellularity in 26% of cases and lymphoid depletion in 6%. The EBV was associated in all cases with the expression of LMP and the absence of EBNA2 [20]. The constant association with EBV and the fact that only

LMP 1 among the EBV encoded latent proteins is expressed is one of the major biologic features of AIDS-related Hodgkin's disease.

References

1. Penn I. The changing pattern of postransplant malignancies. Transplant Proc 1991; 23: 1101–1103.
2. Beral V, Peterman T, Berkelman R, Jaffe H. AIDS-associated non Hodgkin's lymphoma. Lancet 1991; 337: 805-809.
3. Hamilton-Dutoit SJ, Raphaël M, Audouin J et al. *In situ* demonstration of Epstein–Barr virus small RNAs (EBER 1) in acquired immunodeficiency syndrome-related lymphomas: correlation with tumor morphology and primary site. Blood 1993; 82: 619–624.
4. Craig FE, Gulley ML, Banks P. Posttransplantation lymphoproliferative disorders. Am J Clin Pathol 1993; 99: 265–276.
5. Swerdlow SH. Post-transplant lymphoproliferative disorders: a morphologic phenotypic and genotypic spectrum of disease. Histopathology 1992; 20: 373–385.
6. Locker J, Nalesnik M. Molecular genetic analysis of lymphoid tumors arising after transplantation. Am J Pathol 1989; 135: 977–987.
7. Frizzera G, Hanto DW, Galj-Peczalska KJ et al. Polymorphic diffuse B-cell hyperplasia and lymphomas in renal transplant recipients. Cancer Res 1981; 41: 4262–4271.
8. Leblond V, Sutton L, Dorent R et al. Lymphoproliferative disorders after organ transplantation: a report of 24 cases observed in a single center. J Clin Oncol 1995; 13: 961–968.
9. Thomas JA, Hochin NA, Allday MJ et al. Immunohistology of Epstein–Barr-associated antigens in B-cell disorders from immunocompromised individuals. Transplantation 1990; 49: 944–953.
10. Young L, Alfieri C, Hennessy K et al. Expression of Epstein–Barr virus transformation-associated genes in tissues of patients with EBV lymphoproliferative disease. N Engl J Med 1989; 321: 1080–1085.
11. Rea D, Fourcade C, Leblond V et al. Patterns of Epstein–Barr virus latent and replicative gene expression in Epstein–Barr virus-B-cell lymphoproliferative disorders after organ transplantation. Transplantation 1994; 58: 317-324.
12. Knowles D. Post-transplantation lymphoproliferative disorders. Am J Surg Pathol 1994; 18(2): 208–210.
13. Raphaël M, Audouin J, Lamine M et al. Immunophenotypic and genotypic analysis of acquired immunodeficiency syndrome-related non-Hodgkin's lymphomas. Am J Clin Pathol 1994; 101: 773-782.
14. Raphaël M, Genthilomme O, Tulliez M, Bryon PA, Diebold J and the French Study Group of Pathology for HIV-associated Tumors. Histopathologic features of high grade non-Hodgkin's lymphomas in acquired immunodeficiency syndrome. Arch Pathol Lab med 1991; 115: 15–20.
15. Raphaël M, Audouin J, Tulliez M et al. Anatomic and histologic distribution of 448 cases of AIDS-related non Hodgkin's lymphomas. Blood 1993; 82: 56a.
16. Delecluse HJ, Raphaël M, Magaud JP et al. Variable morphology of human immunodeficiency virus-associated lymphomas with the c-myc rearrangements. Blood 1993; 82: 552–563.
17. Ballerini P, Gaidano G, Gong JZ et al. Multiple genetic lesions in acquired immunodeficiency syndrome-related nonHodgkin's lymphoma. Blood 1993; 81: 166–173.
18. Camilleri-Broët S, Davi F, Feuillard J, Bourgeois C, Seilhan D, Hauw JJ, Raphaël M. High expression of latent membrane protein 1 (LMP1) of Epstein–Barr virus and bcl2 oncoprotein in AIDS-related primary brain lymphomas. Blood 1995 (in press).

19. Cesarman E, Chang Y, Moore P, Said JW, Knowles D. Kaposi's sarcoma-associated herpes virus-like DNA sequences in AIDS-related body-cavity-based lymphomas. N Engl J Med 1995; 332: 1186-1191.
20. Prevot S, Audouin J, Raphaël M, Le Charpentier Y, Michiels JF, Diebold J. Association of HIV1-related hodgkin's disease with Epstein–Barr Virus. Cold Spring Harbor Meeting on Cancer Cells. Epstein–Barr virus and Associated Diseases 1994 Sept 7–11.

25. Production and role of cytokines in lymphoproliferations of immune deficiency

D. EMILIE

In order to understand the role of cytokines in the growth of lymphoid malignancies developing in patients with immune deficiency, either related to transplantation or HIV infection, we analyzed in such cases the production of cytokines with potential B lymphocyte stimulating properties. The cytokines studied were mainly IL-13, IL-10 and IL-6. Their production was analyzed combining several methodological approaches: RT-PCR, *in situ* hybridization and/or immunochemistry. This study was usually performed on frozen malignant tissues. In some instances, cell lines or freshly isolated malignant B cells were studied.

Production of IL-13 in B lymphoid malignancies

We studied IL-13 gene expression by RT-PCR in 26 B lymphoid malignancies, 6 of which were from HIV-infected patients (coll: M. Raphael) [1]. IL-13 gene expression was detected in most cases (16 of 26, including 6 of 6 AIDS lymphomas). We could show that malignant B lymphocytes themselves contributed to this IL-13 gene expression, as fresh and highly purified malignant B cells isolated from 2 Burkitt's lymphomas (one of which was from an HIV-infected patient) expressed the gene. This finding was confirmed by the positivity for IL-13 gene expression by several B cell lines, including 6 EBV-infected, 7 Burkitt lymphoid cell lines (2 of which from HIV-infected patients) and 2 cell lines from SIV-infected macaques with a lymphoma.

We then tested whether such an autocrine production of IL-13 could contribute to the autonomous growth of malignant cells. Neither IL-13 nor anti-IL-13 antibodies affected the *in vitro* growth of the cell lines (one Burkitt cell line and one derived from SIV-infected monkeys). Moreover, we detected no binding of radiolabelled IL-13 on the cell lines in an assay able to detect 25 binding sites per cell, indicating that such malignant B cells may not express functional IL-13 receptors. It remains to be determined whether IL-13 production by malignant cells alters the growth of lymphoproliferations by modulating the anti-tumoral immune response.

J.L. Touraine et al. (eds.), Cancer in Transplantation. Prevention and Treatment, 223–228.

IL-10 production in lymphoproliferations from patients with immune deficiency

We also studied IL-10 production in malignancies from patients with immune deficiency. Two conditions were considered.

In transplanted patients with lymphoproliferative diseases (coll: A. Durandy, M. Peuchmaur), no IL-10 gene expression was detected by *in situ* hybridization in frozen tissues, and results from immunochemical experiments were questionable. Although these experiments did not rule out an IL-10 production, they indicated that the level of IL-10 production by such tumors may be limited. However, RT-PCR analysis of either fresh tumors or cell lines derived from the patients consistently showed an amplified band for IL-10.

In HIV-infected patients (coll: M. Raphael), very high amounts of IL-10 were detected in approximately half of the tumors, both by *in situ* hybridization and by immunochemistry [2, 3]. Malignant B lymphocytes were responsible for this production. This dramatic production significantly correlated with the presence of the EBV genome in the tumor. Human IL-10 but not viral IL-10 accounted for this production. Therefore, a strong upregulation of IL-10 production in malignant cells occurs when these latter contain the EBV genome and emerge in an HIV-infected patient. Similar results were observed by studying IL-10 production by B cell lines, showing that Burkitt cell lines derived from HIV-infected patients and containing the EBV genome produce very large amounts of IL-10 [4]. Similar results were also obtained when studying lymphomas developing in SIV-infected monkeys, and in which a simian EBV homologue is present in malignant cells (coll: P. Biberfeld). In this case, malignant cells also contain IL-10, as assessed by either *in situ* hybridization or immunochemistry (unpublished results).

We next asked whether IL-10 contributed to the growth of malignant cells in AIDS lymphomas. The *in vitro* addition of a neutralizing anti-IL-10 antibody did not affect the spontaneous proliferation of the cell lines. More importantly, the same antibody did not affect the *in vivo* growth of the tumor: when cell lines derived from SIV-infected monkeys were injected intraperitoneally or subcutaneously to SCID mice, a tumor developed: the survival of mice was not improved by treating them with an anti-IL-10 mAb. In these experiments, we used the same protocol of treatment and the same antibody as those we used successfully to modulate the function of non malignant B cells in the SCID mice model [5]. Although IL-10 may theoretically stimulate the growth of malignant cells or may decrease the anti-tumoral immune response, our findings question the role of autocrine production of IL-10 in the behaviour of AIDS lymphomas.

Cytotoxic cell activation in AIDS lymphomas

In order to test whether the immune deficiency of AIDS affects the emergence and activation of cytotoxic cells in the tumor, we monitored by *in situ* hybridization the expression of the perforin and of the granzyme B gene, 2 genes coding for enzymes contained in the granules of cytotoxic cells and involved in the lysis of target cells, as shown by the decreased ability of cytotoxic cells from mice with a deletion of either gene to kill target cells. The transcription of both genes is induced upon cytotoxic cell activation. We previously showed that both genes are expressed in lymphoid malignancies emerging in patients without immune deficiency [6].

Unexpectedly, we observed an expression of either gene in AIDS lymphomas, and which did not differ when compared to matched lymphomas from HIV-uninfected patients (coll: M. Raphael). In the same line, the density of activated cytotoxic cells in the tumor was not dependent on the CD4+ cell counts of the patients [7]. Although these results do not allow to conclude whether such cells efficiently fight malignant cells in case of immune deficiency, they nevertheless indicate that cytotoxic cells are present in such tumors and that they are still able to be activated. This finding may have important therapeutic consequences, as it may be possible to potentiate the function of such intratumoral cytotoxic cells by administrating immunostimulating drugs to the patient. A clinical trial (ANRS W045) testing the efficacy of IL-12 in AIDS lymphomas is expected to start in the fall.

IL-6 production and role in lymphoproliferative disorders from transplanted patients

In a collaborative work with the group of A. Fisher and A. Durandy, we showed that in lymphoproliferative disorders from transplanted patients malignant B cells produce IL-6, as do cell lines derived from the patients. This was shown by both RT-PCR and *in situ* hybridization [8]. In this case, we could formally demonstrate that this autocrine production plays a role in the growth of the tumor: when the cell lines are injected to SCID mice, administration of a neutralizing anti-IL-6 antibody delays or even prevent the death of the mice [8]. This observation strongly suggests that neutralizing IL-6 in lymphoproliferative disorders developing in transplanted patients may be curative.

IL-6 production in AIDS lymphomas

We studied IL-6 production in AIDS lymphomas by both *in situ* hybridization and immunochemistry (coll: M. Raphael) [9]. We observed IL-6 gene expression in all cases, but at a variable level. In Burkitt's lymphomas and monomorphic large cell lymphomas, the level of IL-6 gene expression was similar to that observed in follicular hyperplasia from HIV-infected patients. In contrast, the IL-6 gene was expressed at a approximately 100 times higher level in polymorphic large cell lymphomas (containing some immunoblasts) and in immunoblastic lymphomas. IL-6 did not arise from malignant cells, but from stromal cells, either endothelial cells or tumor-infiltrating macrophages. The pattern and the level of expression was similar in lymphomas from HIV-uninfected patients, and it was not dependent on the presence of EBV in malignant cells. Finally, we showed that malignant cells express the p80 chain of the IL-6 receptor. Therefore, these findings show that IL-6 is produced in a paracrine fashion in AIDS lymphomas, and at a high level in the pathological forms containing malignant immunoblasts. These findings are reminiscent of those described in multiple myeloma, indicating that a high production of IL-6 by stromal cells in B lymphoid malignancies is restricted to the pathological forms containing the more differentiated malignant cells. Stimulation of the IL-6 production by the stroma may actually be a property of differentiated B cells, whether malignant or not, and it may involve interactions between adhesion molecules such as VLA-4 expressed by differentiated B cells and VCAM-1 exopressed by the stroma.

Role of IL-6 in AIDS lymphomas

In view of the poor prognosis of AIDS immunoblastic lymphomas, specially in patients at a late stage of the infectious disease, and of the putative role of IL-6 in the growth of malignant cells, we initiated a clinical trial (ANRS 018) (coll: J. Wijdenes) in which was tested the effect of the administration of an anti-IL-6 mAb in such patients [10]. Eleven patients received a 3 week course of mAb (one I.V. injection of 20–80 mg each day).

In half of the patients, the growth of the tumor was unaffected. In 5 other patients, the lymphoma stopped to grow but did not regress. In one additional patient, a partial remission was achieved. When a beneficial effect was obtained, one or 2 additional courses of the mAb allowed a control of the tumor for 8 to 28 weeks, after which a relapse insensitive to the mAb occurred. Therefore, the growth of malignant cells in AIDS immunoblastic lymphomas is partly IL-6 dependent. A synergistic effect of the anti-IL-6 mAb and of chemotherapies in inducing apoptosis of malignant cells is an attracting hypothesis, as shown recently for multiple myeloma, indicating that anti-IL-6 mAb administration may potentiate results obtained with chemotherapies. Survival advantage induced by so-called "growth factors" may actually be as important than their growth promoting activity to explain their *in vivo* effects on malignant cells.

A clear effect on lymphoma-associated systemic manifestations was observed in AIDS lymphoma patients treated with the anti-IL-6 mAb, as shown by a complete disappearance of fever, acute phase reaction and cachexia [10]. Average weight gain in the 11 patients was 1.5 kg in 3 weeks, accompanied by an increased appetite and an improved well-being. Therefore, B clinical manifestations of AIDS lymphomas (and certainly of immunoblastic lymphomas from HIV-uninfected patients as well) are mediated by IL-6.

Conclusion

Therefore, a conjunction of autocrine (for IL-13 and IL-10, and for IL-6 in transplanted patients) and paracrine (for IL-6 in AIDS lymphomas) production of cytokines occurs in lymphoproliferations of patients with immune deficiencies. Whereas the putative role of the cytokines on the growth of the tumor and on anti-tumoral immune defenses remains to be established for IL-13 and IL-10, IL-6 is clearly involved in the growth of malignant cells in patients with immune deficiencies. It is likely that this effect is more complete in transplanted patients than in AIDS lymphomas. Clinical trials performed with an anti-IL-6 mAb in transplanted patients with a LPD should solve this issue. This difference may be explained by the usual involvement of oncogene alterations in AIDS lymphomas but not in LPD from transplanted patients. Therefore, manipulation of the cytokine network, either to starve malignant cells from growth or survival factors or to stimulate the *in situ* anti-tumoral immune response, may represent a new therapeutical approach synergyzing with present chemotherapies and/or substituting for them in case of drug resistance.

References

1. Fior R, Vita N, Raphael M, Minty A, Maillot MC, Crevon MC, Caput D, Biberfeld P, Ferrara P, Galanaud P, Emilie D. Interleukin-13 gene expression by malignant and EBV-transformed human B lymphocytes. Eur Cytok Netw, 1995; 5: 593–600.
2. Emilie D, Touitou R, Raphael M, Peuchmaur M, Devergne O, Rea D, Coumbaras J, Crevon MC, Edelman L, Joab I, Galanaud P. *In vivo* production of IL-10 by malignant cells in AIDS lymphomas. Eur J Immunol , 1992; 22: 2937–2942.
3. Emilie D, Galanaud P, Raphael M, Joab I. IL-10 production in AIDS lymphomas. Blood 1993; 81: 1106–1107.
4. Benjamin D, Knobloch TJ, Dayton MA. Human B-cell interleukin-10: B-cell lines derived from patients with AIDS and Burkitt's lymphoma constitutively secrete large quantities of interleukin-10. Blood 1992; 80: 1289–1297.
5. Llorente L, Zou W, Levy Y, Richaud-Patin Y, Wijdenes J, Alcocer-Varela J, Morel-Fourrier B, Brouet JC, Alarcon-Segovia D, Galanaud P, Emilie D. Role of Interleukin-10 in the B lymphocyte hyperactivity and autoantibody production of human systemic lupus erythematosus. J Exp Med 1995; 181: 839–844.
6. Leger-Ravet MB, Devergne O, Peuchmaur M, Solal-Celigny P, Brousse N, Gaulard P, Galanaud P, Emilie D. *In situ* detection of activated cytotoxic cells in follicular lymphomas. Am J Pathol 1994; 144: 492–499.

7. Devergne O, Raphael M, Autran B, Leger-Ravet MB, Coumbaras J, Crevon MC, Galanaud P, Emilie D. Intratumoral activation of CD8+ cytotoxic lymphocytes in AIDS lymphomas. Hum Pathol 1995; 26: 284–290.
8. Durandy A, Emilie D, Peuchmaur M, Forveille M, Clement C, Wijdenes J, Fischer A. Role of IL-6 in promoting growth of human EBV-induced B-cell tumors in SCID mice. J Immunol 1994; 152: 5361–5367.
9. Emilie D, Coumbaras J, Raphael M, Devergne O, Delecluse HJ, Gisselbrecht C, Michiels JF, Van Damme J, Taga T, Kishimoto T, Crevon MC, Galanaud P. IL-6 production in high grade B lymphomas: correlation with the presence of immunoblasts in AIDS and HIV-unrelated lymphomas. Blood 1992; 80: 498–504.
10. Emilie D, Wijdenes J, Gisselbrecht C, Jarrousse B, Billaud E, Blay JY, Gabarre J, Gaillard JP, Brochier J, Raphael M, Boue F, Galanaud P. Administration of an anti-interleukin-6 monoclonal antibody to patients with acquired immunodeficiency syndrome and lymphoma: effect on lymphoma growth and on B clinical symptoms. Blood 1994; 84: 2472–2479.

26. Interleukin 10 and non Hodgkin's lymphomas

N. VOORZANGER & J.-Y. BLAY

Introduction

Interleukin 10 (IL-10) is a pleiotropic cytokine which plays a central role in several physiological and pathological processes, in particular in infectious diseases and cancer. IL-10 was initially described in three different reports, as cytokine synthesis inhibitory factor (CSIF) which inhibits the production of Th1 derived cytokine [1, 2], as a thymocyte growth factor produced by B lymphoma cells [3] and as a mast cell growth factor [4]. IL-10 regulates the survival, proliferation and differentiation of T, B lymphocytes and monocyte macrophages, and modulates bone formation and erythropoiesis.

In the recent years, several reports have shown that IL-10 may play an important role in the physiopathology of non Hodgkin's lymphomas (NHL) of immunocompromised patients as well as in NHL of patients with no known cause of immunosuppression.

Here, we will review the immunological properties of IL-10 and discuss the possible role of IL-10 in the physiopathology of NHL in man.

Interleukin 10: a cytokine with multiple biological properties

Human IL-10 is a polypeptide of 18.647 kD which comprises 160 amino acids in its mature form, after cleavage of a 18 aminoacid signal peptide [2]. Human IL-10 is unglycosylated and exists as a homodimer *in vivo* [5]. A receptor for hIL-10 (IL-10R) was recently cloned [5–7]. This IL-10R has a molecular weight of 90–100 kD and belongs to the interferon receptor family [6, 7]. Human IL-10 is produced by a large variety of cells including activated monocytes, macrophages, normal and transformed B cells, B NHL fresh tumor cells and cell lines, activated T cells and T cell clones of the Th0, Th1 and Th2 phenotype, keratinocytes, melanoma and carcinoma cell lines.

J.L. Touraine et al. (eds.), Cancer in Transplantation. Prevention and Treatment, 229–241.

There is an important structural homology between hIL-10 and an open reading frame of EBV genome termed BCRF1 [2, 9]. The BCRF1 gene product, also termed vIL-10, share a 84% homology of sequence at the protein level and expresses most but not all properties of hIL-10 [9]. vIL-10 has CSIF activity, induces macrophage deactivation, blocks super oxide anion production by macrophages and modulates B cell growth similarly to hIL-10 [9, 10]. The specific activity of vIL-10 is however 3 to 10 fold lower than hIL-10 on human cells; vIL-10 does not enhance class II MHC expression on mouse B cells, does not stimulate thymocyte and mastocyte growth [8]. Actually, vIL-10 has been reported to not compete effectively for IL-10 binding to rIL-10 [7]. This suggest that vIL-10 may bind to other not reported IL-10 receptors yet not reported. The vIL-10 gene was possibly captured by EBV during evolution and its expression may give a selective advantage to the virus.

IL-10: a cytokine with immunosuppressive and B cell growth factor activities in vitro

IL-10 exerts a potent down-regulatory activity of monocyte macrophage function. IL-10 down regulates MHC class II expression induced by IFNg, IL-4 and IL-13 on monocytes [10, 11]. IL-10 also inhibits the expression of ICAM-1 (CD54), B7 (CD80) and B70 (CD86) on monocytes and ma crophages [12–14]. These biological activities of IL-10 result in a reduction of the APC function of these cells and play a major role in the inhibitory effect of IL-10 on the antigen-specific activation of T lymphocytes [10].

In addition, IL-10 inhibits the production of a large number of cytokines by LPS activated monocytes, in particular proinflammatory cytokines: IL-1a, IL-1b, IL-6, IL-8, MIP1a, TNF, G-CSF, M-CSF, GMCSF, IL-12 [15–18]. NO production by monocytes stimulated by LPS or IFNg is also significantly reduced by hIL-10, in part through an inhibition of TNF production [19–22]. All these properties result in a reduction of the microbicidal activity of monocyte macrophage [20, 21].

IL-10 is normally produced by activated human monocytes, although the maximal mRNA expression occurs later than proinflammatory cytokines [15]. IL-10 production by monocytes is in part induced by TNF and exerts an autoregulatory negative feedback on activated monocytes [15].

In addition, IL-10 induces the production of antagonists of IL-1 and TNF, i.e. IL-1ra, p55 and p75 TNF-R, by activated monocytes [22]. These observations, together with the general inhibition of proinflammatory cytokine production, indicate that IL-10 is a potent anti-inflammatory agent. The *in vivo* observations in mice defective for IL-10 as well as the protective effect of IL-10 on death from endotoxinemia indicate that these antiinflammatory properties play an important role *in vivo* [23, 24]. In man, the high serum IL-10 concentrations observed in patients with septic shock is also in agreement with these observations [25].

hIL-10 exerts also exerts an inhibitory effect on T cell function. In contrast to the mouse model, both Th1, Th2 cells are able to produce hIL-10 as well as CD8+ cells in man [26, 27]. Tumor samples of TNHL produce IL-10 in vitro and *in vivo* [28, N. Voorzanger, unpublished results]. Although IL-10 exerts most of its inhibitory effects on T cells indirectly, via the inhibition of monocyte macrophage activation, it also modulates directly T cell function and proliferation [29, 30]. In man, hIL-10 partially inhibits the proliferation of T cell clones of the Th0, Th1, Th2 phenotype and normal resting T cells induced by cross linking of anti CD2 and CD3 or PHA, in part through an inhibition of IL-2 production [29, 30]. Although IL-10 down regulates both T cell activation and proliferation, it inhibits the apoptosis of activated T cells and T cell clones induced by the deprivation of IL-2 [31]. Finally, IL-10 has chemotactive activity on human peripheral blood CD8+ T cells but not CD4+ T cells [32].

The inhibitory effect of hIL-10 on monocyte-macrophages and T cell function contrasts with its properties on B cells. mIL-10 increases MHC class II expression of splenic B cells [33]. hIL-10 is a potent stimulator of B cell growth and differentiation [33–38]. In mice, IL-10 enhances the survival of splenic B lymphocytes and this effect is associated with an induction of the expression of bcl-2 [34]. IL-10 stimulates DNA synthesis of naive B cell, germinal center B cells and memory B cells [35, 36]. In particular, it increases the proliferation of mature B lymphocytes costimulated with SAC or anti-CD40 Ab, in synergy with IL-4 and IL-2, as well as the proliferation of B cells induced by EBV infection [36, 37]. hIL-10 is produced by B cell during EBV infection and increases the proliferation of B cells through an autocrine/paracrine loop [37, 38]. In contrast, hIL-10 has been reported to specifically decrease the viability and induce apoptosis of B-CLL, whereas the viability of B NHL cells and myeloma cells was not affected [39]. IL-10 is also a potent stimulator of B cell differentiation. IL-10 is a switch factor which induces IgG1–3, IgA and IgM production by naive B cells costimulated with immobilized CD40 [40]. It is also a inducer of IgG1–3, IgA and IgM , but not IgG4 nor IgE, production by already committed B cells [35].

Therefore, IL-10 exert immunosuppressive and antiinflammatory activity on monocyte macrophage function and both indirectly and directly on T lymphocyte differentiation and proliferation *in vitro*. hIL-10 is a survival factor for both B and T lymphocyte, monocyte macrophages and is a potent growth and differentiation factor for B lymphocytes. The potent down regulating activity of IL-10 towards specific and non specific immune responses was confirmed by observations *in vivo* in animals and in man.

Immunosuppressive and anti-inflammatory activities of IL-10 in vivo

Transgenic IL-10-deficient mice have been created and express a characteristic phenotype: these mice develop a wasting syndrome due to chronic inflammatory enterocolitis [23]. IL-10 deficient mice are characterised by an exaggerated production of proinflammatory cytokines in intestinal tissue by macrophages; the administration of IL-10 reduces the incidence and severity of the enterocolitis in this model [23]. This model shows that IL-10 plays a physiological antiinflammatory role *in vivo* in mice.

Observations of experimental infections in animals and clinical observations indicate that IL-10 exerts immunosuppressive and/or antiinflammatory activity *in vivo* in pathological situations. In a mouse model of septic shock due to the administration of endotoxin, the administration of IL-10 prior to LPS reduced LPS-induced TNF production, hypothermia and lethality [24]; this indicates that the anti-inflammatory effect of IL-10 protects the mice from the lethality of LPS challenge. The same group has reported that high levels of IL-10 are detectable *in vivo* in man with septic shock, and that serum IL-10 may be involved in the control of the inflammatory response due to bacterial products [25].

Although these *in vivo* properties of IL-10 could be beneficial, endogenous IL-10 production may play a detrimental role in several infectious disease through an inhibition of an adequate T cell response.

In human leishmaniasis, IL-10 plays a key role in inhibiting T cell proliferation and IFNg production and probably contributes to dissemination of the disease [41, 42].

In the lepromatous form of leprosy, characterised by a disseminated disease with inadequate T cell response, a majority of T cell clones from skin lesions express a Th2 phenotype and produce IL-10 and IL-4. M.leprae directly induces the production of IL-10 by monocyte-macrophages, which inhibits PBMC response, proliferation and cytokine (TNF, IFNg) production and therefore probably contributes to the inadequate host response against mycobacteria [43, 44]. Asymptomatic patients with HIV infection overexpress IL-10 mRNA and protein either spontaneously and after stimulation [45]; the incubation of PBMC with an anti-IL-10 Ab improves the proliferative response of PBMC to different stimuli indicating that endogenous IL-10 is involved in the defective cellular immune responses of these patients [45].

Taken together, these observations clearly indicate that IL-10 exerts immunosuppressive properties *in vivo* in pathological situations and that the level of IL-10 production may influence the clinical presentation and outcome of several infectious diseases.

An *in vivo* immunosuppressive role of hIL-10 has also been documented in man, in patients receiving allogeneic graft. In SCID patients transplanted with allogeneic stem cells, a recent report has demonstrated that tolerance was associated with high levels of production of IL-10 by unstimulated PBMC and alloreactive T cell clones, suggesting an immunosuppressive role of IL-10 *in vivo* in these patients [46].

Production of IL-10 in cancer

The production of hIL-10 is not restricted to cells of the immune system and IL-10 could exert an immunosuppressive role in several tumor types. Several different tumor types have been reported to produce IL-10: in NHL occurring in immunosuppressed and immunocompetent patients [47, 48], colon carcinoma [49], ovarian cancer [50], basal cell carcinoma [51], bronchogenic carcinoma [52], glioblastoma [53], melanoma [54, 55], renal cell carcinomas cell lines [49], neuroblastoma [49]. In ovarian carcinoma, IL-10 and IFNg mRNA production was found exclusively in malignant tissue and not in normal ovaries [49]. IL-10 mRNA expression, and that of other Th2 cytokines, IL-4 and IL-5, were found significantly superior in the malignant basal cell carcinoma lesion as compared to that observed in benign skin lesions [51].

The production of IL-10 does not occur only locally in patients with cancer. Increased serum IL-10 levels have been observed in patients with NHL [47, 48], in multiple myeloma [56], in the ascite and serum of patients with ovarian cancer [57], in patients with malignant melanoma [55]. There is therefore a massive production of IL-10 in several tumor types *in vivo* in patients with cancer. The possible roles of this cytokine in the physiopathology of cancer is discussed under.

Production of IL-10 by non Hodgkin's lymphoma cells in vivo and in vitro

An early report has demonstrated the production of IL-10 by murine B lymphoma cell lines [3]. The possibility that IL-10 may act as an autocrine growth factor for malignant B lymphomas in man was therefore investigated. Emilie et al have studied h-vIL-10 expression in tumor samples of 15 HIV positive lymphomas using in situ hybridization and immunohistochemical staining. h-vIL-10 was found detectable in 8 samples, more than 50% of tumor cells produced IL-10 in most positive samples. vIL-10 was detectable in only 3 of IL-10 positive samples and in minority of cells indicating that the IL-10 detected was hIL-10 in most cases. No correlation was found with histological subtype. h-vIL-10 expression was found highly correlated to the presence of EBV in tumor cells. Of note, none of the 11 non HIV NHL, including 7 cases from transplanted patients were found to produce IL-10 in this study [47].

Several studies have demonstrated the production of hIL-10 by human B cell lines and its relation to the presence of EBV. Burdin et al have shown a constitutive hIL-10 production in medium by ELISA in 25 of the 36 tested mature B cell lines, among which 24 were EBV positive [37]. Benjamin et al have investigated 21 NHL cell lines and 7 normal lymphoblastoid cell lines for IL-10 production [60]. A constitutive hIL-10 production, was observed in all 6 AIDS related BL cell lines and in 6 of the 15 non AIDS with Northern blot analysis. Using RT PCR all 21 EBV positive cell lines were found to have detectable hIL-10 compared to 1 of the 7 EBV negative cell lines. In two other studies, hIL-10 expression in B NHL cell lines was also found highly correlated to EBV status, although a significant number EBV negative cell lines also produced spontaneously IL-10 [61, 62]. In two studies, hIL-10 expression was found correlated to the differentiation status of B NHL cell lines, with a lack of expression in pro-B and pre-B cells lines as well as in myeloma cell lines [37, 61].

We had initially reported that serum IL-10 was detectable in patients with active NHL a no known cause of immunosuppression and correlated to the disease status [56]. The detection of circulating IL-10 in these patients was confirmed latter by 2 different studies which also reported a correlation with disease status for both of them and a correlation with response to treatment and outcome in one [57, 62]. In view of our initial results, IL-10 expression was investigated in the NHL tumor samples of a series of 42 patients with no known cause of immunosuppression. Using immunohistochemistry with the 85 Ab, which recognizes both hIL-10 and vIL-10, 27 samples were found positive for hIL-10 and 9 for viral IL-10. Both tumor cells and infiltrating mononuclear cells were found to stain positively for IL-10 [48]. The most striking difference with the report on HIV+ NHL samples was that only 11% of tumors had more than 50% IL-10+ cells compared to 6/8 (75%) in the paper by Emilie et al [47]. These results suggest that HIV+NHL may produce higher amounts of IL-10 than NHL of immuno-competent patients. HIV may be directly responsible for an increased IL-10 secretion in these patients: the levels of production of hIL-10 by PBMC of patients with asymptomatic HIV infection has been found to be consistently superior to that of normal individuals [45], and transfection of HIV tat gene expression vector has been reported to induce IL-10 production in a T cell line [65, 66].

Taken together, these results indicate that IL-10 is frequently expressed at high levels in B NHL tumor samples obtained from HIV+ and HIV- patients and in B cell lines. IL-10 expression was observed at a lower frequency in B cell lines from non HIV non immunosuppressed patients. A large number of B cell lines produce hIL-10 and in all studies, the presence of IL-10 was highly correlated to the presence of EBV, although IL-10 production is also observed in EBV negative cell lines.

Role of EBV in IL-10 production by NHL cells

The capacity of EBV to induce the production of hIL-10 in normal or malignant B cells is well demonstrated [37, 38]. EBV infection induces the production of hIL-10 by normal tonsillar purified B lymphocytes and an anti-hIL-10 Ab inhibits partially cell growth in this study, indicating that hIL-10 plays an important role in EBV transformation [37]. In another study using a sensitive RT PCR approach for the detection of vIL-10 and hIL-10 mRNA, vIL-10 mRNA was found detectable in the first hours after the infection. Of note, an antisense anti-vIL-10 completely abrogated the transformation of B cells in this study [38].

In vivo, the role of EBV in the induction of hIL-10 production in malignant B cell tumors is strongly suggested by the observations of a correlation between IL-10 expression in tumor sample and the presence of EBV genome in the study by Emilie et al [47]. In our series of 42 non immunosuppressed NHL, a similar correlation was observed since only 2 of 12 EBV negative NHL were IL-10 positive compared to 25 of the 30 EBV positive NHL [48].

A molecular mechanism by which EBV could induce the transcription of the hIL-10 gene has been reported. Transfection of the LMP1 gene in EBV negative BL cell lines which do not constitutively produce hIL-10 has been found to induce IL-10 mRNA expression, whereas EBNA1, 2, 5,6 had no effect in this study [63].

The role of IL-10 in the physiopathology of non Hodgkin's lymphoma in vivo

An immunosuppressive role for IL-10 in cancer?

In vivo in man, IL-10 is detectable in fresh tumor samples in several different tumor models: HIV+ lymphoma, non HIV NHL, basal cell carcinoma, bronchogenic carcinoma, glioblastoma [47–55]. In view of its potent immunosuppressive effects *in vitro*, IL-10 may influence tumor growth through an inhibition of immune response.

The capacity of IL-10 to modulate an immune response directed towards the tumor has not been reported in animal models of B or T cell lymphoma. Actually, the capacity of IL-10 produced by tumor cells to inhibit the autologous immune response towards the tumor *in vivo* has not yet been demonstrated in any tumor and inconsistent observations have been made concerning this point in different animal models of cancer.

In mice, the capacity of local IL-10 produced by the tumor to block CTL activation or to inhibit local cytokine production, including cytokines with growth-inhibitory effects has been reported in several reports. IL-10 produced by colon carcinoma and melanoma cell lines was capable to inhibit DNA synthesis in MLR and to block IL-2, TNF and IFNg production by PBL [50, 54]. This inhibition was partially abrogated by an anti-IL-10 Ab [50, 54]. In an allogeneic tumor model, the local expression of IL-10 by allogeneic tumor cells was found able to abrogate the response towards class I determinants through an inhibition of CD4+ T cell function [67]. The local production of IL-10 induced by UV in skin modulates the local production of IFNg and

TNF and is essential to the growth of a transplanted melanoma cell line in mice [68]. In these animal models, the local production of IL-10 may interfere with local immune responses directed towards tumors and thus be involved in tumor progression.

In other models of mouse tumors, in particular mammary carcinoma, IL-10 appear to play an opposite role. In Balb/c mice, TSA, a mammary carcinoma cell line, transfected with IL-10 elicited a protective and curative immune response against the parental untransfected cell line [69]. A reduction in the incidence of metastasis was observed in a different model of mouse mammary carcinoma using a similar approach [70]. In a different model, IL-10 transfected CHO cells have been reported to be able to suppress the growth of their parental untransfected countertype when injected locally [71]; in this model, IL-10 may inhibit macrophage infiltration and production of cytokines which could act as growth factor for tumor cells.

Therefore, the role of local IL-10 in the modulation of the response to the tumor is probably variable among tumor types. Animal experiments *in vivo* suggest that IL-10 may exert a defavorable role in melanoma and colon carcinoma in mice and a favorable role in mammary carcinoma. The role of the local IL-10 production in the modulation of the immune response against B lymphomas in man, in particular in HIV+ NHL is not known. hIL-10 is overproduced in asymptomatic patients with HIV and induces a defective T cell response in these patients. T cell immunosuppression is a well known risk factor for the development of B cell tumors. The massive local IL-10 production in tumor samples in these patients is therefore likely to play a detrimental role on local immune response , and could contribute therefore to tumor progression along with the direct growth promoting activity of IL-10 on tumor cells.

IL-10 as a growth factor for NHL

IL-10 is a potent growth factor for normal B cells. The observation of a local production of IL-10 in tumor samples of patients with B NHL made it tempting to speculate that IL-10 could be an autocrine or a paracrine growth factor for these tumor *in vivo*. Indeed, this possibility is supported by several reports in the mouse model and in man.

In a mouse model of CLL, the transformation of a B-1 tumor cell line into an aggressive NHL (a model comparable to the Richter's syndrome in man) was found associated with dramatic increase of IL-10 production by the malignant transformed cloned as compared to the parental B-1 cell line [72]. The autocrine role of IL-10 was further demonstrated in experiment showing that antisense anti-IL-10 inhibit the growth of B-1 tumor cells in this model [73].

In man, the capacity of IL-10 to act as an autocrine growth factor has been demonstrated in cell lines derived from AIDS NHL [74]. In this study, an antisense anti-IL-10 was capable to inhibit partially thymidine incorporation by these cell lines demonstrating its activity as an autocrine growth factor [74]. In another study, incubation in the presence of anti-IL-10 antibodies induced a significant cell growth inhibition and sensitized the tumor to the cytotoxic agents and cytokine [75].

We have also investigated the possible role of IL-10 as an autocrine growth factor in nonimmunosuppressed patients. Purified B NHL tumor cells were obtained from tumor samples of immunocompetent patients with NHL. Upon costimulation with CD40, the addition of exogenous IL-10 significantly increased 3HTdR incorporation of all 11 tumor tested, indicating that IL-10 may also promote the growth of non HIV NHL in a paracrine or an autocrine manner [Voorzanger et al, unpublished results].

Taken together, these results indicate that IL-10 may act as growth factor for NHL cells *in vivo* in man.

Conclusion

IL-10 is produced at high levels in B cell lines *in vitro* and in NHL tumor samples of immunosuppressed and immunocompetent patients *in vivo*. IL-10 production in these tumors is highly correlated to the presence of EBV and the LMP1 gene of EBV is capable to trigger IL-10 secretion in B cell lines. In NHL of HIV positive patients, HIV could contribute to the increased IL-10 production. IL-10 promotes the growth of B cell tumors *in vivo* through its direct growth promoting activity on tumor cells and possibly through an inhibition of local immune reaction directed towards the tumor cells.

References

1. Fiorentino DF, Bond MW, Mosman TR: Two types of mouse T helper cell. IV. Th2 clones secrete a factor that inhibits cytokine production by Th1 clones. J Exp Med 1989; 170: 2081.
2. Vieira P, de Waal-Malefyt R, Dang MN, et al. Isolation and expression of human cytokine synthesis inhibitory factor (CSIF/IL10) cDNA clones: homology to Epstein–Barr virus open reading frame BCRF1. Proc Natl Acad Sci USA 1991; 88: 1172–76.
3. Suda T, O'Garra A, MacNeil I, et al. Identification of a novel thymocyte growth promoting factor derived from B cell lymphomas Cell Immunol 1990; 129: 228–40.
4. O'Garra A, Stapleton G, Dhar V, et al. Production of cytokines by mouse B cells: B lymphomas and normal B cells produce interleukin 10. Int Immunol 1990; 2: 821–32.
5. Tan JC, Indelicato S, Narula SK, et al. Characterisation of IL-10 receptors on human and mouse cells. J Biol Chem 1993; 268: 21053–59.
6. Liu Y, Wei SH, Ho AS, de Waal Malefyt R, Moore KW. Expression cloning and characterization of a human IL-10 receptor. J Immunol 1994; 152: 1821–1829.
7. Ho AS-Y, Liu Y, Khan TA, et al. A receptor for IL-10 is related to interferon receptors. Proc Natl Acad Sci USA 1993; 90: 11267–11271.

8. Moore KW, Ho AS-Y, Xu-Amano J. Molecular biology of interleukin 10 and its receptor. In: JE deVries, R de Wall Malefyt eds. Molecular Biology Intelligence Unit. Interleukin 10. RG Landes, 1995: 1–6.
9. Hsu DH, de Waal Malefyt R, Fiorentino DF, et al Expression of interleukin-10 activity by Epstein–Barr virus protein BCRF1. Science 1990; 250: 830–832, 1990.
10. de Waal Malefyt R, Haanen J, Spits H, et al. Interleukin 10 (IL-10) and viral IL-10 strongly reduce antigen specific human T cell proliferation by diminishing the antigen- presenting capacity of monocytes via downregulation of class II Major Histocompatibility Complex expression. J Exp Med 1991; 174: 915–924.
11. De Waal Malefyt R, Figdor CG, Huijbens R, et al. Effects of IL-13 on phenotype, cytokine production, and cytotoxic function of human monocytes. Comparison with IL-4 and modulation by IFNg or IL-10. J Immunol 1993; 151: 6370–6381.
12. Ding L, Linsley PS, Huang LY, et al. IL-10 inhibits macrophage costimulatory activity by selectively inhibiting the upregulation of B7 expression. J Immunol 1993; 151: 1224–1234.
13. Willems F, Marchant A, Delville JP, et al. IL-10 inhibits B7 and intercellular adhesion molecule 1 expression on human monocyte. Eur J Immunol 1994; 24: 1007–1009.
14. Kubin M, Kamoun M, Trinchieri G. IL-12 synergizes with B7/CD28 interaction in inducing efficient proliferation and cytokine production of human T cells. J Exp Med 1994; 180: 211–222.
15. de Waal Malefyt R, Abrams J, Bennett B, Figdor CG, de Vries JE. Interleukin 10 (IL-10) inhibits cytokine synthesis by human monocytes: an autoregulatory role of IL-10 produced by monocytes. J Exp Med 1991; 174: 1209.
16. Ralph P, Nakoinz I, Sampson JA, et al. IL-10, T lymphocyte inhibitor of human blood cell production of IL-1 and TNF. J Immunol 1993; 151: 5574–5585.
17. Fiorentino DF, Zlotnik A, Mosmann TR, Howard M, O'Garra A. IL-10 inhibits cytokine production by activated macrophages. J Immunol 1991; 147: 3815.
18. D'Andrea A, Aste-Amezaga M, Valiante NM, Ma X, Kubin M, Trinchieri G. Interleukin 10 (IL-10) inhibits human lymphocyte interferon gamma-production by suppressing natural killer cell stimulatory factor/IL-12 synthesis in accessory cells. J Exp Med 1993; 178: 1041–1048.
19. Bogdan C, Vodovotz Y, Nathan C. Macrophage deactivation by IL-10. J Exp Med 1991; 1549–1555.
20. Gazzinelli RT, Oswald JP, James SL, et al. IL-10 inhibits parasite killing and NO production by IFNg activated macrophages. J Immunol 1992; 148: 1792–1796.
21. Oswald IP, Wynn TA, Sher A, et al. IL-10 inhibits macrophage microbicidal activity by blocking the endogenous production of TNF required as a costimulatory factor for IFNg-induced activation. Proc Natl Acad Sci USA 1992; 89: 8676–8680.
22. DeWaal Malefyt Figdor C, deVries JE. Regulation of human monocyte function by IL-10. In: JE deVries, R de Wall Malefyt eds. Molecular Biology Intelligence Unit. Interleukin 10. RG Landes 1995: 37–52.
23. Kuhn R, Lohler J, Rennick D, Rajewsky K, Muller W. Interleukin-10-deficient mice develop chronic enterocolitis. Cell 1993; 75: 263–274.
24. Gerard C, Bruyns C, Marchant A, et al. Interleukin 10 reduces the release of tumor necrosis factor and prevents lethality in experimental endotoxemia. J Exp Med 1993; 177: 547–552.
25. Marchant A, Deviere J, Byl B, De Groote D, Vincent JL, Goldman M. Interleukin-10 production during septicaemia. Lancet 1994; 343: 707–709.
26. Del Prete G, De Carli M, Almerigogna F, Giudizi MG, Biagiotti R, Romagnani S. Human IL-10 is produced by both type 1 helper (Th1) and type 2 helper (Th2) T cell clones and inhibits their antigen-specific proliferation and cytokine production. J Immunol 1993; 150: 353–360.

27. Yssel H, DeWaal Malefyt R. IL-10 and human T cells. In: JE deVries, R de Wall Malefyt eds. Molecular Biology Intelligence Unit. Interleukin 10. RG Landes 1995: 19–27.
28. Saed G, Fivenson DP, Naidu Y, Nickoloff BJ. Mycosis fungoides exhibits a Th1-type cell-mediated cytokine profile whereas Sezary syndrome expresses a Th2-type profile. J Invest Dermatol 1994; 103: 29–33.
29. DeWaal Malefyt R, Yssel H, de Vries JE. Direct effects of IL-10 on subsets of human CD4+ T cell clones and resting T cells: specific inhibition of IL-2 production and proliferation. J Immunol 1993; 150: 4754–4765.
30. Taga K, Mostowski H, Tosato G. Human interleukin-10 can directly inhibit T-cell growth. Blood 1993; 81: 2964–2971.
31. Taga K, Cherney B, Tosato G. Interleukin-10 inhibits apoptotic cell death in human T cell starved of IL-2. Int Immunol 1993; 5: 1599–1506.
32. Jinquan T, Larsen CG, Gesser B, Matsushima K, Thestrup-Pedersen K. Human IL-10 is a chemoattractant for CD8+ T lymphocytes and an inhibitor of IL-8-induced CD4+ T lymphocyte migration. J Immunol 1993; 151: 4545–4551.
33. Go NF, Castle B, Barrett R, et al. IL-10, a novel B cell stimulatory factor: unresponsiveness of X chromosome-linked immunodeficiency B cells. J Exp Med 1990; 172: 1625–1631.
34. Levy Y, Brouet JC. IL-10 prevents the apoptotic cell death of germinal center B cells by the induction of the bcl-2 protein. J Clin Invest 1994; 93: 424–428.
35. Rousset F, Garcia E, Defrance T, et al. Interleukin 10 is a potent growth and differentiation factor for activated human B lymphocytes. Immunology 1992; 89: 1890.
36. Saeland S, Duvert V, Moreau I, et al. Human B cell precursors proliferate and express CD23 after CD40 ligation. J Exp Med 1993; 178: 113–120.
37. Burdin N, Peronne C, Banchereau J, Rousset F. Epstein–Barr virus transformation induces B lymphocytes to produce human interleukin 10. J Exp Med 1993; 177: 295–304.
38. Miyazaki I, Cheung RK, Dosch HM. Viral interleukin 10 is critical for the induction of B cell growth transformation by Epstein–Barr virus. J Exp Med 1993; 178: 439–447.
39. Fluckiger AC, Durand I, Banchereau J. Interleukin 10 induces apoptotic cell death of B-chronic lymphocytic leukemia cells. J Exp Med 1994; 179: 91–99.
40. Brière F, Servet Delprat C, Bridon J-M, et al. HIL-10 induces naive sIgD+ B cells to secrete IgG1 and IgG3. J Exp Med 1994; 179: 757–762.
41. Ghalib HW, Piuvezam MR, Skeiky, YA et al. Interleukin 10 production correlates with pathology in human Leishmania donovani infections. J Clin Invest 1993; 92: 324–329.
42. Holaday BJ, Pompeu MM, Jeronimo S, et al. Potential role for interleukin-10 in the immunosuppression associated with kala azar. J Clin Invest 1993; 92: 2626–2632.
43. Yamamura M, Uyemura K, Deans RJ, et al. Defining protective responses to pathogens: cytokine profiles in leprosy lesions. Science 1991; 254: 277–279.
44. Sieling PA, Abrams JS, Yamamura M, et al. Immunosuppressive roles for IL-10 and IL-4 in human infection. In vitro modulation of T cell responses in leprosy. J Immunol 1993; 150: 5501–5510.
45. Clerici M, Wynn TA, Berzofsky JA, et al. Role of interleukin-10 in T helper cell dysfunction in asymptomatic individuals infected with the human immunodeficiency virus. J Clin Invest 1994; 93: 768–775.
46. Bacchetta R, Bigler M, Touraine JL, et al. High levels of interleukin 10 production *in vivo* are associated with tolerance in SCID patients transplanted with HLA mismatched hematopoietic stem cells. J Exp Med 1994; 179: 493–502.
47. Emilie D, Touitou R, Raphael M, et al. In vivo production of interleukin-10 by malignant cells in AIDS lymphomas. Eur J Immunol 1992; 22: 2937–2942.
48. Voorzanger N, Touitou R, MC Favrot, et al. Correlation between IL-10 expression and the presence of EBV in non Hodgkin's lymphoma. Blood 1994; 84: 159a (abstract).
49. Pisa P, Halapi E, Pisa EK, et al. Selective expression of IL-10, IFNg and GM-CSF in ovarian cancer biopsies. Proc Natl Acad Sci USA 1992; 89: 7708–7712.

50. Gastl GA, Abrams JS, Nanus DM, et al. Interleukin-10 production by human carcinoma cell lines and its relationship to interleukin-6 expression. Int J Cancer 1993; 55: 96–101.
51. Yamamura M, Modlin RL, Ohmen JD, Moy RL. Local expression of anti-inflammatory cytokines in cancer. J Clin Invest 1993; 91: 1005–1010.
52. Smith DR, Kunkel SL, Burdick MD, et al. Production of interleukin-10 by human bronchogenic carcinoma. Am J Pathol 1994; 145: 18–25.
53. Nitta T, Hishii M, Sato K, Okumura K. Selective expression of interleukin-10 gene within glioblastoma multiform. Brain Res 1994; 649: 122–128.
54. Chen Q, Daniel V, Maher DW, Hersey P. Production of IL-10 by melanoma cells: examination of its role in immunosuppression mediated by melanoma. Int J Cancer 1994; 56: 755–760.
55. Sato T, Takao Y, Berd J. IL-10 production in metastatic melanoma. Proc Am Assoc Cancer Res 1995; 36: 466 (abstract).
56. Blay JY, Burdin N, Rousset F, et al. Serum interleukin-10 in non-Hodgkin's lymphoma: a prognostic factor. Blood 1993; 82: 2169–2174.
57. Stasi R, Zinzani L, Galieni P, et al. Detection of soluble interleukin-2 receptor and interleukin-10 in the serum of patients with aggressive non-Hodgkin's lymphoma. Identification of a subset at high risk of treatment failure. Cancer 1994; 74: 1792–1800.
58. Gotlieb WH, Abrams JS, Watson JM, Velu TJ, Berek JS, Martinez-Maza O. Presence of interleukin 10 (IL-10) in the ascites of patients with ovarian and other intra-abdominal cancers. Cytokine 1992; 4: 385–390.
59. Merville P, Rousset F, Banchereau J, et al. Serum IL-10 in earlystage multiple myeloma. Lancet 1992; 340: 1544–1545.
60. Benjamin D, Knobloch TJ, Dayton MA. Human B-cell interleukin-10: B-cell lines derived from patients with acquired immunodeficiency syndrome and Burkitt's lymphoma constitutively secrete large quantities of interleukin-10. Blood 1992; 80: 1289–1298.
61. Stewart JP, Behm FG, Arrand JR, Rooney CM. Differential expression of viral and human interleukin-10 (IL-10) by primary B cell tumors and B cell lines. Virology 1994; 200: 724–732.
62. Finke J, Ternes P, Lange W, Mertelsmann R, Dolken G. Expression of interleukin 10 in B lymphocytes of different origin. Leukemia 1993; 7: 1852–1857.
63. Nakagomi H, Dolcetti R, Bejarano MT, Pisa P, Kiessling R, Masucci MG. The Epstein–Barr virus latent membrane protein-1 (LMP1) induces interleukin-10 production in Burkitt lymphoma lines. Int J Cancer 1994; 57: 240–244.
64. Cortes JE, Talpaz M, Cabanillas F, et al. Serum levels of IL-10 in patients with diffuse large cell non Hodgkin's lymphoma: lack of correlation with prognostic. Blood 1994; 84: 160a (abstract).
65. Akridge RE, Oyafuso LK, Reed SG. IL-10 is induced during HIV-1 infection and is capable of decreasing viral replication in human macrophages. J Immunol 1994; 153: 5782–5789.
66. Masood R, Lunardi-Iskandar Y, Moudgil T, Zhang Y, Law RE, Huang CL, Puri RK, Levine AM, Gill PS. IL-10 inhibits HIV-1 replication and is induced by tat. Biochem Biophys Res Commun 1994; 202: 374–383.
67. Wang L, Goillot E, Tepper RI. IL-10 inhibits alloreactive cytotoxic T lymphocyte generation *in vivo*. Cell Immunol 1994; 159: 152.
68. Donawho CK, Bucana CD, Kripke ML. Enhanced growth of murine melanoma by UVB is dependent on IL-10. Proc Am Assoc Cancer Res 1995; 36: 475 (abstract).
69. Allione A, Consalvo M, Nanni P, et al. Immunizing and curative potential of replicating and non replicating murine mammary adenocarcinoma cells engineered with IL-2, IL-4, IL-6, IL-7, IL-10, TNFa, GM-CSF and IFNg gene or admixed with conventional adjuvants. Cancer Res 1994; 54: 6022–6026.

70. Kundu N, Beaty T, Jackson MJ, Fulton AM. IL-10 inhibits mammary tumor growth and metastasis. Proc Am Assoc Cancer Res 1995; 36: 465 (abstract).
71. Richter G, Kruger-Krasagakes S, Hein G, et al. Interleukin 10 transfected into Chinese hamster ovary cells prevents tumor growth and macrophage infiltration. Cancer Res 1993; 53: 4134–4137.
72. Peng B, Sherr DH, Mahboudi F, et al. A cultured malignant B-1 line serves as a model for Richter's syndrome. J Immunol 1994; 153: 1869–1880.
73. Peng B, Raveche E. Regulation of malignant B-1 cells by IL-10 antisense oligonucleotides. Proc Am Soc Cancer Res 1995; 36: 495 (abstract).
74. Masood R, Bond M, Scadden D, Kaplan M, Levine AM, Gill PS. IL-10: an autocrine B-cell growth factor for human B cell lymphoma and their progenitors. Blood 1992; 80: 115a (abstract)
75. Demidem A, Lam D, Gan X-H, Levine A, Sallahuddin Z, Bonavida B. Endogenous IL-10 is a protective factor in drug resistant AIDS related lymphoma. Proc Am Assoc Cancer Res 1995; 36: 323 (abstract).

27. Serum monoclonal immunoglobulins in renal transplant recipients: A study using high resolution electrophoresis and western blotting

GUY TOUCHARD, THIERRY PASDELOUP, THIERRY HAUET, MARC BAUWENS, GENEVIÈVE DUMONT, PIERRE AUCOUTURIER & JEAN-LOUIS PREUD'HOMME

Introduction

Transplant patients are prone to develop B cell lymphomas with a frequency increased by "high-dose" immunosuppressive regimens. Some studies suggest that transplant patients should be carefully screened to detect the occurrence of serum monoclonal immunoglobulins (moIg) which could be the first step of a patent immunoproliferative disorder.

Known frequencies of apparently benign serum monoclonal immunoglobulins (moIg) in renal transplant recipients vary from 12 to 30%, when conventional methods of detection are used [1–5]. This frequency strikingly increases (up to 79%) when recently available sensitive methods, such as high resolution agarose zone electrophoresis (HRE) are used [6]. We have applied HRE and immunoelectrophoresis to the study of sera from 84 renal transplant recipients. In 72 of them, a sensitive western blot technique coupled to HRE was also performed to characterize moIg. Their evolution and the predictive factors or clinical correlates were also studied. The incidence of serum moIg was much higher than in previous reports. Their isotypic distribution resembled that found in healthy individuals over 60 years of age and in other immunodeficient conditions.

J.L. Touraine et al. (eds.), Cancer in Transplantation. Prevention and Treatment, 243–248.

Material and methods

Sera and patients

Serum samples were collected just before, six months, one year and then yearly after renal transplantation in 84 patients; in all cases the graft had been functional for at least one year. The mean age of patients was 44.6 ± 13.4 years (16–70 years) at the time of the study and 40.7 ± 13.6 years (15–69 years) at the time of transplantation. The sex ratio was 0.6. The mean follow-up was 47.6 ± 24.9 months (12–101 months). The mean dialysis duration before transplantation was 23.9 ± 36.1 months. The initial immunosuppressive therapy was a sequential association of azathioprine (AZA), corticosteroids (Cs) and anti-lymphocyte globulins (ALG) with ciclosporine (CsA) introduced at the end of ALG therapy. At the time of the study, the maintenance regimen was a CsA monotherapy in 35 patients (41.6%), a bitherapy (CsA + AZA: 30 cases or AZA + Cs: 2 cases) in 32 patients (38.1%) and tritherapy (CsA + AZA + Cs) in 17 patients (20.2%). Sixty three patients were steroid free (75%). No patient had clinical or biological feature suggestive of immunoproliferative disorder.

Electrophoresis, immunoelectrophoresis and immunoblotting

Serum moIg were searched for by HRE in all serum samples. One microlitre of serum was deposited on thin layer (0.4 mm) agarose (Paragon^{TM}, Beckman, Brea, CA) and migrated during 25 mn at 100 V in 50 mM barbital buffer, pH 8.6. Electrophoresis were fixed with a methanolacetic acid solution, desiccated and stained by amido black.

A single pressure western blot technique [7] was used for moIg isotype characterization in 72 patients. Briefly, sera diluted at 1:50 to 1:500 were fractionated by HRE as before; proteins were then transferred onto a nitrocellulose sheet (HAHY, Millipore, Bedford, MA) under a pressure of 15 g/cm^2 during 10 mn. After a saturation step in 5% non-fat milk, the blots were incubated with appropriate isotype specific anti-human Ig. Alkaline phosphatase-conjugated polyclonal antibodies to kappa and lambda light chains were purchased from Sigma (St Louis, MO); anti-gamma, alpha, and mu heavy chains were from Biosys (Compiègne, France).

Standard immunoelectrophoresis was performed on 1.2% agarose in 50 mM barbital buffer, pH 8.2, with antisera against human serum proteins (Sebia, Issy-les-Moulineaux France) and each Ig isotype (Silenus, Hawthorn, Australia).

Statistical analysis

Percentages were compared using the Chi^2 test; mean values were compared with the Student's t test.

Results

HRE and immunoblotting allowed to demonstrate moIg, generally in small amount, in the serum of 56 patients before transplantation (66.6%). In 72 patients (85.5%) moIg were detected 6 months to 8 years after transplantation. By comparison, immunoelectrophoresis allowed to detect moIg (most often transient) in the serum of 18 recipients only (21.4%). Twenty moIg were detected (IgG: 7, IgM: 13) with a κ:λ ratio of 2.

The sex ratio was identical in patients with moIg before graft, in patients with moIg after graft and in the whole group of studied patients (0.59, 0.6 and 0.59 respectively). After graft moIg were more frequent in patients over 50 years (96.8%) than in younger patients (78.8%) ($p = 0.025$). Before graft this difference was not significant (< 50 years: 65.4%, > 50 years: 68.7%, $p = 0.75$). The incidence of serum moIg was not significantly higher after than before graft (85.5 versus 66.5%, $p = 0.18$). However, occurrence of new moIg after graft was significantly more frequent in older patients (< 50 years: 62%, > 50 years: 88%, $p = 0.006$).

Before grafting the incidence of moIg was not significantly correlated with the duration of dialysis (27 ± 40 months versus 18 ± 27 months for patients with and without moIg, $p = 0.27$). No correlation was found between the incidence of serum moIg and the maintenance immunosuppressive regimen, HLA A, B, DR incompatibilities, the occurrence of acute rejection episode and its treatment regimen or CMV infection episodes. However new moIg after graft were more frequent in patients suffering from CMV infections (90 versus 64% in patients without CMV infection, $p = 0.027$).

Immunoblotting demonstrated one or several moIg in the serum from 60 recipients out of 72 after transplantation . A single moIg was found in 14 patients (23.3%), 2 moIg in 7 (11.7%) 3 or 4 moIg in 21 (35%), 5 or 6 moIg in 9 (15%), 7 or more moIg in 9 (15%) including two Hbs antigen positive patients. A total of 224 moIg were characterized; the κ/λ ratio was 1.1; 141 moIg were IgG (κ/λ ratio of 0.8) and 82 were IgM (κ/λ ratio of 1.5). Only one moIgA was detected.

Discussion

This study of serum Ig from renal transplant recipients using HRE and immunoblotting revealed a striking frequency of moIg present in small amount both before and after the graft. Older patients were more prone to develop new serum moIg after grafting. In most sera (76.7%) moIg were multiple and different light chain types were often found in the same sample suggesting that they were secreted by distinct clones. The incidence of serum moIg is known to increase markedly in aging generally without any significant pathological manifestation. We found moIg in 57% of sera from healthy individuals aged 70 years or more using the same sensitive methods [8]. This frequency increased to 77% after 90 years and was 4.5% before 50 years. Using similar methods, Radl and associates found that 76% healthy individuals aged 95 years or more and 79% kidney graft recipients bore serum molg [9, 10]. Using agar electrophoresis and immunofixation they found serum molg in 30% of renal graft recipients and in 3% of the patients with chronic renal failure treated by dialysis [6].

The sensitivity of immunoblotting is greater than that of immunofixation. molg concentrations as low as 0.5 mg/l can be detected by immunoblotting as compared with approximately 50 mg/l for immunofixation, 100 mg/l for HRE and 2 to 5 g/l for cellulose acetate electrophoresis [7]. Using immunoblotting after HRE, Beaume et al [11] reported a 80% frequency of molg in sera from patients with B chronic lymphocytic leukemia while only 7.6% were detected by immunoelectrophoresis. The isotypic distribution of molg was different from that found in immunoproliferative disorders [11, 12], but was similar to that found in sera of healthy aged people [8–10] and patients with T cell-related immunodeficiencies including HIV infection [13] with the predominance of IgM, IgG1 and IgG3 and a relatively high proportion of λ-type molg. This isotypic distribution was also demonstrated after allogeneic bone marrow transplantation [12, 14, 15] as after renal transplantation [6]. IgG3 is a rare isotype in normal plasma cells [16] and among myeloma proteins [9, 12]. The decreasing order of frequency of molg isotypes in immunodeficiency nearly follows the $5'$-$3'$ heavy chain constant region gene sequence except for $C\delta$ and $C\alpha 1$. In our series IgG class was more frequent than IgM by immunoblotting but less frequent by immunoelectrophoresis.

In renal transplant recipients the molg detected by immunoelectrophoresis or immunofixation were most often transient and found generally six months to two years post transplant [1–5]. It is noteworthy that in our series the HRE pattern was stable in most patients who were followed six years or more.

None of our 84 selected patients developed a post transplant lymphoproliferative disorder (PTLD). The great incidence of molg hamper their clinical interest in terms of diagnostic value for the B cell PTLD. We observed two further patients who developed PTLD localized in the renal graft. They were treated successfully by transplantectomy and immunosuppressive therapy withdrawal during the first year posttransplant and they could not be included in the series described herein. In both patients serum immunoblotting demonstrated oligoclonal patterns similar to those of most patients without PTLD. Comparable findings were noted in the serum of transplant recipients with or without infectious EBV-related lymphoproliferative syndrome by Touraine et al [17, 18] and by Deteix et al [19] using isoelectrofocusing and immunofixation. A longer follow up period is needed to determine the exact significance of molg. Monoclonal or oligoclonal antibody responses may be a quite normal finding without clinical significance under certain conditions featuring excess of antigen stimulations. In transplant recipients the viral infections

(EBV, CMV ...) and the allograft act as the source of chronic antigenic stimulation. The antibody response is altered by immunosuppressive therapy, aging and virus themselves which may result in altered T and B cell function.

References

1. Radl J, Valentijn RM, Haaijman JJ and Paul LC. Monoclonal gammapathies in patients undergoing immunosuppressive treatment after renal transplantation. Clin Immunol Immunopathol 1985; 37: 98–102.
2. Stanko CK, Jeffery JR and Rush DIN. Monoclonal and multiclonal gammapathies after renal transplantation. Transplant Proc 1989; 21: 3330–3332.
3. Pollock CA, Mahony JF, Ibels LS, Caterson RJ, Waugh DA, Wells JV and Ross Sheil AG. Immunoglobulin abnormalities in renal transplant recipients. Transplantation 1989; 47: 952–956.
4. Chakalarovski C, Lang Ph, Buisson Cl, Weil B. Immunoglobulines monoclonales en transplantation rénale. Caractérisation, évolution et facteurs de risque. Presse Med 1991; 20: 2033–2035.
5. Modesto A, Rostaing L, Abbal M, Niquet L, Tkaczuk J, Durand D and Ohayon E. Long term follow-up of de novo monoclonal gammapathies. Transplant Proc 1994; 26: 282.
6. Radl J, Weis J and Hoogeven CM. Immunoblotting with (sub) class-specific antibodies reveals a high frequency of monoclonal gammapathies in persons thought to be immunodeficient. Clin Chem 1988; 34: 1839–1842.
7. Aucouturier P, Capella M, Briault S, Danon F, Intrator L, Preud'homme JL. Caractérisation des immunoglobulines monoclonales dans les liquides biologiques par immunoempreinte sur nitrocellulose. Rev Inst Pasteur Lyon 1987; 20: 147–153.
8. Connault L, Preud'homme JL, Gombert J, Aperce JM and Aucouturier P. Serum monoclonal immunoglobulins in healthy aged people: a study of incidence and isotype using a sensitive immuno-blotting method. Aging Immunol Infect Dis 1991; 3: 37–42.
9. Radl J, Weis J and Hoogeveen CM. Representation of IgG and IgA subclasses within monoclonal gammapathies of different origin. A minireview. In Poulik M.D Editor, Protides of the biological fluids, Oxford UK, Pergamon Press 1989; 143–146.
10. Radl J. Age-related monoclonal gammapathies: clinical lessons from aging C57 BL mouse. Immunol Today 1990; 11: 234–236.
11. Beaume A, Brizard A, Dreyfus B and Preud'homme JL. High incidence of serum monoclonal Ig detected by a sensitive immunoblotting technique in B-cell chronic lymphocytic leukemia. Blood 1994; 84: 1216–9.
12. Aucouturier P and Preud'homme JL. Subclass distribution of human myeloma proteins as determined with monoclonal antibodies. Immunol Letters 1987; 16: 55–57.
13. Walker S, Riches P and Hobbs JR. IgG subclasses of human monoclones differ between myeloma and post bone-marrow graft patients. In Poulik MD Editor. Protides of the biological fluids, Oxford UK Pergamon Press 1989; 36: 121–125.
14. Briault S, Courtois-Capella M, Duarte F, Aucouturier P and Preud'homme JL. Isotype of serum monoclonal immunoglobulins in human immunodeficiency virus-infected adults. Clin Exp Immunol 1988; 74: 182–184.
15. Hammarström L and Smith CIE. Frequent occurrence of monoclonal gammapathies with an imbalanced light-chain ratio following bone-marrow transplantation. Transplantation 1987; 43: 447–449.
16. Riches P, Polce B and Hong R. Isotype analysis of specific antibody responses in long term survivors of bone-marrow transplantation. In Poulik MD Editor. Protides of the biological fluids, Oxford UK, Pergamon Press 1989; 36: 167–171.

17. Fischer AM, Simon F, Le Deist F, Blanche S, Griscelli C and Fischer A. Prospective study of the occurrence of monoclonal gammapathies following bone marrow transplantation in young children. Transplantation 1990; 49: 731–5.
18. Mayumi M, Kuritani T, Kubagawa H and Cooper MO. IgG subclass expression by human B lymphocytes and plasma cells: B lymphocytes precommited to IgG subclass can be preferentially induced by polyclonal mitogens with T cell help. J Immunol 1983; 130: 671–677.
19. Touraine JL. Immunoglobulin abnormalities and infectious lymphoproliferative syndrome in cyclosporin treated transplant patients. Transplant Proc 1983; 15: 2798–2804.
20. Touraine JL, Deteix P, El Yafi M. Virus induced lymphomas in transplant patients under immunosuppressive therapy. Transplant Proc 1987; 19: 4087–4088.
21. Deteix P, Chapuis-Cellier C, Ghais Z, Lefrançois N, Brusa M, Touraine JL and Traeger J. Systematic survey of immunoglobulin abnormalities; frequency and evolution in organ transplant recipients. Transplant Proc 1985; 17: 2651–2654.

28. Increased risk of lymphoproliferative disorders following the use of OKT3: Association with cumulative dose

LODE J. SWINNEN

Introduction

Post-transplantation lymphoproliferative disorder (PTLD) is a frequently fatal complication of immunosuppression [1]. The term describes Epstein–Barr virus associated B-lymphoproliferations occurring after organ transplantation. The disease has assumed increasing clinical importance in view of the constantly rising number of organ transplant recipients and the development of highly potent and specific immunosuppressive drugs. Continued, uncontrolled EBV-driven proliferation of B-cells in the absence of adequate T-cell control has been proposed as a mechanism for the development of PTLD by Klein and others [2, 3]. As proliferation continues, clones with a growth advantage emerge, and a monoclonal population eventually predominates. This model is capable of at least partially explaining many of the otherwise puzzling clinical and pathologic features of this disease.

The incidence of PTLD has varied with the organ transplanted; ranging from about 1% of renal transplant recipients to about 4% of heart or heart-lung recipients [1, 4]. Although PTLD has been seen with all forms of antirejection therapy to date, the risk of developing the disease is strongly influenced by the nature of the immunosuppressive regimen used, a not unexpected observation in view of the above mentioned pathogenetic model. Comparison of one institution's experience with that of another is often complicated by the fact that different regimens were used; individual components of the immunosuppressive regimen nevertheless appear to specifically influence both the risk for PTLD and its clinical pattern. Associations of this type were first identified when cyclosporine (CsA), a potent and relatively specific anti-T-cell agent, was first introduced. The particularly high incidence of PTLD noted in early studies furthermore diminished when blood levels were monitored and lower CsA doses were used [5, 6]. CsA has also been noted to shorten

J.L. Touraine et al. (eds.), Cancer in Transplantation. Prevention and Treatment, 249–258.

the interval between transplantation and the appearance of PTLD, from an average of 30 months to an average of 6 months [7], with similar observations being reported from other series [8, 9]. The most recently introduced agents, monoclonal antibodies directed against the human CD3 receptor-T-cell complex, profoundly deplete circulating CD3+ T-lymphocytes [10]. A course of the highly potent and selective immunosuppressive antibody OKT3 is very effective at reversing rejection episodes refractory to other measures [11]. OKT3 had come into extensive use between about 1985 and 1990 for the prophylaxis of rejection in cardiac transplantation [12]. The value of such prophylactic immunotherapy, whether with OKT3 or with polyclonal preparations such as ATG, was poorly defined at the time [13]. Indications that the use of anti-CD3 monoclonal antibodies might influence the risk for PTLD first appeared in the allogeneic bone marrow transplant setting, following use of the monoclonal antibody known as 64.1 [14].

A strong temporal and statistical association between the use of OKT3 and an increase in the incidence of PTLD has been established in the Loyola University Chicago series of cardiac transplant recipients. The results of that clinical study have been reported in detail elsewhere [15]. An update, and a summary of the methods and principal findings of the original study are presented, as are preliminary data on the effect that discontinuation of prophylactic immunotherapy has had on the incidence of PTLD.

Study summary and update

Patient population

162 consecutive orthotopic cardiac transplants, performed at a single institution over a six year period, were studied retrospectively. Data from three repeat transplants were cumulated within the individual patients; five patients who died of post-operative complications within 3 days of transplantation were deleted from the analysis. No other patients were censored from the study. 154 patients were therefore analyzed for risk of developing PTLD. 75 percent of patients were male, 84 percent were white, mean age was 46 ± 13 years, and there was an even distribution of dilated (47%) and ischemic (44%) cardiomyopathy.

Immunosuppressive regimens

86 patients received ATG prophylaxis (ATGAM, Upjohn, Kalamazoo MI; 5 mg per kg per day for 9 days), and 65 patients received OKT3 prophylaxis (Orthoclone OKT3, Ortho Pharmaceutical, Raritan NJ; 5 mg per day for 14 days). 3 patients received no prophylactic immunotherapy. OKT3 was introduced in November 1985, initially only for the treatment of refractory rejection (14 patients); subsequently also for prophylaxis. A total of 79

patients therefore received OKT3 for one or both indications. The immunosuppressive regimen further consisted of: methylprednisolone 500 mg i.v. pre-operatively and intra-operatively, and 125 mg i.v. every 8 hours for 3 doses post-operatively; azathioprine 2 mg/kg i.v. pre-operatively followed by 2 mg/kg/day orally, adjusted to maintain the white cell count $> 3.5 \times 10^9$ per liter; prednisone 1 mg/kg per day orally, tapered by 0.1 mg/kg every other day to 0.2 to 0.3 mg/kg/day, and reduced to 0.1 mg/kg/day after 1 year; cyclosporin (CsA) 5 to 8 mg/kg per day, adjusted to maintain serum CsA level within a specified target range. Until July 22, 1988 the Sandoz polyclonal antibody assay for CsA was used, with a target range of 120 to 160 ng per ml for the first year following transplantation, 80 to 120 ng per ml for year 2, and 50 to 80 ng per ml for year 3 and subsequent years. After July 22, 1988, the Abbott TDx assay was used, with a target range of 180 to 220 ng per ml for year 1, 140 to 180 ng per ml for year 2, and 100 to 140 ng per ml for year 3 and subsequent years. As the results of these two assays are not readily convertible, all CsA levels were expressed as a multiple of the number corresponding to the middle of the target range for the applicable assay and year following transplantation.

Endomyocardial biopsies were histologically graded according to a standard system [16], and rejection episodes were treated in a uniform manner. Intensified immunosuppression was used only for moderate or severe rejection. In the absence of hemodynamic compromise, the oral steroid dose was increased; if hemodynamic compromise was present, 1 gram methylprednisolone per day was given i.v. for 3 days. Refractory rejection was treated with either OKT3 5 mg i.v. per day for 10 days, or ATG 5 mg/kg/day i.v. for 5 days. If rejection was not reversed, increased doses of OKT3 (up to 10 mg per day) or ATG (up to 15 mg per kg per day) were used.

Statistical methods

Univariate analysis using Fisher's exact test or the chi square test, and Student's t-test were conducted on categorical and continuous variables respectively. Cumulative OKT3 dosage was expressed as an ordinal variable (none, ≤ 75 mg, > 75 mg) for multivariate analysis. Multiple logistic regression was used to identify factors associated with PTLD while adjusting for possible confounding variables.

Pathology

Diagnosis of PTLD was based on histologic examination of biopsy material in all cases. Lesions were classified according to the Working Formulation scheme [17]. Immunophenotyping by immunoglobulin staining, immunogenotyping by DNA analysis for clonal immunoglobulin-gene rear-

Table 1. Incidence of PTLD according to cumulative OKT3 dose

OKT3	PTLD		
None	1 / 75 (1.4%)	P=.03 (None vs. < 75 mg)	P<.0001 (None, < 75 mg, > 75 mg)
< 75 mg	6 / 65 (9.2%)		
> 75 mg	5 / 14 (35.7%)		

rangements, and Southern blot analysis for the presence of EBV-DNA, were performed on tumor specimens whenever technically feasible.

Effect of OKT3 on the risk of developing PTLD

The only factor demonstrated to be statistically different between patients developing PTLD and those not developing PTLD was the use of OKT3. The following factors were assessed by univariate analyses: sex, race, indication for transplantation, age, body weight, use of OKT3, the number of rejection episodes requiring intensified immunosuppression, cumulative ATG, cumulative methylprednisolone, and mean CsA level.

Of 75 transplant recipients who had not received OKT3, 1 developed a lymphoproliferative disorder, an incidence of 1.3%. Of 79 patients who had received OKT3 for prophylaxis and/or treatment of rejection, 9 developed PTLD, an incidence of 11.4%. This represented a 9.5 fold greater risk (odds ratio 9.5, 95% confidence interval 1.65–54.72, Fisher's exact test $P = 0.018$).

The cumulative dose of OKT3 furthermore showed a clear relationship to the incidence of PTLD. A course of OKT3 generally amounted to a total of 70 mg (5 mg/day for 14 days). All OKT3 recipients who developed PTLD had received at least a prophylactic course of the drug. Cumulative doses in excess of 75 mg were the result of an additional, later course of OKT3 for treatment of refractory rejection. Of 65 patients receiving ≤ 75 mg cumulative OKT3, 4 developed PTLD (6.1%), while 5 of 14 patients (35.7%) receiving > 75 mg developed the disease ($P < 0.01$). An analysis of PTLD risk at cumulative OKT3 exposures ranging from none to > 75 mg demonstrated a highly significant trend of increasing disease incidence with increasing dosage (Mantel Haenszel chi square: 16.0, $P < 0.0001$). In order to adjust for possible confounding variables, a multivariate analysis was performed using logistic regression techniques. The factors analyzed were: use of OKT3 (designated as none, $\leq$ 75 mg, or $>$ 75 mg cumulative dose), race, sex, cumulative ATG, cumulative methylprednisolone, mean CsA level, number of rejection episodes requiring treatment, and the etiology of the pre-existing cardiac disease. The only factor significantly predictive for the development of PTLD while controlling for all other factors in the model was the use of OKT3 ($P < 0.001$).

Thirty patients had, over the course of time, received both OKT3 and ATG; this combination of agents was specifically assessed as a possible risk factor for PTLD. However, only two patients who had received both drugs developed PTLD (6.7%), whereas 7 of the remaining 49 patients who had received OKT3, but no ATG, developed the disease (14.3%, $P = 0.47$).

Over the 5 years since that study was completed, two more patients in the original group of OKT3 recipients have developed PTLD, both after a single prophylactic course, resulting in a current overall incidence of 13.9%, eleven-fold higher than in patients who had not received the drug (Table 1). The updated incidence among patients receiving a single course of OKT3 is therefore 6/65 (9.2%), also significantly higher than in patients who had never received the drug ($P = 0.03$).

Effect of OKT3 on the clinical presentation of PTLD

The interval between transplantation and the appearance of PTLD was very short, on the order of one to two months, in patients who had received $>$ 75 mg OKT3. The correlation between higher dose and shorter interval was statistically significant ($r = -0.91$, $P = 0.0006$, $N = 10$), and that pattern has persisted as more cases have appeared.

Only one of six patients who had received a single course of OKT3 ($\leq$ 75 mg) presented with organ failure, systemic sepsis, and a fulminant clinical course. Three of four patients who had received two courses of OKT3 ($>$ 75 mg) presented with very extensive PTLD, characterized by organ failure and/or systemic sepsis and a very rapid clinical course.

Relationship to EBV

Since primary EBV infection has been identified as carrying a higher risk than reactivated infection [18], it was important to determine whether the higher incidence of PTLD in OKT3 treated patients might have been due to an incidental clustering of primary EBV infections in that group. This did not however prove to be the case. IgG antibody titers to EBV capsid antigen had been obtained prior to and at intervals following transplantation. Overall, 93% of patients had a positive pre-transplant titer ($\geq$ 1:10). All but two initially seronegative patients became seropositive after transplantation, indicating that primary infection occurred in virtually all initially seronegative patients. While only 5% of patients who did not develop PTLD were initially seronegative, 30% of patients who did develop PTLD had negative EBV serology pre-transplant, a significant difference (P = 0.025) indicating a higher frequency of primary infection in the PTLD group. However, when patients were grouped according to whether they had or had not received OKT3, no difference in the rate of initial seronegativity was found. The high rate of PTLD in the group of patients who had received OKT3 could therefore not be attributed to a disproportionate number of primary EBV infections in that group. The frequency of reactivated infection, defined as a $\geq$ 4-fold rise in titer, did not differ significantly between patients who did and patients who did not develop PTLD (P = 0.21).

Elimination of prophylactic immunotherapy: impact on PTLD incidence

Prophylactic immunotherapy was discontinued at our institution in January of 1990 based on the results of the study summarized above. The impact of this policy change on the incidence of PTLD was assessed in September 1993, at which point 113 additional patients had been transplanted, with a mean follow-up of 23 $\pm$ 13 months. The mean time to lymphoma development in patients transplanted prior to the policy change had been 7 $\pm$ 6 months. The incidence of lymphoma had dropped following elimination of OKT3 prophylaxis, to a level not statistically different from that observed prior to its introduction. No other changes had been made, and this was verified by analyzing such potentially significant variables as mean CsA levels and the frequency of rejection episodes [19].

Discussion

A substantial increase in the incidence of PTLD was identified following the addition of OKT3 to a conventional cardiac transplant immunosuppressive regimen. No other risk factor could be associated with the increased incidence. The concomitant use of other immunosuppressive agents was quantitated to the fullest extent possible, and rigorous statistical analyses were applied. The use of CsA in particular was analyzed extensively; the increased risk of PTLD seen with OKT3 was clearly independent of mean CsA level. Elimination of OKT3 prophylaxis resulted in a reduction in PTLD incidence to baseline levels, strongly supporting a cause and effect relationship for the previously reported association between the use of OKT3 prophylaxis and an increased risk of PTLD.

One could speculate about whether mechanisms specific to OKT3 might account for the increased incidence or whether this could simply be the result of greater total immunosuppression [15, 20]. The answer to such mechanistic questions cannot be determined from these data nor, probably, from any other retrospective clinical study. Certain observations are nevertheless worth reviewing in this context, particularly if one considers a model of inadequate T-cell control as the mechanism for the emergence of this disease. PTLD is uncommon (incidence less than 1%) in the allogeneic bone marrow transplant setting, despite the intensive immunosuppression involved, in the absence of certain risk factors [21]. Use of the monoclonal anti-CD3 antibody 64.1 was found to be associated with a 14% incidence of PTLD, and T-cell depletion of donor marrow resulted in a 12% incidence [14]; in a separate series, T-cell depletion of mismatched donor marrow resulted in a 24% incidence of the disease [22]. Subsequent observations in organ transplant recipients at a number of centers are in keeping with our findings regarding OKT3, both in terms of an increased incidence of PTLD and of differences in the clinical pattern of disease [23–27]. Interestingly, a re-analysis of the University of Cincinnati tumor registry prompted by our observations in heart recipients revealed that CsA, and to an even greater extent OKT3, disproportionately increase the frequency of lymphomas as a proportion of all post-transplant tumors. Specifically, lymphomas accounted for 11% of tumors after immunosuppression with azathioprine and prednisone; for 28% of tumors in patients immunosuppressed with a CsA-containing regimen; and for 64% of tumors in patients who had received OKT3 [28]. Registry data cannot of course provide incidence figures, but unless CsA and OKT3 prevent other tumors in the post-transplant setting, which is highly unlikely, those registry data imply an increase in the incidence of PTLD in association with CsA and especially with OKT3. All these observations are in keeping with the hypothesis that progressively more potent and selective anti T-cell agents also progressively increase the risk of PTLD.

The strong correlation between cumulative OKT3 dose and PTLD risk may represent a dose-response phenomenon. However, the duration of OKT3-induced immunosuppression may be as or more important in this context. This cannot be determined from our data as the two parameters (time and cumulative dose) were equivalent in our series of patients. Since cumulative dose = dose/day × number of days treated, using the number of days as an indicator of exposure would affect the analysis only if dose/day varied among patients. All but 7 patients received a uniform daily OKT3 dose of 5 mg. None of the exceptions would be reclassified, in terms of "high" or "low" exposure, if the number of days were used as the indicator of exposure rather than cumulative dose. Exchanging one parameter for the other would not affect the results of our analysis. However, some indirect data suggest that the duration of continuous OKT3 exposure may be important, in that the interval between courses in the five patients who developed PTLD at cumulative OKT3 doses greater than 75 mg was generally much shorter (median 13 days, range 0–33) than in the nine patients receiving > 75 mg who did not develop PTLD (median 115 days, range 8–884; Mann Whitney

U test P = 0.02). Firm conclusions cannot however be drawn from analysis of such small numbers.

High cumulative OKT3 dosage furthermore corresponded with very short intervals between transplantation and PTLD, and other clinical features also strongly suggested that the pattern of disease was influenced by such doses. Although previously described, presentation with widespread tumor, organ failure and/or systemic sepsis, followed by a fulminant clinical course, has been considered rare [1]. Such presentations were common in the Loyola University series, and were strongly associated with the use of OKT3 at high cumulative doses. An increased incidence of fulminant PTLD in association with OKT3 therapy has since been noted at other centers [23–27]; similar observations have been made in the bone marrow transplant setting [22]. Either prolonged immunosuppression due to short intervals between courses, and/or the specific immune defects induced by OKT3 might predispose to this type of presentation. The increased incidence of PTLD seen up to a year or more after a single course of prophylactic OKT3 is more difficult to explain in terms of overall intensity of immunosuppression. There are *in vitro* indications that anti T-cell agents such as OKT3, and perhaps CsA also, can directly affect the outgrowth of EBV-transformed B-cells [29, 30]. Regardless of the exact mechanisms involved, it is likely that the composition of the immunosuppressive regimen as a whole is significant. Data from the Minneapolis Heart Institute are of interest in that regard [31]. The incidence of PTLD was found to be low in cardiac transplant recipients treated with OKT3 and triple drug immunosuppression with early weaning of steroids, but was found to be high in heart and heart-lung recipients in whom steroids were not weaned.

In view of past experience with CsA, the possible contribution of that drug is particularly worth investigating. In addition to studying the effect of mean CsA level, it was possible in our series to assess the impact of delaying the initiation of CsA during the administration of prophylactic OKT3. CsA was delayed to between day 8 and day 11 in 24 of the 65 patients who received prophylactic OKT3. The remaining 41 patients started CsA on day 1 or day 4. There was no difference in the incidence of PTLD between the two groups (12.5 versus 14.6%, P = 0.81), indicating that the simple expedient of reducing other immunosuppressive drugs during OKT3 administration may not obviate the problem.

From a practical point of view, it can be concluded that the addition of OKT3 to a standard triple-drug immunosuppressive regimen significantly increases the incidence of PTLD after cardiac transplantation. Repeated courses at short intervals should be avoided, and the advisability of OKT3 prophylaxis should be reassessed, particularly since the value of prophylactic immunotherapy in cardiac transplantation is not clearly established.

References

1. Nalesnik MA, Makowka L, Starzl TE. The diagnosis and treatment of posttransplant lymphoproliferative disorders. Current Problems In Surgery 1988; 25: 367–472.
2. Purtilo DT. Epstein–Barr-virus-induced oncogenesis in immune-deficient individuals. Lancet 1980; 1: 300–303.
3. Klein G. Lymphoma development in mice and humans: diversity of initiation is followed by convergent cytogenetic evolution. Proceedings of the National Academy of Sciences of the United States of America 1979; 76: 2442–2446.
4. Armitage JM, Kormos RL, Stuart RS et al. Posttransplant lymphoproliferative disease in thoracic organ transplant patients: ten years of cyclosporine-based immunosuppression. Journal of Heart & Lung Transplantation 1991; 10: 877-886.
5. Starzl TE, Nalesnik MA, Porter KA et al. Reversibility of lymphomas and lymphoproliferative lesions developing under cyclosporin-steroid therapy. Lancet 1984; 1: 583–587.
6. Beveridge T, Krupp P, McKibbin C. Lymphomas and lymphoproliferative lesions developing under cyclosporin therapy [letter]. Lancet 1984; 1: 788.
7. Penn I. Malignant lymphomas in organ transplant recipients. Transplantation Proceedings 1981; 13: 736–738.
8. Cleary ML, Warnke R, Sklar J. Monoclonality of lymphoproliferative lesions in cardiac-transplant recipients. Clonal analysis based on immunoglobulin-gene rearrangements. New England Journal of Medicine 1984; 310: 477-482.
9. Nalesnik MA, Jaffe R, Starzl TE et al. The pathology of posttransplant lymphoproliferative disorders occurring in the setting of cyclosporine A-prednisone immunosuppression. American Journal of Pathology 1988; 133: 173–192.
10. Bach JF, Chatenoud L. Immunologic monitoring of Orthoclone OKT3-treated patients: the problem of antimonoclonal immune response. Transplantation Proceedings 1987; 19: 17–20.
11. Costanzo-Nordin MR, Silver MA, O'Connell JB et al. Successful reversal of acute cardiac allograft rejection with OKT monoclonal antibody. Circulation 1987; 76: V71–V80.
12. Renlund DG, O'Connell JB, Gilbert EM et al. A prospective comparison of murine monoclonal CD-3 (OKT3) antibody-based and equine antithymocyte globulin-based rejection prophylaxis in cardiac transplantation. Decreased rejection and less corticosteroid use with OKT3. Transplantation 1989; 47: 599–605.
13. Barr ML, Sanchez JA, Seche LA, Schulman LL, Smith CR, Rose EA. Anti-CD3 monoclonal antibody induction therapy. Immunological equivalency with triple-drug therapy in heart transplantation. Circulation 1990; 82: IV291–IV294.
14. Witherspoon RP, Fisher LD, Schoch G et al. Secondary cancers after bone marrow transplantation for leukemia or aplastic anemia [see comments]. New England Journal of Medicine 1989; 321: 784–789.
15. Swinnen LJ, Costanzo-Nordin MR, Fisher SG et al. Increased incidence of lymphoproliferative disorder after immunosuppression with the monoclonal antibody OKT3 in cardiac-transplant recipients. New England Journal of Medicine 1990; 323: 1723–1728.
16. Billingham ME. Some recent advances in cardiac pathology. Human Pathology 1979; 10: 367–386.
17. National Cancer Institute sponsored study of classifications of non-Hodgkin's lymphomas: summary and description of a working formulation for clinical usage. The Non-Hodgkin's Lymphoma Pathologic Classification Project. Cancer 1982; 49: 2112–2135.
18. Ho M, Miller G, Atchison RW et al. Epstein-Barr virus infections and DNA hybridization studies in posttransplantation lymphoma and lymphoproliferative lesions: the role of primary infection. Journal of Infectious Diseases 1985; 152: 876–886.

19. Swinnen LJ, Fisher SG, Fisher RI, Koch D, Costanzo MR. Elimination Of OKT3 Induction Therapy: Impact On The Incidence Of Lymphoma Following Cardiac Transplantation. J Heart Lung Transplant 1994; 13 No. 1(2)(abs 148): S68 (abstract).
20. Swinnen LJ, Fisher RI. OKT3 monoclonal antibodies induce interleukin-6 and interleukin-10: a possible cause of lymphoproliferative disorders associated with transplantation. [Review]. Current Opinion in Nephrology & Hypertension 1993; 2: 670–678.
21. Zutter MM, Martin PJ, Sale GE et al. Epstein–Barr virus lymphoproliferation after bone marrow transplantation. Blood 1988; 72: 520–529.
22. Shapiro RS, McClain K, Frizzera G et al. Epstein-Barr virus associated B cell lymphoproliferative disorders following bone marrow transplantation. Blood 1988; 71: 1234–1243.
23. Alfrey EJ, Friedman AL, Grossman RA et al. A recent decrease in the time to development of monomorphous and polymorphous posttransplant lymphoproliferative disorder. Transplantation 1992; 54: 250–253.
24. Cockfield SM, Preiksaitis J, Harvey E et al. Is sequential use of ALG and OKT3 in renal transplants associated with an increased incidence of fulminant posttransplant lymphoproliferative disorder? Transplantation Proceedings 1991; 23: 1106–1107.
25. Renard TH, Andrews WS, Foster ME. Relationship between OKT3 administration, EBV seroconversion, and the lymphoproliferative syndrome in pediatric liver transplant recipients. Transplantation Proceedings 1991; 23: 1473–1476.
26. Rosenthal JT, Wilkinson AH, Canfield CW. Fulminant Epstein–Barr Virus-Associated Post-Transplant lymphoproliferative Disorders Following OKT3 Therapy. ASTP Annual Meeting 1991; 74 (abs).
27. Rinde-Hoffman D, Cintron GB, Ferguson JE, Toole JC, Bugni WB. Lymphoproliferative disorder early after cardiac transplantation [published erratum appears in Am J Cardiol 1992 Mar 15; 69(8): 844]. American Journal of Cardiology 1991; 68: 1724–1725.
28. Penn I. The changing pattern of posttransplant malignancies. Transplantation Proceedings 1991; 23: 1101–1103.
29. Ren EC, Chan SH. Possible enhancement of Epstein–Barr virus infections by the use of OKT3 in transplant recipients. Transplantation 1988; 45: 988–989.
30. Bird AG, McLachlan SM, Britton S. Cyclosporin A promotes spontaneous outgrowth in vitro of Epstein-Barr virus-induced B-cell lines. Nature 1981; 289: 300–301.
31. Emery RW, Lake KD. Post-transplantation Lymphoproliferative Disorder and OKT3 (let.). N Engl J Med 1991; 324: 1437.

29. Clinical characteristics of lymphoproliferations after renal transplantation. Nantes experience

J. DANTAL, A. MOREAU, M. HOURMANT, D. CANTAROVICH, M. GIRAL-CLASSE, G. BLANCHO, F. BUZELIN, F. GAILLARD & JP. SOULILLOU

It is well known that patients who have undergone organ transplantation (Tx) have an increased risk of developing de novo malignancies (100 times what is observed in the general population). The more frequent malignancies after Tx are carcinoma of the skin and lips, lymphoproliferative disorders and Kaposi's sarcoma. All of them are strongly associated with viral infections (Epstein Barr virus, Human Papilomas virus, Human herpes virus 8) [1, 2].

The diverse lymphoid disorders found in organ recipients belong to a spectrum of disease processes [3], from indolent proliferation to an aggressive and fatal infiltration of tumoral cells, and are grouped as Post Transplant Lymphoproliferative Disorders (PTLD). This severe complication, of B lymphocyte origin at least in 85% of the cases, is associated with the duration and the type of immunosuppression and EBV infection [4]. The risk for a renal allograft recipient to develop PTLD is 40 times greater than expected in the general population.

We present here the analysis of the clinical characteristics of patients with PTLD in our population of patients who underwent renal Tx during a 23 year period. Therapeutic approach and response are the subject of an other presentation in this issue.

Patients and methods

Patients

Between 1972 and 1994, among 1692 renal Tx, 21 patients were diagnosed as having PTLD.

J.L. Touraine et al. (eds.), Cancer in Transplantation. Prevention and Treatment, 259–266.

Immunosuppressive regimen, during this period, has included different protocols. Conventional therapy by corticosteroids and azathioprine (CS-AZA) was used until 1982, with the addition of antilymphocyte or thymocyte globulins (ALG, ATG, Pasteur Merieux, France) after 1981. The sequential therapy was the more widely used, with ATG/ALG or more recently with monoclonal antibodies (anti-interleukine2 receptor monoclonal antibody: 33B3.1, anti-CD11a: 25–3 or anti-CD4: BF-5) and delayed introduction of Cyclosporine A (CsA). Few patients received CsA since the first day post Tx. All these treatments were given in combination with CS and AZA with the goal to withdraw CS after the first months post-Tx.

Rejection episodes were treated with steroid boluses as first line and in case of corticoresistance with ATG/ALG. Only few patients have received anti-CD3 monoclonal antibody (OKT3) in rescue therapy.

Histopathology

Histologic evaluation was done on formalin-fixed, paraffin embedded histologic sections for the 21 patients, stained with haematoxylin-eosin, Giemsa, periodic acid Schiff and silver stains. All material has been reviewed by a single pathologist (A.M.). Lymphoproliferations were classified into 1) polymorphous PTLD (including both B-cell hyperplasia and lymphoma), represented by an infiltrate of various cells including small lymphocytes, plasma cells, follicular center cells and immunoblasts, and 2) monomorphous PTLD defined as an infiltrate with the cytology of diffuse large cell lymphoma.

Immunohistochemical analysis was performed on paraffin embedded sections and on frozen sections (when available) using the streptavidin-biotin complex method. Antibodies against B cells (L26, kappa and lambda light chains), T cells (UCHL1, CD3) and CD30 were used on parafin-embedded sections, and additional anti-B cell (CD19, 21, 22, 37, 10) and anti-T cell antibodies (CD2, 4, 8, 7, 5) for the frozen sections analysis.

The presence of EBV virus was detected on paraffin embedded sections by immunohistochemistry with antibodies against EBV latent membrane protein (LMP1). In situ hybridization for EBV was performed using EBER1+2 and BHLF oligonucleotide probes and/or non isotopic DNA probe (BamH1w fragment).

Results

Incidence

Since the first case diagnosed in our unit in 1986, 21 patients have presented PTLD among 1692 renal transplantations (1.24%). PTLD is the third type of neoplasia (14.8% of all de novo cancers) encountered after skin/lip carcinomas and "frequent cancers in the general population". The outcome of PTLD is poor, 11 patients died (52.3% of patients with PTLD, representing 40% of death from all the malignancies).

Clinical characteristics

There is no significant difference on clinical parameters between our general transplanted population and the patients suffered of PTLD. At the time of transplantation patient's age ranged from 20 to 66 years (39.6 ± 16.5 years). Eight patients were female and 13 male. Renal failure was due to a large variety of causes, 47% were from glomerulonephritis, but no patient had received immunosuppressive therapy before renal transplantation. All the patients received a first cadaveric kidney graft.

Excepted for 2 patients who have received CsA since the first day post-transplantation and 2 a conventional therapy, all the others have been treated by sequential therapy with either ATG/ALG (n = 16, 76.2%) or anti-IL2R monoclonal antibody (n = 3, 14.3%) with delayed introduction of CsA between day 2 to 44 (13 ± 10 days). The maintenance therapy was conventional (CS-AZA) in 2 patients and for the others included CsA, alone (n = 3, 14.3%), in association with AZA (n= 10, 47.6%) or in triple therapy with CS and AZA (n = 6, 28.6%).

Nine patients have never presented rejection (43%). Twenty acute cellular rejection episodes were treated in 12 patients mainly with steroid boluses (70%) and 4 patients required ATG. OKT3 was used in rescue one time only and one patient had been involved in a pilot study using 33B3.1 in the treatment of ongoing rejection. The interval between the last episode of rejection and the diagnosis of PTLD was 54 ± 41 months.

The PTLD was diagnosed 4 to 149 months after Tx (62.4 ± 39.5 months). In 3 patients this interval was less than 1 year. At the time of PTLD diagnosis patient age ranged from 23 to 72 years (44.7 ± 15.6 yrs).

The clinical symptoms at the diagnosis frequently involved an abnormal examination of tonsil or lymph nodes (9 patients, 42.8%). Isolated extra nodal disease was also common. Four patients presented with an abdominal mass and/or unspecific symptoms (pains, diarrhea). In two patients the diagnosis was done on abnormal kidney graft function with the discovery of a tumor mass at the ultrasound examination. Only one patient in our series presented neurologic abnormalities, revealing isolated central nervous system lymphoma. In 5 patients (23.8%) the first symptom was an isolated unexplained fever. In addition, fever was frequently associated with the other clinical presentations (6 patients, 28.6%)

Clinical presentation after complete staging of the disease showed frequent isolated extranodal disease (n = 8, 38%) but involved the brain in only one patient (4.7%). Disease confined to the lymphoreticular system was present in 7 patients (33.3%) and 6 patients had disease in both sites. Only two patients (9.5%) had bone marrow involvement. Dosages of LDH were obtained in

10 patients and were elevated in 50% of them, CRP levels were high in all the patients tested (n = 9) from 1.2 to 20 fold increase. No monoclonal immunoglobulin was detected in these patients.

No patients were seronegative for EBV at the time of PTLD diagnosis, but two of them had presented a primoinfection during the first months of transplantation, 8 and 24 months prior PTLD diagnosis. The EBV serologic profile remained, compared to pre transplantation status, stable in 6 patients or suggestive for reactivation in 7 patients.

Histopathology

Four patients presented a polymorphous B PTLD pattern, 2 with polymorphic hyperplasia and 2 with polymorphic lymphoma. The predominant PTLD recognized was monomorphous B PTLD (9 cases of large B cell lymphoma, 2 cases of Burkitt's lymphoma and one case of T cell rich B lymphoma). In addition we have diagnosed 2 cases of Hodgkin's disease and T cell lymphoma in 2 others. One patient suffered from MALT lymphoma (gastric).

Lymphoid cells showed a B immunophenotype in 76.2% and are monoclonal in 66.7% of the cases. The research for EBV in the tumor tissue was positive in all cases of polymorphic hyperplasia and in the two cases of Hodgkin's disease (LMP, EBER1+2, BamH1w) and in 83% of the large B cell lymphoma. The two T cell lymphomas were negative.

Comments

The increased incidence of PTLD in immunosuppressed organ transplant recipients is well established, ranging from 1 to 2% after renal Tx to 4.6% for heart-lung Tx [5]. PTLD represents 21% of the tumors in immunosuppressed patients versus the 5% expected in the non immunosuppressed population (2). The increased incidence of "reticulum cell sarcoma" was first recognized in renal transplant patients [6] and still remains today a feared and frequently lethal disease [7].

PTLD rate was especially high during the first year post Tx (0.2% in renal recipients) but this incidence drops for the other years to 0.04% per year [8]. The same tendency is observed after heart Tx but with a higher incidence than after kidney Tx (first year: 1.2%, after the first year: 0,3%) [8]. Earlier reports described two clinical subgroups of patients with PTLD [9]. The first group is represented by young patients with a widespread mononucleosis-like syndrome at a mean of 9 months post Tx and the second is a group of older patients (middle age) with more localized and with frequently extra nodal tumors, a mean of 6 years following renal Tx.

The risk of PTLD is related, at least, to the aggressiveness of immunosuppressive therapies and the optimisation of induction therapies and the lowering of acute rejection episodes are important factors that could explain the difference observed with the different organ Tx. The beginning of CsA era in renal Tx was associated with a high and unacceptable incidence of PTLD (more than 10%), but a reduction in the CsA doses led to a decrease in PTLD incidence [10]. The recent conclusions showing that the use of CsA is associated with a high incidence of PTLD are due to the increased number of non renal Tx treated by CsA and it seems that there is no increased incidence of PTLD in renal Tx as compared to conventional therapy [8, 11]. Nevertheless CsA has a dramatic effect on the time of onset of PTLD (1–12 months) compared to that known with CS-AZA (42–45 months) [7, 12]. The anti-CD3 monoclonal antibody led to an increased incidence of PTLD [13, 14] with a correlation with its cumulative dose. Swinnen [15], in cardiac transplant recipients has shown, using a multivariate analysis, that OKT3 was the only factor to be significantly linked with the increased incidence of PTLD from 1.3 to 11.4% before and during the OKT3 era. In addition, the incidence raised from 6.2 to 35.7% with a total dose of OKT3 below or above 75 mg. In pediatric liver Tx the use of OKT3 in steroid resistant rejection episodes was associated with a 3 fold increase in the PTLD frequency [16].

In our experience, PTLD have occurred late after renal Tx and the induction or anti-rejection therapy has consisted in OKT3 for only one patient. It is noteworthy that 4 patients were treated by a monoclonal antibody against interleukine-2 receptor (19%). The incidence of PTLD for this treatment is 3.33%, twice more than that observed in our general population, but no significant increase in PTLD has been reported with others anti interleukine-2 receptor monoclonal antibodies (Lo-Tac-1: D. Latinne and B. Charpentier, BB10: J. Wijdenes and anti-Tac: RL Kirkman, personal communications) If it is evident that PTLD may occur only above a certain threshold of immunosuppression and especially during the first months post Tx, it is also important to consider the level of maintenance therapy. It is not clear if triple therapy induces a higher incidence of PTLD, as the few publications on this topic are contradictory [17, 18]. In addition, on a large cohort of patients, Opelz [8] has shown an increased incidence of PTLD for patients treated with CsA and AZA as compared to all other combinations, on the other hand, this combination gives a better graft survival (but a longer exposition to immunosuppression). In a randomized trial, we have studied the effect of two CsA blood trough level ranges and it seems that patients receiving a high dose CsA regimen (more than 150 ng/ml) present an increased risk for malignancies and PTLD (manuscript in preparation).

EBV has been implicated in malignant transformation; it is associated with nasopharyngeal carcinoma, Burkitt's lymphoma and Hodgkin's disease. In immunodeficient patients EBV genome has been found in most of the PTLD [12, 19, 20, 21] and more recently in smooth-muscle tumors [22]. The outgrowth of B infected cells is under control of specific T-cell immunity. Impairment of this response due to the immunosuppressive therapies in organ

Tx leads to the disruption of the host-virus balance, allowing uncontrolled B-cell proliferation and further transformation [23, 24]. EBV primary infection during Tx, is of course, strongly associated with PTLD, especially in a setting of high CsA levels. Although, paediatric patients are at risk for primary infection (19 vs 2.7% in liver Tx) [25], we have not observed any case of PTLD in our series of 60 paediatric renal Tx contrasting with other organ Tx. In addition, serologic evidence of an active EBV infection after Tx is very common (more than 30%) [26] and is not diagnostic of a PTLD. EBV genome is detectable in 89% of PTLD [27] and it was shown recently that EBV-related B-cell PTLD exhibited the 3 types of EBV latent infection [20, 23].

The clinical presentation of PTLD can vary from a moderate illness of viral type to a rapidly fatal disease. The extra nodal involvement at the presentation is frequent, unlike lymphomas that occur in immunocompetent patients. Localization to central nervous system is especially common and represent the more frequent primary intracranial neoplasm encountered in transplanted patients (22 vs 0.5–2% in general population) [28]. The reason of this presentation is not known and in our small series we have not reported such disequilibrium. The gastro intestinal infiltration is also frequent herald by non specific symptoms and the practice of early systematic fibroscopic and/or radiologic examinations is able to establish the diagnosis. Isolated involvement of solid organs is less predominant, with a preference for graft infiltration mimicking acute rejection [8]. Adenopathies are strongly suggestive of PTLD; they tend to involve the head and neck as well as tonsil abnormalities but this is not always the rule. As shown in our series, isolated fever without common infectious agent is also strongly evocative of PTLD. Biopsies are required with routine and immunohistochemical analysis to establish the diagnosis. The histological appearance of PTLD is that of a diffuse proliferation of lymphoid cells with a spectum of histopathologic findings reported by Frizzera [3], from polymorphic diffuse B-cell hyperplasia to large cell lymphoma with an increasing malignant potential. In general the polymorphic lesions could be either monoclonal or polyclonal, while the monomorphic lesions appeared monoclonal. The determination of clonality was done by staining for heavy and light-chain surface and cytoplasmic immunoglobulins and by cytogenetic analysis [29], more recently, by immunoglobulin gene rearrangement [30] and by the analysis of the genomic termini fragments of EBV [31]. It was shown that the tumor clonality was not absolutely linked to a poor outcome and especially to a resistance to antiviral therapy [32]. Although most of the PTLD are B cell processes, T cell lymphoma [33] and Hodgkin disease [34] have been also described representing less than 10% of PTLD [4] and few cases were from donor origin [35, 36].

In conclusion, PTLD remains a severe and lifethreatening complication after organ Tx. There is a frail equilibrium between the two main parameters involved in the pathogenesis of PTLD, the level of immunosuppression administered and the EBV infection. It is important to minimize as much as possible the level of immunosuppressive therapy or to discuss its interest in case of poor graft outcome, not only for the induction/antirejection therapy but also in maintenance therapy as suggested in our study concerning the CsA used after the first year post Tx. We should consider the EBV seronegative patients as a high risk patients and give preference to a seronegative donor or contraindicate intensive immunosuppressive therapy like OKT3 for them.

References

1. Sheil AGR. Development of malignancy following renal transplantation in Australia and New Zealand. Transplant Proc 1992; 24: 1275–1279.
2. Penn I. The changing pattern of posttransplant malignancies. Transplant Proc 1991; 23: 1101–1103.
3. Frizzera G, Hanto DW, Gajl-Peczalska KJ et al. Polymorphic diffuse B-cell hyperplasias and lymphomas in renal transplant recipients. Cancer Res 1981; 41: 4262–4279.
4. Penn I. Lymphomas complicating organ transplantation. Transplant Proc 1983; 15: 2790–2797.
5. Nalesnick MA, Makowka L, Starzl TE. The diagnosis and treatment of post-transplant lymphoproliferative disorders. Curr Prob Surg 1988; 25: 371–382.
6. Penn I. Tumor incidence in human allograft recipients. Transplant Proc 1979; 11: 1047–1051.
7. Morisson VA, Dunn MD, Manivel JC et al. Clinical characteristics of post-transplant lymphoproliferative disorders. Am J Med 1994; 97: 14–24.
8. Opelz G, Henderson R. For the collaborative transplant study. Incidence of non-Hodgkin lymphoma in kidney and heart transplant recipients. Lancet 1993; 342; 1514–1516.
9. Hanto DW, Gajl-Peczalska KJ, Frizzera G et al. Epstein–Barr virus (5EBV) induced polyclonal and monoclonal B-cell lymphoproliferative diseases occurring after renal transplantation. Ann Surg 1983; 198: 356–368.
10. Starzl TE, Porter KA, Iwatsuki S. Reversibility of lymphomas and lymphoproliferative lesions developing under cyclosporine-steroid therapy. Lancet 1984; 1: 583–587.
11. Stephanian E, Gruber SA, Dunn DL et al. Posttransplant lymphoproliferative disorders. Transplant Rev 1991; 5: 120–129.
12. Nalesnik Ma, Jaffe R, Starzl et al. The pathology of posttransplant lymphoproliferative disorders occurring in the setting of cyclosporine A-prednisone immunosuppression. Am J Pathol 1988; 133: 173–192.
13. Cockfield SM, Preiksaitis J, Harvey E et al. Is sequential use of ALG and OKT3 in renal transplants associated with an increased incidence of fulminant posttransplant lymphoproliferative disorder? Transplant Proc 1991; 23: 1106–1107.
14. Zutter MM, Martin PJ, Sale GE et al. Epstein–Barr Virus lymphoproliferation after bone marrow transplantation. Blood 1988; 712: 520–529.
15. Swinnen LJ, Costanzo-Nordin MK, Fischer SG et al. Increased incidence of lymphoproliferative disorder after immunosuppression with the monoclonal antibody OKT3 in cardiac transplant recipients. N Engl J Med 1990; 323: 1723–1728.
16. Renard T, Andrews W, Foster ME. Relationship between OKT3 administration, EBV seroconversion and lymphoproliferative syndrome in pediatric liver transplant recipients. Transplant Proc 1991; 23: 1473–1476.
17. Lopatin WB, Hickey DP, Nalesnik MA et al. Post-transplant lymphoproliferative disease and triple therapy. Clin Transplant 1990; 4: 47–52.

18. Wilkinson AH, Smith JL, Hunsicker LG et al. Increased frequency of post-transplant lymphomas in patients treated with cyclosporine, azathioprine, and prednisone. Transplantation 1989; 47: 293–296.
19. Randhawa PS, Jaffe R, Demetris AJ et al. Expression of Epstein–Barr virus-encoded small RNA (by the EBER-1 gene) in liver specimens from transplant recipients with post-transplantation lymphoproliferative disease. N Engl J Med 1992; 327: 1710–1714.
20. Rea D, Fourcade C, Leblond V et al. Patterns of Epstein–Barr virus latent and replicative gene expression in Epstein–Barr virus B cell lymphoproliferative disorders after organ transplantation. Transplantation 1994; 58: 317–324.
21. Young L, Alfieri C, Hennessy K et al. Expression of Epstein Barr Virus transformation-associated genes in tissues of patients with EBV lymphoproliferative disease. N Engl J Med 1989; 321: 1080–1085.
22. Lee ES, Locker J, Nalesnik M et al. The association of Epstein–Barr virus with smooth-muscle tumors occurring after organ transplantation. N Engl J Med 1995; 332: 19–25.
23. Rowe M, Young S, Crocker J et al. Epstein Barr Virus associated lymphoproliferative disease in the SCID mouse model: implication of EBV-positive lymphomas in man. J Exp Med 1991; 173: 147–156.
24. Bird AG, McLachlan SM, Britton S. Cyclosporine A promotes spontaneous outgrowth in vitro of Epstein–Barr virus induced B-cell lines. Nature 1981; 289: 300–301.
25. Cox KL, Lawrence-Miyasaki, Garcia-Kennedy R et al. An increased incidence of Epstein–Barr virus infection and lymphoproliferative infection and lymphoproliferative disorder in young children on FK 506 after liver transplantation. Transplantation 1995; 59: 524–529.
26. Ho M, Miller G, Atchison RW et al. Epstein Barr Virus infections and DNA hybridization studies in posttransplantation lymphoma and lymphoproliferative lesions. The role of primary infection. J Infect Dis 1985; 152: 876–886.
27. Ferry JA, Jacobson JO, Conti D et al. Lymphoproliferative disorders and hematologic malignancies following organ transplantation. Mod Pathol 1989; 2: 583–592.
28. Penn I, Porat G. Central nervous system lymphomas in organ allograft recipients. Transplantation 1995; 59: 240–244.
29. Nalesnik MA, Jaffe R, Starzl TE et al. The pathology of posttransplant lymphoproliferative disorders occurring in the setting of Cyclosporine A-Prednisone immunosuppression. Am J Pathol 1988; 133: 173–192.
30. Hanto DW, Birkenbach M, Frizzera G et al. Confirmation of the heterogeneity of post-transplant Epstein–Barr virus-associated B cell proliferations by immunoglobulin gene rearrangement analyses. Transplantation 1989; 47: 458–464.
31. Patton DF, Wilkowski CW, Hanson CA et al. Epstein–Barr virus-determined clonality in postransplant lymphoproliferative disease. Transplantation 1990; 49: 1080–1084.
32. Alfrey EJ, Friedman AL, Grossman RA et al. A recent decrease in the time to development of monomorphous and polymorphous posttransplant lymphoproliferative disorders. Transplantation 1992; 54: 250–253.
33. Griffith RC, Saha BK, Janney CM et al. Immunoblastic lymphoma of T-cell type in a chronically immunosuppressed renal transplant recipient. AJCP 1990; 93: 280–285.
34. Garnier JL, Lebranchu Y, Dantal J, et al. Hodgkin disease after renal transplantation. Transplantation 1995; (in press).
35. Hjelle B, Evans-Holms M, Yen TSB et al. A poorly differentiated lymphoma of donor origin in a renal allograft recipient. Transplant Proc 1989; 47: 945–948.
36. Meduri G, Fromentin L, Vieillefond A et al. Donor-related non-Hodgkin's lymphoma in a renal allograft recipient. Transplant Proc 1991; 23: 2649.

30. Therapeutic issues in lymphoproliferative disorders: Treatment and outcome of 28 cases observed in a single center

VÉRONIQUE LEBLOND, RICHARD DORENT,
MARC-OLIVIER BITKER, CAROLE SOUSSAIN,
DIDIER SAMUEL, JACQUES-LOUIS BINET & MARTINE RAPHAEL

Immunosuppressed organ transplant recipients have an increased risk of developing cancer such as Kaposi's sarcoma and posttransplant lymphoproliferative disorders (PTLDs) [1–3]. After organ transplantation, about 40% of patients with PTLDs survive, either because of spontaneous resolution after the cessation of immunosuppressive therapy, or possibly because of the efficacy of antiviral drugs, monoclonal antibodies and chemoradiotherapy [4]. Determination of the best treatment is difficult because of the limited number of published series, and because of the morphologic spectrum of the lymphoproliferative disorders which appears to range from a benign reactive lymphoid process to a malignant lymphoma. We reexamined our experience of 28 transplant recipients with a PTLD observed at our institution in an attempt to determine the response to therapy in 25 treated patients with reduction of immunosuppressants, monoclonal antibodies, surgery and/or chemotherapy after a median of follow-up of 60 months (range 4–84 months).

Patients and methods

Patients and methods

As shown in Table 1, the study population comprised 19 men and 9 women, who underwent 13 heart, 2 lung, 2 liver and 11 kidney transplants. All patients in whom PTLD was diagnosed before death underwent a thorough work-up to detect lymphoproliferative sites, which included CT scans of the chest, abdomen and central nervous system, together with bone marrow biopsy and aspiration. Tumors were classified according to Frizzera and Locker [5, 6]. The clonality was assessed by the detection of intracytoplasmic

J.L. Touraine et al. (eds.), Cancer in Transplantation. Prevention and Treatment, 267–278.

Table 1. Patient population, Pathological findings, clonality, and EBV studies of posttransplant lymphoproliferative disorders

UPN #	Age	Sex	Organ transplanted	Delay between graft-PTLD (days)	Morphology	Immuno-phenotype	CIg/ SIg	Genotypic clonality	EBV
1	45	M	Heart	150	Polymorphic	B	M	ND	+
2	43	M	Heart	750	Polymorphic	B	M	JHR	+
3	50	M	Heart	90	Polymorphic	B	M	ND	ND
4	38	F	Heart	150	Polymorphic	B	M	JHR	+
5	68	F	Heart	210	Polymorphic	B	M	JHR	+
6	50	F	Heart	180	Polymorphic	B	M	JHR	–
7	39	M	Kidney	180	Polymorphic	B	M	ND	ND
8	43	F	Liver	900	Polymorphic	B	M	JHR	–
9	22	F	Liver	640	Polymorphic	B	M	JHR	ND
10	20	M	Heart	150	Polymorphic	B	NM	ND	+
11	52	M	Heart	150	Polymorphic	B	NM	GL	+
12	46	M	Heart	120	Polymorphic	B	NM	GL	+
13	33	F	Lung	60	Polymorphic	B	NM	ND	+
14	51	M	Lung	180	Polymorphic	B	NM	GL	+
15	62	M	Kidney	3 450	Monomorphic	B	M	ND	–
16	40	M	Kidney	1 800	Monomorphic	B	M	ND	+
17	45	M	Heart	1 980	Monomorphic	B	M	ND	–
18	59	M	Heart	900	Monomorphic	B	M	JHR	–
19	54	M	Kidney	910	Monomorphic	B	M	JHR	+
20	35	F	Kidney	360	Monomorphic	B	M	ND	–
21	32	M	Kidney	420	Monomorphic	B	M	JHR	+
22	57	M	Kidney	450	Monomorphic	B	M	JHR	–
23	51	M	Kidney	180	Monomorphic	B	M	ND	+
24	63	M	Kidney	680	Monomorphic	B	M	JHR	+
25	58	F	Kidney	4 140	Polymorphic	T (CD4)	–	TCR R	–
26	67	M	Heart	1 380	Polymorphic	T (CD8)	–	TCR R	–
27	15	M	Heart	120	Polymorphic	T (CD8)	–	TCR R	+
28	49	M	Kidney	10220	Polymorphic	T (CD3)	–	TCRR	–

UPN: unique patient number.

JHR: rearrangement of immunoglobulin gene.

TCR R: rearrangement of T-cell receptor.

NM: non monotypic.

M : monotypic.

GL: germ line.

ND: not done.

immunoglobulin (CIg), surface immunoglobulin (SIg) and genotypic studies. Immunoglobulin gene and TCR rearrangements were detected by Southern blot using a heavy-chain joining region (JH) and the T-cell receptor β chain constant region complementary probe labelled with 32P by random priming. Epstein–Barr virus (EBV) was detected either by Southern blot, or by in situ hybridization on routinely processed sections with fluorescein isothiocyanate (FITC)-labelled EBER1+2 specific oligonucleotides [7].

Treatment

The treatment modalities varied during the years 1980 to 1995. The immunosuppressive regimen was modified in 23 patients after diagnosis of PTLD, azathioprine being withdrawn in 20 cases. In more recent patients (from 1988 through 1992), treatment consisted of infusions of anti-B cell monoclonal antibodies (specific for CD 21 and CD 24) every day at a dose of 0.2 mg/kg intravenously (10 patients) or by the intraventricular route at a daily dose of 2.5 mg (2 patients) for central nervous system (CNS) PTLD, as described by Fischer [8, 9], and/or polychemotherapy (11 patients). The first line chemotherapy was a CHOP regimen in 6 patients [10], CCNU, high-dose methotrexate (5 g/m^2) and holoxan in 3 patients with CNS involvement, and ESAP in two patients [11]. Two patients with localized PTLD were treated surgically.

Results

Time to tumor diagnosis

The time interval between organ allografting and tumor diagnosis ranged from 60 to 10220 days, with a median of 360 days. Thirteen patients developed a PTLD within the first year after the graft and 15 developed a late-onset of PTLD (> 1 year).

Clinical presentation (Tables 2, 3, 4)

One patient (#27) had a mononucleosis-like syndrome with fever and splenomegaly. PTLD developed on the allograft in two cases (#13, 14). Seven patients had lung involvement, 7 had small or large bowel involvement, 5 had liver involvement and 5 had central nervous system (CNS) involvement with a brain involvement. Ten patients had bone marrow and/or lymph node involvement. PTLD was diagnosed post mortem in two patients (#16, 22).

Pathological findings and clonality

Diffuse proliferation of lymphoid cells was observed in all cases. In 10 cases, tumors were classified as monomorphic. In the other cases, the lesions were polymorphic. All but four of the PTLDs expressed immunological markers of the B-cell lineage, as assessed by immunophenotyping of B-cell differentiation antigens and/or surface immunoglobulin analysis (SIg). Four tumors expressed T-cell markers (#25, 26, 27, 28) (Table 1). Monotypic B-cell PTLDs were observed in 19 cases and polymorphic PTLD in 5 cases respectively. Genotypic studies were performed in 18 cases and confirmed the monoclonality of the tumor in 15 cases. There were Ig gene rearrangements in 11 cases and a TCR rearrangement in four (Table 1).

EBV studies

The presence of the EBV genome and/or EBER 1+2 mRNAs was demonstrated in 15 of the 25 patients tested. In the remaining 10 cases we failed to detect EBV despite the use of Southern blot and *in situ* hybridization techniques in four cases. Most of EBV-negative PTLDs were observed in the monomorphic B-cell PTLD group. In the four cases of T-cell PTLD, EBV was associated with the tumor in one (Table 1).

Clinical outcome

Ten patients received 0.2 mg of CD21-specific and CD24-specific antibodies intravenously for 10 days with their oral informed consent (Tables 2, 3). Immunosuppressive therapy was always reduced before anti-B cell antibody therapy, but was usually considered unsuccessful because of disease progression. Tolerance was excellent, despite transient neutropenia in every case. Complete remission was defined as the disappearance of all clinical manifestations of PTLD, as well as a significant reduction in monoclonal serum components and normalization of LDH. As shown in Tables 2 and 3, infusion of anti-B cell antibodies led to complete remission in 8 patients. Complete remission was achieved within 15 to 90 days, not only in patients with an oligoclonal B-cell lymphoproliferative syndrome (#10, 11, 13, 14) but also in three patients with monoclonal lymphoproliferative disorders (#4, 5, 21). Salvage chemotherapy of two unresponsive patients (#6, 19) was successful in one case (#19). No relapse was observed in responders, but one patient died in complete remission of a second malignancy at 37 months (#12). Two patients with CNS PTLDs were treated via the intraventricular route using an Ommaya reservoir, as previously described [8]; one patient entered partial remission but died 4 months later of relapse, while the other was resistant to this treatment and died of disease progression after salvage chemotherapy. Eight patients were treated initially with chemotherapy (#2, 3, 8, 17, 18, 20,

Table 2. Clinical features, treatment and outcome of patients with B-cell polymorphic lymphoproliferative disorders

UPN #	Tumor sites	Surgical treatment	Change in immunosuppression (drug stopped)	Anti-B monoclonal antibodies	Chemotherapy (number of cycles)	Outcome
1	Lung Liver	Lung biopsy	Azathioprine	–	–	CR + 84 months
2	Lymph nodes Brain Kidney	Lymph node biopsy	Azathioprine	–	MTX Holoxan (1) CCNU	Died from infection at 1 month
3	Lung Liver Lymph nodes Small bowel	Lymph node biopsy	Azathioprine	–	CHOP (2)	Died from progression at 3 months
4	Liver Lung Uterus	Biopsy	Azathioprine	+	–	CR + 60 months
5	Lung	Biopsy	Azathioprine	+	–	CR + 60 months
6	Large bowel Bladder Peritoneum	Large bowel resection	Azathioprine	+	ESAP (1)	Died from infection at 1 month
7	Brain	Biopsy	↓ CSA	+ (IT)	–	Died from progression at 4 months
8	Lymph nodes	Biopsy	Azathioprine	–	CHOP (6)	CR+ 18 months
9	Lymph nodes	Biopsy	↓ FK 506	–	–	CR + 24 months
10	Liver	Liver biopsy	Azathioprine	+	–	CR + 84 months
11	Lung	Biopsy	Azathioprine	+	–	CR + 60 months
12	Large bowel	Biopsy	Azathioprine	+	–	Died in CR from lung carcinoma at 37 months
13	Transplanted lung	Biopsy	Azathioprine	+	–	CR + 60 months
14	Transplanted lung	Biopsy	Azathioprine	+	–	CR + 48 months

CHOP: cyclophosphamide, adriamycine, vincristine, prednisone.
MTX: high dose methotrexate.
ESAP: etoposide, cisplatin, high dose cytarabine, prednisolone.
IT: intrathecal.
CR: complete remission.

Table 3. Clinical features, treatment and outcome of patients with B-cell monomorphic lymphoproliferative disorders

UPN #	Tumor sites	Surgical treatment	Change in immunosuppression (drug stopped)	Anti-B monoclonal antibodies	Chemotherapy (number of cycles)	Outcome
15	Native Kidney	Nephrectomy	Azathioprine	–	–	Died from infection at 1 month
16	Brain	–	–	–	–	Autopsy findings
17	Lymph nodes Small bowel	–	Azathioprine	–	CHOP (6)	CR + 16 months
18	Skin Testis Breast	Orchidectomy	Azathioprine	–	ESAP (3)	Died in CR form heart failure at 30 months
19	Native kidney	Nephrectomy	Ciclosporine	+	CHOP (6)	CR + 24 months alive in relapse
20	Brain CSF Bone marrow	–	–	– Holoxan CCNU	MTX	Died from infection at 1 month
21	Bladder	Biopsy	Azathioprine	+	–	CR + 60 months
22	Small bowel Large bowel	Biopsy	–	–	–	Autopsy findings
23	Brain	Biopsy	–	+ (IT)	MTX Holoxan CCNU	Died from progression at 1 month
24	Large bowel Lymph nodes Spleen	Biopsy	Azathioprine	–	CHOP (4)	Died from infection at 4 months

CHOP: cyclophosphamide, adriamycine, vincristine, prednisone.
MTX: high dose methotrexate.
ESAP: etoposide, cisplatin, high dose cytarabine, prednisolone.
IT: intrathecal.
CR: complete remission.

24, 28). There were three toxic deaths after one month; three patients was cured but one of them died in remission 30 months later of chronic rejection (#18), one patient died in failure 4 months later and the last patient is under evaluation (#28).

Two patients died within a month of diagnosis without receiving treatment (#15,26); three patients were improved by reducing the doses of immunosuppressive agents (#1,9,27) but one died from infection at 3 months (#27). Both patients treated surgically died of sepsis (#15) or relapse (#26).

According to the pathological findings, death related to PTLD occurred in six of the ten patients with B-cell monomorphic PTLD and four of the fourteen patients with B-cell polymorphic PTLD. All patients with B-cell polyclonal tumors were cured (Tables 2, 3). Only one patient with T-cell PTLD is alive under evaluation (Table 4). As shown on the survival curve (Figure 1), a plateau has been reached at 45.7%, with a median follow-up of 60 months (range 4–84 months) among the survivors, and a median survival of 36 months for the whole group.

Discussion

We report 28 cases of lymphoproliferative disorders in allograft recipients on various posttransplant immunosuppressive regimens. The histopathological observations in this group concur with the general concept that the entire morphologic spectrum of B-cell differentiation from nonspecific reactive hyperplasia to large cell lymphoma can be observed in PTLD lesions. A wide spectrum of morphological and genotypic aspects was observed in this series, ranging from polyclonal polymorphic to monoclonal monomorphic tumors, as extensively described in the literature [6, 12]. Immunoglobulin and TCR-gene rearrangement studies show that most tumors have clonal rearrangements, despite a polymorphic morphology [6, 13, 14].

Epstein–Barr virus is often associated with PTLD [15–17]. In seven out of 21 tested B-cell PTLDS (33%), we failed to detect EBV in the tumor. Among the seven cases of EBV-negative B-cell PTLDs in this series, all except one appeared one year after the graft, raising the possibility that the number of EBV-negative PTLDs in organ transplant recipients might increase with time and suggesting that lymphomagenesis in such tumors requires other genetic changes.

The frequency of T-cell PTLD in our series was similar to that reported in the literature (14%) [2]. In the majority of cases, tumors that develop in transplant patients are monoclonal and oligoclonal B-cell lymphomas [13, 14, 18]. In this series of 28 PTLDs, we found four tumors that expressed T-cell surface markers and lacked expression of surface Ig, and CD20; three tumors had TCR gene rearrangements, one TCR$\gamma\delta$ gene rearrangements and one had EBV DNA sequences, as first described by Waller [19].

Table 4. Clinical features, treatment and outcome of patients with T-cell polymorphic lymphoproliferative disorders

UPN #	Tumor sites	Surgical treatment	Change in immunosuppression (drug stopped)	Anti-B monoclonal antibodies	Chemotherapy (number of cycles)	Outcome
25	Small bowel	Small bowel excision	Azathioprine	–	–	Died from relapse at 6 months
26	Lymph nodes Blood spleen	–	–	–	–	Died from infection at 1 month
27	Blood	–	Azathioprine	–	–	Died from infection at 3 months
28	Bone marrow Spleen Liver	Biopsy	Azathioprine	– ESAP (2)	CHOP (3)	Alive under evaluation + 4 months

CHOP: cyclophosphamide, adriamycine, vincristine, prednisone.
ESAP: etoposide, cisplatin, high dose cytarabine, prednisolone.

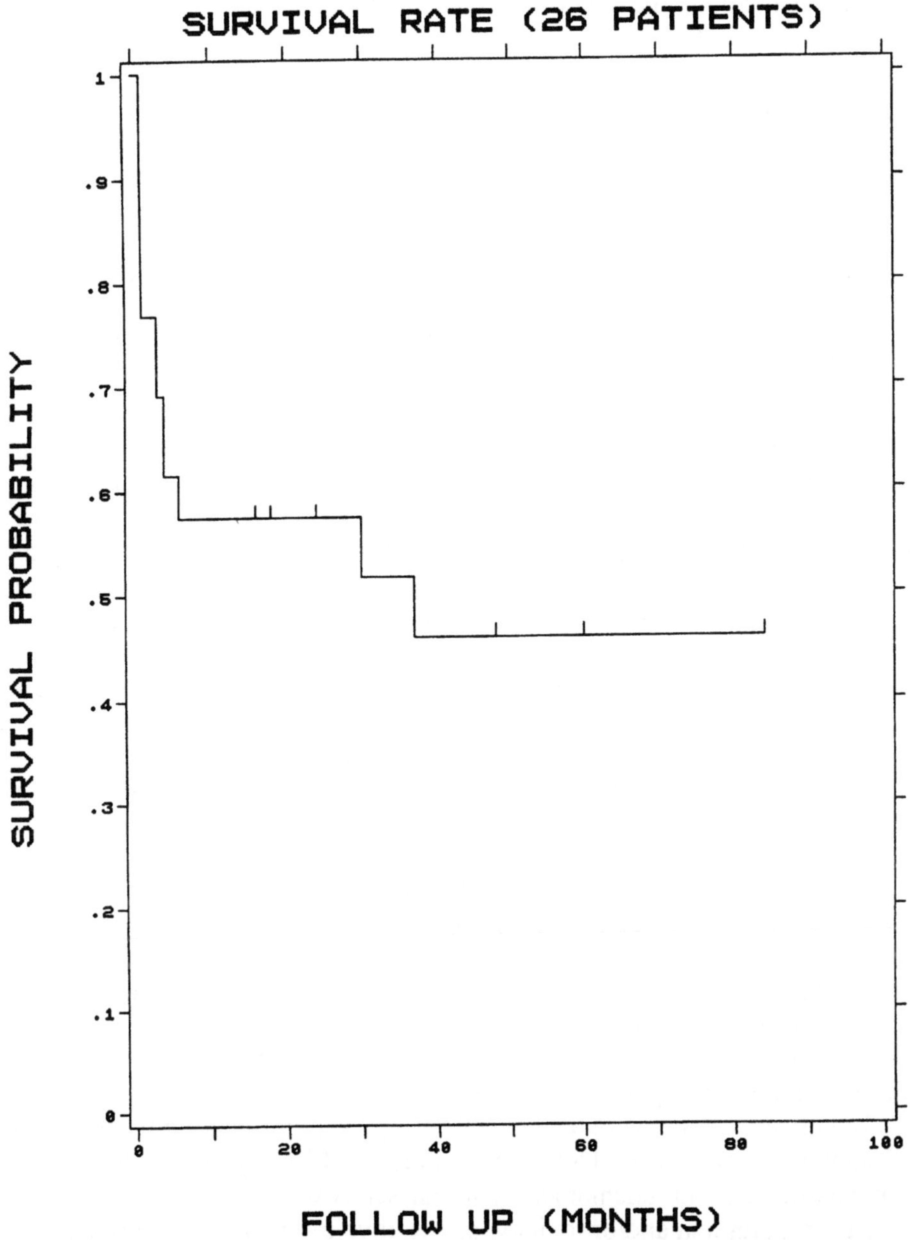

Fig. 1. Overall survival rate of the 26 patients in whom posttransplant lymphoproliferative disorder was diagnosed before death: 45.7% (13 alive, 15 dead), median survival time: 36 months.

The outcome of our patients was poor, as in previous reports: only 13 patients are alive, 11 in complete remission, one in relapse and the last patient is under evaluation. The overall survival rate is 45.7%, with a median overall survival time of 36 months.

Recognition of the polyclonal nature of many of these tumors has fostered approaches that preserve or enhance the host's innate capacity to suppress proliferation. Withdrawal or reduction of immunosuppressants has resulted in significant tumor regression and resolution of lymphoma in many patients with a minimal risk of rejection [7, 15, 20]. Theoretically, a reduction in immunosuppression would be most successful when the tumor expresses LMP1 and EBNA2, latency proteins which have been shown to facilitate interactions between EBV-infected B cells and cytotoxic T cells and to serve as antigenic targets for the EBV-specific T cell response [21]. Azathioprine was withdrawn from most patients in our study, with no manifestations of graft rejection and 3 patients were cured by reducing immunosuppression. Treatment with antiviral agents such as acyclovir and ganciclovir, in addition to reduction of immunosuppressants, has been reported to be effective in polyclonal disease [22]. Antiviral drugs inhibit viral replication in productive cells, but do not affect episomal EBV in non-productive, transformed lymphocytes; restoration of host immunity is therefore probably the most effective way of controlling lymphoid proliferation in these patients. Similarly, in a limited number of cases, recombinant -interferon plus immunoglobulin has been effective, with long-term cures in a few cases [23]. Low doses of interleukin 2 (IL2) prevent EBV-associated lymphoproliferative disorders in the SCID-human mouse, but the use of IL2 in organ transplantation could lead to rejection [24]. Theoretically, such treatments could be successful only in PTLD associated to EBV but in our series we failed to detect EBV in 30% of B-cell PTLD.

Results published by Fischer et al indicated that anti-B cell antibodies might be effective in controlling B-cell lymphoproliferative disorders [9]. Our results confirm this, even in the case of monoclonal B-cell proliferative disorders. However, no response was obtained in cases of CNS lymphoproliferation, despite intraventricular administration. Neither relapse nor graft loss occurred in the patients treated with anti-B cell antibodies, despite a reduced dosage of immunosuppressive agents.

Treatment with conventional chemotherapy and/or radiation therapy was disappointing, with several toxic deaths [12, 13, 20]. Only three of the eleven patients treated with chemotherapy in our series were cured; six died from disease progression and/or toxicity, one is alive in relapse after a remission of 24 months and the last in under-evaluation.

Optimal management approach and treatment of PTLDs are unknown. In the future, immunological treatment of PTLDs such as monoclonal antibodies specific for B, T-cell antigens or cytokines or expansion and infusion of EBV-cytotoxic T cells should be a good alternative to chemoradiotherapy [21–

23]. As spontaneous resolution of lymphoproliferative syndromes has been reported, randomized controlled trials of candidate treatments for PTLD are now required.

References

1. Penn I. Cancers after cyclosporine therapy. Transplant Proc 20 1988; suppl 1: 276–279.
2. Penn I. Cancers complicating organ transplantation. N Engl J Med 1990; 323: 1767–1769.
3. Opelz G, Henderson R, for the Collaborative Transplant Study: Incidence of non-Hodgkin lymphoma in kidney and heart transplant recipients. Lancet 1993; 342: 1514–1516.
4. Leblond V, Sutton L, Dorent R et al. Lymphoproliferative disorders after organ transplantation: a report of 24 cases observed in a single center. J Clin Oncol 1995; 13: 961–968.
5. Frizzera G, Hanto DW, Gajl-Peczalska KJ et al. Polymorphic diffuse B-cell hyperplasias and lymphomas in renal transplant recipients. Cancer Res 1981; 41: 4262–4271.
6. Locker J, Nalesnik M. Molecular genetic analysis of lymphoid tumors arising after organ transplantation. Am J Pathol 1989; 135: 977–987.
7. Brousset P, Chittal S, Schlaifer, and al. Detection of Epstein–Barr virus messenger RNA in Reed–Steinberg cells of Hodgkin's disease by in situ hybridization with biotynylated probes on specially processed modified acetone methyl benzoate xylene (ModAMeX) sections. Blood 1991; 77: 1781–1786.
8. Stephan JL, Le Deist F, Blanche S et al. Treatment of central nervous system B lymphoproliferative syndrome by local infusion of a B cell-specific monoclonal antibody. Transplantation 1992; 54: 246–248.
9. Fischer A, Blanche S, Le Bidois J et al. Anti-B-cell monoclonal antibodies in the treatment of severe B-cell lymphoproliferative syndrome following bone marrow and organ transplantation. N Engl J Med 1991; 324: 1451–1456.
10. Elias L, Portlock CS, Rosenberg SA. Combination chemotherapy of diffuse histiocytic lymphoma with cyclophosphamide, adriamycin, vincristine and prednisone (CHOP). Cancer 1978; 42: 1705–1710.
11. Velasquez WS, Swan F, Redman JR et al. Combination of Etoposide, high-dose Ara-C and Solumedrol with or without Platinol in relapsing or resistant lymphoma. Proc ASCO 1988; 256A (abst).
12. Nalesnik MA, Jaffe R, Starzl TE et al. The pathology of posttransplant lymphoproliferative disorders occurring in the setting of cyclosporine A – prednisone immunosuppression. Amer J Path 1988; 133: 173–192.
13. Hanto DW, Frizzera G, Galj-Peczalska et al. Epstein–Barr virus, immunodeficiency, and B-cell lymphoproliferation. Transplantation 1985; 39: 461–472.
14. Cleary ML, Warnke F, Sklar J. Monoclonality of lymphoproliferative lesions in cardiac-transplant recipients. N Engl J Med 1984; 310: 477–482.
15. Hanto DW, Galj-Peczalska KJ, Frizzera G et al. Epstein–Barr virus (EBV) induced polyclonal and monoclonal B-cell lymphoproliferative diseases occurring after renal transplantation. Ann Surg 1983; 198: 356–369.
16. Cleary ML, Nalesnik MA, Shearer WT et al. Clonal analysis of transplant-associated lymphoproliferations based on the structure of the genomic termini of the Epstein–Barr virus. Blood 1988; 72: 349–352.
17. Young L, Alfieri C, Henessy K et al. Expression of Epstein–Barr virus transformation associated genes in tissues of patients with EBV lymphoproliferative disease. N Engl J Med 1989; 321: 1080–1085.

18. Ho M, Jaffe R, Miller G et al. The frequency of Epstein–Barr virus infection and associated lymphoproliferative syndrome after transplantation and its manifestations in children. Transplantation 1988; 45: 719–727.
19. Waller EK, Ziemianska M, Bangs CD et al. Characterization of posttransplant lymphomas that express T-cell-associated markers: immunophenotypes, molecular genetics, cytogenetics, and heterotransplantation in severe combined immunodeficient mice. Blood 1993; 82: 247–261.
20. Starzl TE, Nalesnik MA, Porter KA et al. Reversibility of lymphomas and lymphoproliferative lesions developing under cyclosporine-steroid therapy. Lancet 1984; i: 583–588.
21. Murray RJ, Kurilla MG, Griffin HM et al. Human cytotoxic T-cell responses against Epstein–Barr virus nuclear antigens demonstrated by using recombinant vaccinia viruses. Proc Natl Acad Sci USA 1990; 87: 2906–2910.
22. Pirsch JD, Stratta RJ, Sollinger HW et al. Treatment of severe Epstein–Barr virus induced lymphoproliferative syndrome with ganciclovir: two cases after solid organ transplantation. Am J Med 1989; 86: 241–244.
23. Shapiro RS, Chauvenet A, McGuire W et al. Treatment of B-cell lymphoproliferative disorders with interferonα and intravenous gammaglobulin. N Engl J Med 1988; 318: 1334 (letter).
24. Baiocchi RA, Caligiuri A. Low dose IL2 prevents the development of Epstein–Barr virus-associated lymphoproliferative disorder in the SCID-human mouse. Blood 1993; 82: suppl 1, 385A (abst.).
25. Buchsbaum RJ, Lieberman J. EBV-specific CTL protect against human lymphoma in SCID mice. Blood 1994; 84, suppl 1: 2074 (abst).
26. Heslop HE, Smith CYK, Loftu S et al. Use of genetically marked virus specific T cytotoxic T lymphocytes to control Epstein–Barr virus related lymphoproliferative. Blood 1994; 84, suppl 1: 426 (abst).
27. Papadopoulos EB, Ladanyi M, Emmanuel D et al. Infusions of donor leucocytes to treat Epstein–Barr virus-associated lymphoproliferative disorders after allogeneic bone marrow transplantation. N Engl J Med 1994; 330: 1185–91.

31. Anti-B-cell MAb therapy of transplant-related lymphoproliferative diseases

ANNE DURANDY, MALIKA BENKERROU & ALAIN FISCHER

Introduction

When Epstein–Bar virus (EBV) infects B lymphocytes, it results in either full viral replication and B cell lysis or partial gene expression associated with cell transformation. Cell transformation is associated with B cell activation and continuous proliferation. Under ordinary circumstances, such B cells are suppressed or destroyed by cytotoxic/suppressor cells of the immune system. However, if severe T cell immune deficiency occurs, for instance, after organ transplantation or in patients with primary or acquired immune deficiencies, transformed B cells may proliferate in an uncontrolled fashion [1,2,6,7,9,11,13,15,17,19,20,26,27]. This uncontrolled proliferation may result in tumor formation. Assessment of cell surface immunoglobulin light chain expression or analysis of immunoglobulin gene rearrangements indicate that the tumors are initially polyclonal, but they may progress through an oligoclonal, and finally a monoclonal malignant transformation. This spectrum of EBV-induced proliferation of B lymphocytes is called B cell lymphoproliferative disorder (BLPD).

The overall frequency of BLPD after transplantation varies from 1–2% in kidney and bone marrow transplant recipients up to 10% in heart recipients. Clinical manifestations of BLPD range from a spontaneously resolving mononucleosis-like syndrome to an aggressive lymphoma with a proclivity for extranodal spread [6].

Prognostic factors

The B cell proliferation can be localized to a single nodal site or to several extranodal sites including the gastrointestinal tract or central nervous system. Pathological examination usually shows a polymorphic lymphoblastic proliferation. Cytologic features considered to predict an agressive course include

J.L. Touraine et al. (eds.), Cancer in Transplantation. Prevention and Treatment, 279–288.

the presence of necrosis, atypical nuclei, and extension of the lymphoblastic infiltrate beyond the capsule of the involved organ. Other adverse prognosis factors include a longer interval after transplantation, monoclonality, karyotype abnormalities, multiple extranodal sites of disease, and the occurrence of BLPD after bone marrow or heart transplantation [6]. In general, experience with BLPD has confirmed the serious nature of this disease. In a retrospective analysis of 102 cases having occurred, following organ or marrow transplantation 74 patients (72,5%) have died [1,6,11,17,20,21,22,24,27].

Treatment strategies (Table 1)

Complete regression of BLPD occurs in approximately 42% of patients when immunosuppressive drugs are reduced or eliminated [1,6,11,17,20,21,22,24,27]. Eliminating immunosuppression is primarily feasible after renal transplantation, where the re-institution of dialysis is a viable alternative if the kidney is rejected. No similar alternatives exist if a liver or heart transplant is rejected. Immunosuppression is intrinsic to marrow transplantation and discontinuation of immunosuppression is likely to result in flares of graft-versus-host disease without significant recovery of T cell mediated immunity.

EBV-transformed B cells have a circular viral DNA that is not very susceptible to inhibition with thymidine kinase inhibitors, such as acyclovir or ganciclovir. Nevertheless, there are anecdotal reports of tumor regressions with both acyclovir and ganciclovir therapy [8,16].

Chemotherapy and irradiation have not proven useful in controlling BLPD. In contrast, surgical resection has proven effective when the BLPD is limited to single sites and in one series, 74% of patients have survived [6]. A logical approach to patients developing BLPD after marrow grafting was the use of irradiated, peripheral blood mononuclear cells obtained from the marrow donor, who may also EBV immunity. However, in a small number of patients, mononuclear cell infusions did not appear to be useful [21]. More interestingly, a interferon given with high dose intravenous gammaglobulin induced remission in 5 patients and 3 patients appeared to have a lasting benefit [21]. These promising results warrant further studies for confirmation; however, we have chosen to attempt to reduce the B cell burden by using B cell specific monoclonal antibodies.

Rationale for the use of anti-B cell monoclonal antibodies

Prior studies of B cell lymphomas demonstrated that in a small number of cases, infusions of anti-idiotypic antibodies were able to reduce remissions [4]. Based on this observations and on separate observations of the ability of anti-T cell antibodies to efficiently kill T cells in vivo, we proposed using two murine monoclonal antibodies of the IgG_1 isotype specific for CD21 and CD24. These monoclonal antibodies were chosen because they bound B cells at most stages of differentiation. The two antibodies were used in combination, because EBV transformed B lymphocytes express membrane molecules defectively [25]. We have indeed found that B cells expressed both CD21 and CD24 in only 50% of the specimens studied. Furthermore, in 2 of 45 cases, B cells were detected that expressed neither CD21 nor CD24 (see below).

Results of therapy

An open trial was initiated in July 1985 including patients with high risk BLPD. The entrance criteria included patients with: (1) rapidly progressing multiorgan B cell proliferation, (2) BLPD refractory to a decrease in immunosuppression with or without acyclovir administration, or (3) poor prognosis characteristics by pathology criteria, i.e. necrosis and nuclear atypia. Patients received a daily intravenous dose of 0.2 mg/kg of each antibody for 10 days.

From July 1985 to May 191, 45 consecutive patients have been enrolled from 20 different centers in France, Belgium, Canada and the USA. Nineteen patients have received a bone marrow transplantation either from a matched unrelated donor or from a mismatched related donor. Eleven patients were kidney recipients, 9 received an heart transplant, 2 heart and lung, 2 lung, 1 liver and 1 a mesentric cluster transplant. In the participation centers, enrollment included 95% of bone marrow recipients that developend BLPD and 65% of organ transplant recipients who developped BLPD.

Results of the treatment in the 26 first patients have been reported previously [3,12]. Characteristics of BLPD are very similar in these 45 cases compared to the first 26. The median interval between organ transplantation and the onset of BLPD is 180 days compared with 109 days in the first cohort. Multiple sites of BLPD were present in 40 patients. Among organ transplant recipients who developped a BLPD, 21 had severe injection episodes that required aggressive immunosuppression.

Tolerance of the treatment has been acceptable. Transient neutropenia occurred in all patients. One patient who received therapy for longer than 10 days developed anti-idiotypic immunoglobulin antibodies that induced transient hypotension. In most of the patients, neither normal nor abnormal B cells were detectable in the circulation after 2 days of treatment. This criterion was used as a minimal index of target saturation at least in the circulation. Twenty percent of the patients required doubling of antibody doses to eliminate circulating B lymphocytes. In two patients with high B cell counts (up to 10,000/mL), antibody doses up to 2 mg/kg/infusion were insufficient to eradicate B cells from the blood. In twenty six out of 45 patients, a complete remission was achieved within 10 days to 2 months with a 10-day course

Table 1. B-cell lymphoproliferative disorders after transplantation: therapy and outcome related to syndrome

Type	Treatment	Survival (%)
Localized	Reduce immunosuppression, surgical resection	74
"Mononucleosislike syndrome" (kidney-liver)	Reduce immunosuppression, a cyclovir	>50
Multivisceral	Reduce immunosuppression, acyclovir, chemotherapy, irradiation	<10
Lymphomas (abnormal karyotype)	Chemotherapy, irradiation	<10

Table 2. Survival of patients with B-cell lymphoproliferative disorders based on tumor clonality

	Number Patients	Number Surviving
Marrow		
Oligoclonal	11	6
Monoclonal	6	0 } 6
Undetermined	2	0
Total	*19*	
Organ		
Oligoclonal	12	10
Monoclonal	11	5 } 17
Undetermined	3	2
Total	*26*	

of anti-B cell monoclonal antibodies (Table 1). In three additional patients, additional infusions of monoclonal anti-B cell antibodies were required (see below). Partial responses occurred in 5 patients. Interestingly, in 3 of 5 the BLPD progressed in the central nervous system but was no longer detectable in the peripheral blood. In 11 patients, there was no response to treatment. Neither prolongation of the duration of treatment in 2 patients, nor increasing the dose in 2 others resulted in control of the disease. These patients also failed to respond to other treatment such as a-interferon or chemotherapy.

As shown in Table 2, BLPD that was oligoclonal (detection of B lymphoblasts with distinct but limited immunoglobulin gene rearrangements or immunoglobulin isotypes expression) were more likely to respond than patients with monoclonal BLPD. These data must be interpreted cautiously, since clonality studies in one or a limited number of tumor sites may not reflect the general behavior of the disease and sampling artifact may lead to confusion [8]. Despite this limitation, patients with monoclonal BLPD can be effectively treated with anti-B cell antibodies, in contrast to our preliminary observations [12]. However, BLPD occurring in marrow transplant recipients appears more resitant to therapy.

Only 2 relapses occurred in the 29 patients who achieved a complete remission.

Interestingly, these two patients had prolonged immunodeficiency – one developped grade IV graft-versus-host disease that required the use of further immunosuppression, and the second had a primary immunodeficiency (Wiskott-Aldrich syndrome) and rejected his transplant. In the latter patient, 4 additional infusions of the ant-B cell antibodies effectively controlled the B cell proliferation.

In two patients, failure of the treatment was associated with defective expression of both CD21 and CD24 molecules on the surface of the B cell lympoblasts. One of these patients received an infusion of a CD23 specific murine monoclonal antibody (IOB8) (0,2 mg/kg/day/12 days), and a complete remission was induced within 4 weeks.

Central nervous system (CNS) involvement with the BLPD was detected in 5/45 patients. Intravenous infusion of anti-B cell antibodies failed to induce regression of CNS infiltration, while the other tumor sites responded to therapy. a-Interferon was used in one patient, but it was also ineffective. Neither anti-B cell antibodies nor a-Interferon could be detected in the cerebrospinal fluid [23] indicating that the integrety of the blood brain barrier was maintained. Thus, another approach was necessary to allow drug delivery to brain lesions. Cerebral lympomas can be successfully treated with local infusion of chemotherapy through an Ommaya reservoir. Similarly, enterovirus meningoencephalitis in agammaglobulinemic patients has been successfully treated with gammaglobulin infusions into the third ventricle delivered through the same device. Therefore, an Ommaya reservoir was placed in two of these five patients, and they received daily infusions of anti/CD21 antibody with an escalating dose protocol from 0.1 mg and 2 mg, respectively. This treatment was not associated with any side effects (the antibody was not reactive in vitro with any cerebral structure), and it resulted in CSF antibody concentrations of approximately 40 mg/ml. Progressive shrinkage of intracerebral tumors was observed [23], and both patients are still in complete remission 16 and 3 months, respectively, after the completion of the treatment.

As shown in Figure 1, a majority of the patients in whom a CR was achieved have survived. The median follow-up is 20 months. Organ transplant recipients had a better survival rate than marrow transplant recipients (Table 3). Five of 21 patients with oligoclonal BLPD in complete remission

Table 3. Outcome of patients with B-cell lymphoproliferative disorders after transplantation

	No. Patients	Complete Remission	Survival
Marrow	19	10	6
Kidney	11	7	6
Heart	9	6	6
Heart/lungs	2	2	2
Lung	2	2	2
Liver	1	1	1
Cluster	1	1	0
Totals	*45*	*29*	*23*

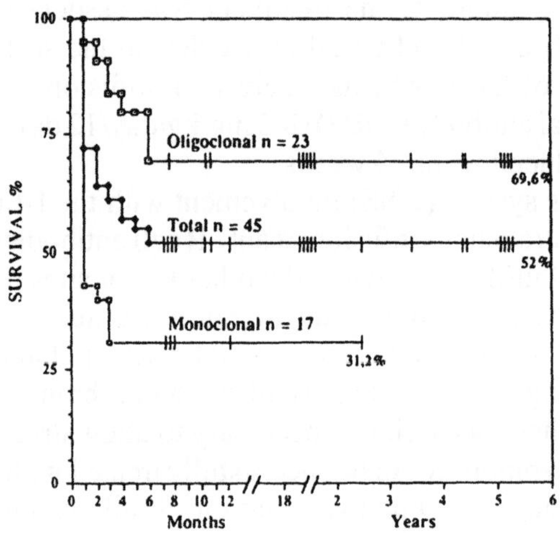

Fig. 1. Treatment of B-cell lymphoproliferative disorders by anti-B cell antibodies.

in the context of graft rejection (n = 1), graft-versus-host disease with recurrence of BLPD (n = 1). One of six patients monoclonal BLPD in complete remission died two months later from severe cytomegalovirus infection. All other patients (n = 23) are alive in unmaintained complete remission. Most of them have developed a normal profile of anti-EBV antibodies (presence of anti-Epstein Barr virus nuclear antibodies -anti-EBNA-) and have normal blood gammaglobulin levels with the exception of two marrow transplant recipients who have a persistent hypogammaglobulinemia.

Deaths in patients who enter complete remission cannot be considered as toxicity of the treatment, since they occurred after a significant disease-free interval in patients who had a persisting T cell immunodeficiency. One of the patients who died sepsis was still receiving intravenous gammaglobulin replacement for infection prophylaxis after bone marrow transplantation. None of them where neutropenic.

Compared to the known poor prognosis of patients with severe BLPD (multiorgan involvement, monoclonal phenotype, lack of response to reduction of immunosuppression or BLPD occurring after marrow transplantation), it appears that anti B cell monoclonal antibody therapy is very effective. (Figure 1, Table 2). For instance, no more than 3 out of 37 marrow transplant recipients with BLPD and no more than 4 out of 23 heart transplant recipients with BLPD reported in the literature have survived, compared with 6/19 and 6/9 respectively who received anti-B cell antibodies [1,11,17,20,24,27]. In our series, four prognostic factors could be defined: (1) clonality (with the limitations discussed above), (2) marrow transplantation (6/19 survivors versus 17/26 among organ transplant recipients), (3) central nervous system involvement, and (4) the presence of large numbers of circulating B lymphoblasts.

Mechanism of action and the scid mouse model

One of the obvious advantages of this therapy is its limited toxicity. Similarly, a-Interferon and high dose gammaglobulin has limited toxicity, but its efficacy requires confirmation. A major advantage of these treatments and a key component of their ability to control BLPD is that they do not increase the patient's immunoincompetence. Antibodies induce B cell destruction, as demonstrated by the disappearance of B cells from the bood in treated patients. B cell destruction cannot be due to complement dependent cytotoxicity, since murine IgG1 antibodies do not bind human complement. It is more likely that B lymphocytes are cleared by opsonization and/or antibody dependent cellular cytotoxicity. These antibodies per se are not able to block B cell proliferation in vitro. Infusions of these anti-B cell antibodies may recuce the B cell tumor burden to a point were the cytotoxic T cells other effector's ability to kill residual transformed B cells is restored. This hypothesis is supported by several lines of evidence. As discussed above, BLPD relapses only occurred in patients in whom immunodeficiency persisted for prolonged periods. Similarly, in a small group of patients with primary BLPD, initial remissions were followed by relapses (unpublished data), presumably because no cell-mediated immunity was capable of permanently suppressing the B cell clones.

EBV transformed B cells can grow in vivo in scid mice, resulting in a fatal lymphoproliferative disease 5. Taking advantage of this system, we asked whether murine anti-human B cell antibodies can control human B cell proliferation in vivo in scid mice. Scid mice were infused with 5×10^6

cells from three different B cells lines which were obtained from 3 patients with BLPD. The tumor development is invariably fatal within 60 days. For two of the B cell lines used, infusion of either CD21, CD24 or CD23-specific antibodies intravenously caused the tumor disappearance in at least 80% of the mice with peritoneal tumors [10]. The third line gave rise to resistant disease, similar to the pattern observed in the patient donor. Following remission 30 to 50% of mice relapsed within 30 to 70 days, providing a very strong indication that persistence of low number of residual B cells can provoke a second tumor ave in the absence of efficient cytotoxic cells [10]. Correlation of findings in scid mice and in humans is important, because it allows further usage of this model as a test system for therapeutic agents against human B cell tumors.

Perspectives

The use of monoclonal antibodies in the treatment of BLPD can be developed in several directions. The selection of antibodies with higher affinity to B cell antigens, the use of combinations of antibodies for distinct specifities, and use of antibodies as a carrier for toxins or radionuclides to increase their efficacy. Combination with a-interferon and/or cytotoxic T cells and other non-T effector cells are also worth testing. The scid mouse model offers an opportunity for such screening of valuable therapeutic agents.

Acknowledgements

We are gratefully indebted to the following physicians who took care of the patients in this multicenter study:

Dr. M. Hallé (Hôpital de la Reine Fabiola, Brussels), Dr. J. Lazarovits (London, Ontario), Dr. G. Souillet (Hematology, Hôpital E. Herriot, Lyon), Dr. J. S. Mercatello (Intensive Care, Hôpital E. Herriot, Lyon), Dr. J. L. Garnier (Nephrology, Hôpital E. Herriot, Lyon), Dr. J. F. Mornex (Pneumology, Hôpital L. Pradel, Lyon), Dr. A. Mahmoud (St Jude Hospital, Memphis), Dr. P. Bordigoni (Pediatrics, Nancy), Dr. Y. Blanloeil (Intensive Care, Bichat, Paris), Dr. J. Le Bidois, Dr. S. Blanche, Dr. J. L. Stéphan, Dr. F. Le Deist, Dr. N. Brousse, Dr. P. Niaudet, Dr. J. De Block (Hôpital des Enfants-Malades, Paris), Dr. C. Legendre (Hôpital Necker, Paris), Dr. V. Leblond, Dr. M. Raphaël, Dr. L. Sutton (Hematology, Pitié, Paris), Dr. Benz-Lemoine (Hematology, CHR, Strasbourg).

We also thank Dr. M. Hirn, Immunotech, Marseilles, for providing the anti-B cell antibodies.

This work has been supported by an institutional grant from INSERM and a grant from La Ligue Nationale contre le Cancer.

References

1. Ash RC, Casper JT, Chitambar CR, et al. Successful allogeneic transplantation of T-cell-depleted bone marrow from closely HLA-matched unrelated donors. N Engl J Med 1990; 322: 485–494.
2. Birx DL, Redfields RR, Tosato G. Defective regulation of EBV infection in patients with acquired immunodeficiency syndrome or AIDS-related disorders. N Engl J Med 1986; 314: 874–879.
3. Blanche S, L Deist F, Veber F, et al. Treatment of severe Epstein–Bar virus-induced polyclonal B-lymphocyte proliferation by anti-B-cell monoclonal antibodies. Ann Intern Med 1988; 108: 199-203.
4. Brown SL, Levy R. Treatment of B cell lymphomas with antiidiotype antibodies alone and in combination with a-IFN. Blood 1989; 73: 651–657.
5. Cannon MJ, Pisa P, Fox RI, Cooper NR. Epstein–Bar virus induces aggressive lymphoproliferative disorders of human B cell origin in SCID/hu chimeric mice. J Clin Invest 1980; 85: 1333–1337.
6. Cohen JI. EBV lymphoproliferative disease associated with acquired immunodefiency. Medicine 1991; 70: 137–160.
7. Crawford DH, Mulholland N, Iliescu V, Hawkins R, Powles R. Epstein–Bar virus infection and immunity in bone marrow transplant recipients. Transplantation 1986; 42: 50–54.
8. D'Amore ESG, Manivel JC, Gajl-Peczalska KJ, Litz CE, Copenhauer CM, Shapiro RS, Strickler JG. B-cell lymphoproliferative disorders after bone marrow transplant. Cancer 1991; 68: 1285–1295.
9. Deeg HJ, Storb R, Thomas ED. Bone marrow transplantation: a review of delayed complications. Br J Haematol 1984; 57: 185–208.
10. Durandy A, Brousse N, Rosenberg F, de Saint Basile G, Fischer Am, Fischer A. Control of human B cell tumor growth in SCID mice by monoclonal anti-B cell antibodies, J Clin Invest 1992; 90: 945–952.
11. Fischer A, Griscelli C, Friedrich W, et al. Bone marrow transplantation for immunodeficiencies and osteopetrosis: European survey, 1968–1985. Lancet 1986; 2: 1980–1084.
12. Fischer A, Blanche S, Le Bidois J, et al. Anti-B-cell monoclonal antibodies in the treatment of severe B-cell lymphoproliferative syndrome following bone marrow and organ transplantation. N Engl J Med 1991; 324: 1451–1456.
13. Frizzera G, Hanto DW, Gajl-Peczalska KJ, et al. Polymorphic diffuse B cell hyperplasias and lymphomas in renal transplant recipients. Cancer Res 1981; 41: 4642 4279.
14. Hanto DW, Frizzera G, Gajl-Peczalska KJ, Simmons Rl. Epstein–Barr virus, immunodeficiency, and B-cell lymphoproliferation. Transplantation 1985; 39: 461–472.
15. Hanto DW, Birkenbach M, Frizzera G, Gajl-Peczalska KJ, Simmons RL, Schubach WH. Confirmation of the heterogeneity of posttransplant Epstein–Barr virus-associated B cell proliferation by immunoglobulins gene rearrangement analyses. Transplantation 1989; 47: 458–464.
16. Hanto DW, Frizzera G, Gajl-Peczalska KJ, Balfour HH Jr, Simmons RL, Naharian JS. Acyclovir therapy of Epstein–Barr virus induced posttransplant lymphoproliferative diseases. Transplant Proc 1985; 17: 89–92.
17. Ho M, Jaffe R, Miller G, et al. The frequency of Epstein–Barr virus infection and associated lymphoproliferation syndrome after transplantation and its manifestations in children. Transplantation 1988; 45: 719–727.
18. Pirsch JD, Stratta RJ, Sollinger HW, et al. Treatment of severe Epstein–Barr virus-induced lymphoproliferative syndrome with ganciclovir: two cases after solid organ transplantation. Am J Med 1989; 86: 241–244.

19. Schubach WH, Miller G, Thomas ED. Epstein–Barr virus genomes are restricted to secondary neoplastic cells following bone marrow transplantation. Blood 195; 65: 525–538.
20. Shapiro RS, McClain K, Frizzera G, et al. Epstein–Barr virus associated B cell lymphoproliferative disorders following bone marrow transplantation. Blood 1988; 71: 1234–1243.
21. Shapiro RS, Chauvenet A, McGuire W, et al. Treatment of B-cell lymphoproliferative disorders with interferon alpha and intravenous gamma globulin. N Engl J Med 1988; 318: 1334.
22. Starzl TE, Nalesnick MA, Porter KA, et al. Reversibility of lymphomas after lymphoproliferative lesions developing under cyclosporin-steroid therapy. Lancet 1984; 1: 583–587.
23. Stephen JL, Le Deist F, Blanche S, et al. Treatment of central nervous system B lymphoproliferative syndrome by local infusion of a B cell-specific monoclonal antibody. Transplantation 1992; 3: 83–100.
24. Swinnen LJ, Constanzo-Nordin MR, Fisher SG, et al. Increased incidence of lymphoproliferative disorder after immunosuppression with the monoclonal antibody OKT3 in cardiac transplant recipients. N Engl J Med 1990; 323: 1723–1728.
25. Thomas JA, Hotchin NA, Aliday MJ, et al. Immunohistology of Epstein–Barr virus-associated antigens in B cell disorders from immunocompromised individuals. Transplantation 1990; 49: 944–953.
26. Young L, Alfieri C, Hennesy K, et al. Expression of Epstein–Barr virus transformation-associated genes in tissues of patients with EBV lymphoproliferative disease. N Engl J Med 1989; 321: 1080-1085.
27. Zutter MM, Martin PJ, Sale GE, et al. Epstein–Barr virus lymphoproliferation after bone marrow transplantation. Blood 1988; 72: 520–529.

32. Antibody treatment of lymphoma: experience and prospects

GEORGE T. STEVENSON, MARTIN J. GLENNIE &
TERRY J. HAMBLIN

Introduction

Lymphomas which appear after transplantation fare poorly with standard chemotherapeutic regimes, so a report on the therapeutic use of antibody in these cases has aroused considerable interest [1]. We present here our experience with antibody treatment of lymphomas in general, and discuss the prospects for applying some of our newer antibody derivatives to treating the post-transplantation tumours.

Most lymphomas treated with antibody have been tumours which recurred after two or more courses of chemotherapy. They are necessarily long-standing, and likely to be driven by multiple oncogenic lesions. In contrast most lymphomas which appear after transplantation must be of relatively recent onset: if the risk of lymphoma in transplant recipients is raised some 20-fold [2], then it follows that the transplantation and its associated immunosuppression have had a major role in oncogenesis in 95% of cases. Consistent with this view is the fact that many of the tumours on presentation are overtly polyclonal, and so presumably at an early stage of evolution. The fact that it is these which have done best when treated with native monoclonal antibody [1,3] is an encouragement to developing more potent antibodies in order to attack the monoclonal lymphomas.

Two modes of attack by antibody are considered in this paper: the recruitment of natural effectors (complement, and cells bearing Fc-receptors (FcR)) by the Fc component of the antibody; and delivery by the antibody of a ribosome-inactivating protein (RIP) such as ricin or saporin. Note that in general different antigenic targets are required for these functions. Thus in the case of B-cell lymphomas an attack on CD22 but not on CD19 or CD37 will deliver saporin effectively [4], whereas we have found the opposite to be true for recruitment of natural effectors. These differences are believed

J.L. Touraine et al. (eds.), Cancer in Transplantation. Prevention and Treatment, 289–298.

to reflect different modes and rates of internalization involved in the normal turnover of these antigens at the cell surface.

Chemical engineering at the antibody hinge

For some years we have engaged in chemical engineering of antibody molecules in order to supplement monoclonal and recombinant technologies in the search for better therapeutic derivatives. Our earliest venture was simply to remove one of the Fab arms from an anti-idiotype antibody which was being used to treat an animal lymphoma [5]. The resulting univalent antibody, consisting of a single Fabγ joined to Fcγ (a molecule known as Fab/c), had considerably enhanced anti-tumour activities both in vitro and in vivo. This reflects the fact that the target molecule involved (surface Ig) was one with considerable ability to undergo antigenic modulation, a term referring to the rapid aggregation and internalization of surface antigen-antibody complexes which thwarts the recruitment of cytotoxic effectors by the antibody Fc region. Further work on chemical engineering led to chimeric [6] and multi-Fc [7] antibodies. We can now present a set of antibody modules (Fig. 1) which may be combined in a variety of stoichiometries and geometries [8]. The central module is antibody Fab$'\gamma$, of monoclonal or recombinant origin. Sulphydryl(SH) groups on cysteine residues at the Fab$'\gamma$ hinge are made available by reduction of interchain disulphide (SS) bonds. They can then be used to form links to other modules, either via thioether bonds, which are stable in vivo, or via SS bonds, which are readily cleaved by reduction in vivo (particularly in the intracellular milieu). As shown in the figure, Fab$'\gamma$ from mouse IgG1 and IgG2a may be prepared with either five or one SH group available for linking [8]. The loss of the normal heavy-light SS bond in Fab(SH)$_5$ does not affect the integrity of the molecule, nor cause any detectable loss of antibody affinity.

In Fig. 2 we depict four antibody derivatives arising from chemical engineering: the mouse/human chimeras FabFc$_2$ and *bis*FabFc; bispecific Fab$_2$ designed to deliver the type I RIP saporin [9]; and the immunotoxin Fab$_2$-Saporin$_2$. The chimeric molecules have dual Fc regions designed to enhance the recruitment of complement and effector cells, all of which require a multiplicity of weak interactions for adequate activation. Fig. 3a demonstrates that the presence of a second Fc region on an anti-CD37 antibody enhances the titre for ADCC (antibody-dependent cellular cytotoxicity) some 10-fold. A similar enhancement is seen in the titre for complement lysis [7]. The univalent FabFc$_2$ is designed to avoid antigenic modulation, reflecting our experience with Fab/c. It should be noted, however, that univalency does not wholly avoid modulation in vivo [10]. It appears that the interaction of FcR-bearing cells with antibody-coated targets effectively cross-links the antibody, so signalling the cell under attack to clear its surface of antigen-antibody complexes [11]. Choice of a suitable molecular target – non-modulating or only

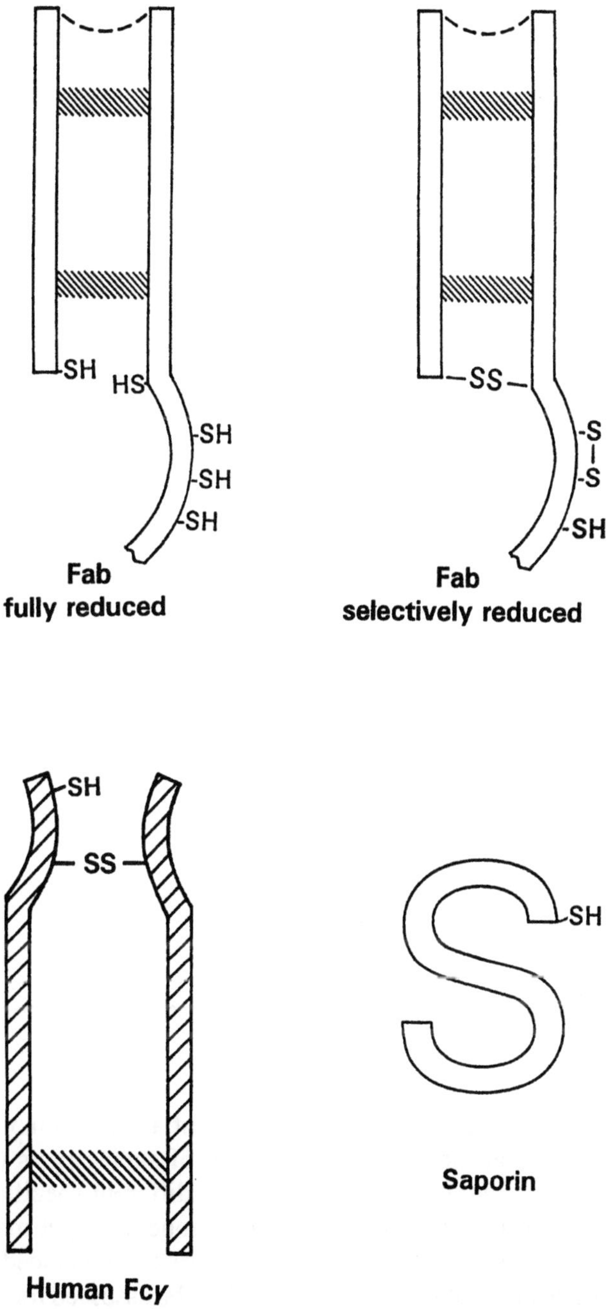

Fig. 1. Modules which form the basis of the chemical engineering discussed in this paper. The two depicted varieties of Fab are derived from mouse IgG1 or IgG2a, which is digested by pepsin to give $F(ab'\gamma)_2$, and then reduced to give $Fab(SH)_5$ or (with additional SS-interchange) $Fab(SH)_1$ [8]. Saporin contains no endogenous SH group: it must be added by reaction with 2-iminothiolane, or with a linker such as SMPT [14].

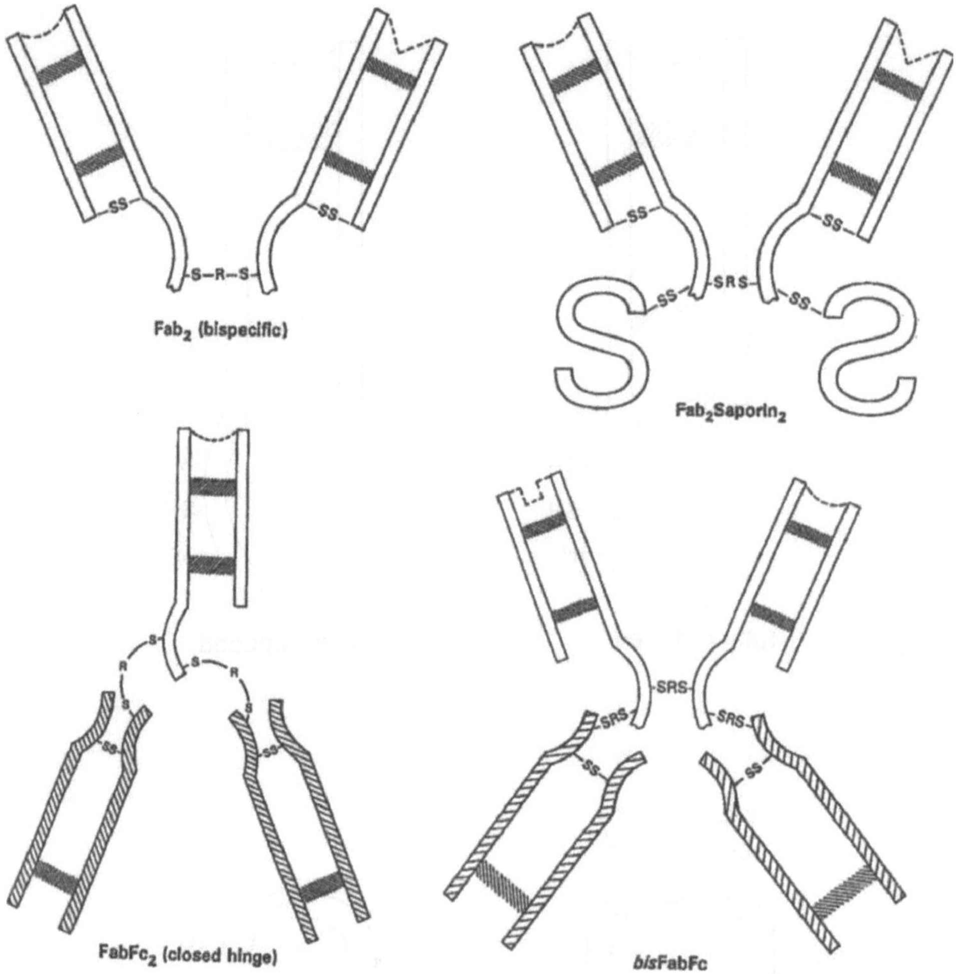

Fig. 2. Four antibody derivatives constructed by chemical engineering which have been examined in our laboratory.

slowly modulating – is possibly just as important as univalency in avoiding modulation, and we are investigating a group of such targets (CD 19, 20, 37, 38). Addition to $FabFc_2$ of a second Fab of different specificity, to form the bispecific, dual-Fc *bis*FabFc, expands the range of target molecules and further enhances the ADCC titre (Fig. 3b). The risk of enhanced modulation attending the presence of the second Fab needs to be assessed for each antigen pair involved.

Bispecific Fab_2 (anti-tumour/anti-saporin) best delivers saporin to the cell when a mixture of two derivatives, containing different anti-saporin Fabs directed at non-overlapping epitopes on the toxin molecule, is used [12]. In this way two cell-bound antibodies are able to chelate a single saporin

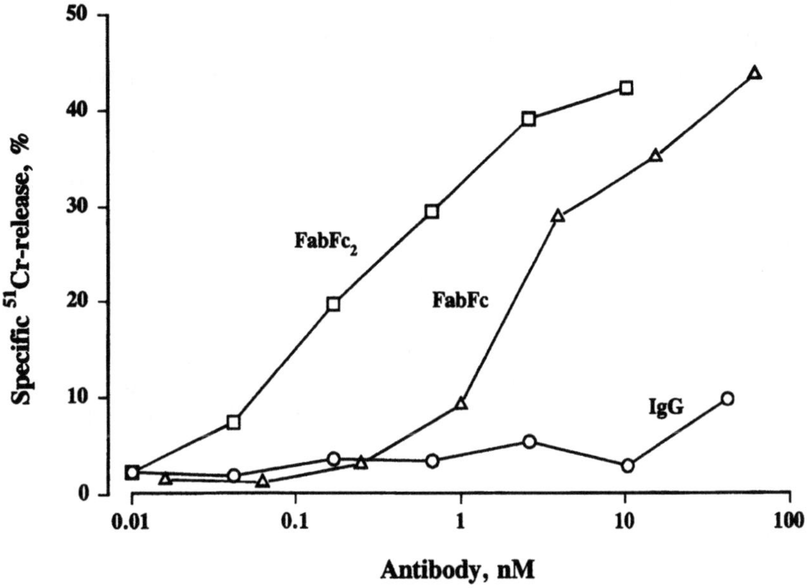

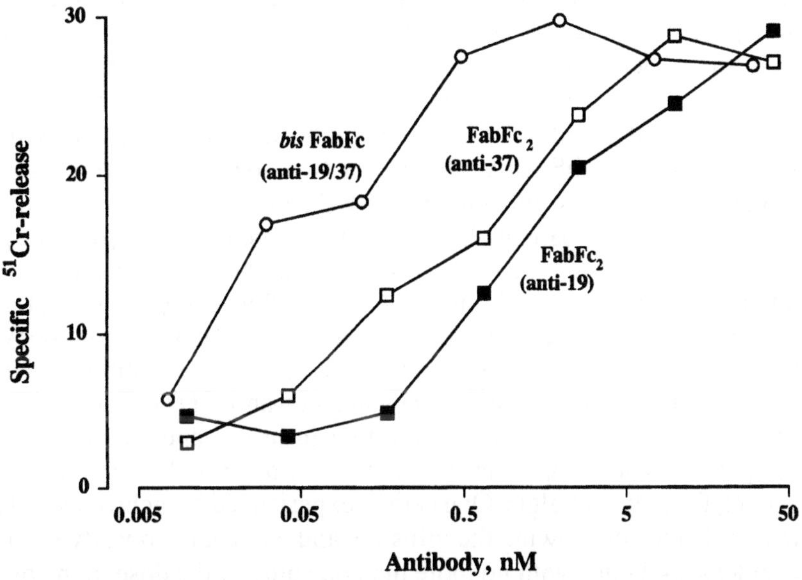

Fig. 3. Antibody-dependent cellular cytotoxicity. The Daudi B-cell line was coated with antibody for 60 min at 20°, effector cells (normal human blood mononuclears) were added at an effector: target ratio of 50:1, and the cell suspension was incubated at 37°. The antibody concentrations given are those in the final cell suspension. The extent of killing was quantified by release of ^{51}Cr from the Daudi cells after 3.5 hours: the killing is then at a low level but the random error is small. The points are averages of duplicates, and allowance has been made for release of ^{51}Cr in the absence of antibody. (a) Univalent chimeric antibodies with one or two Fc modules are compared with the parent mouse monoclonal IgG. (b) *Bis*FabFc is compared with its two univalent equivalents.

molecule with their outwardly oriented Fab arms, binding it firmly to the cell prior to internalization. Delivery of the toxin in this way avoids the need to subject it to chemical manipulation, and avoids also the complication seen with conventional immunotoxins of delivery being influenced by Fc-FcR interactions [13]. Our use of the antibody in animal and human lymphoma has entailed prior incubation of antibody and saporin in vitro, so that preformed immune complexes are infused into the subject. The immunotoxin $Fab_2Saporin_2$ (Fig. 2) also avoids the problem of Fc-directed routing in vivo, and presents less complicated pharmacokinetics than the bispecific antibody. The possibility of reduction of the Fab-saporin SS bond in extracellular fluid before delivery to the target cell is minimized by having it hydrophobically shielded [14]. We have as yet not reached a decision as to whether the bispecific or immunotoxin approach to delivery of RIP is preferable.

Therapeutic experience

It is interesting to compare our results in the clinical use of two of the derivatives in Fig. 2, the chimeric $FabFc_2$ and the RIP-delivery system Fab_2/saporin. Although the experience is limited it is broadly in line with that of others [15,16] and provides hints of a strategy for antibody therapy of tumour.

Table 1 sets out details of ten patients who have been treated with the chimeric derivative $FabFc_2$. Antibodies of two specificities were used for each patient: anti-CD37, plus either anti-CD19 or anti-CD38 according to tumour phenotype. All patients had had extensive chemotherapy apart from patient 3, who requested an initial trial with antibody, and patient 9 who presented with a pelvic lymphoma 19 months after receiving a renal graft. The antibody was usually given over three weeks, with two infusions per week of alternating specificities; in patient 9 the availability of antibody dictated successive 3-week courses of anti-CD38 and then anti-CD37. Toxicity tended to manifest shortly after beginning the first infusion, and was more likely in those patients with neoplastic cells present in the blood. Commonly there were rigors, fever and myalgia. One patient experienced bronchospasm. These problems subsided on slowing the infusion, and we would now advise giving it over at least 24 hours, with no more than one quarter the dose in the first 12 hours. Two patients experienced arthralgia for 2 days post-infusion without apparent arthropathy. Symptoms rarely attended the second and subsequent infusions. Post-infusion falls in platelet count could cause concern if the initial count was less than 40 000/μl. No long-term problems were encountered, and only one anti-antibody response was noted (an anti-idiotype response to one only of the antibodies in patient 3).

In all patients the numbers of antigen-positive cells in the blood fell rapidly, and any B symptoms (malaise, sweats, fever) subsided. However reductions in the size of solid tumour which could qualify as complete or partial responses

Table 1. Patients treated with $FabFc_2$ antibody.

Patient	Age & sex	Diagnosis[a]	Stage	Neopl. cells in blood (10^9/l)	Courses of chemo-therapy	$FabFc_2$ Specif.	Doses	Total mg	Toxicity[b]	Outcome[c]
1	57M	SLL	4B	24	>2	CD37	4	400	2	MR[d]
						CD19	4	400		
2	67M	FCL, I	4A	0	>2	CD37	3	400	1	Stable
						CD19	3	400		
3	56F	FCL, II	3B	0	0	CD37	3	400	2	Progression
						CD19	3	400		
4	62M	FCL, II	4B	4	>2	CD37	3	400	2	MR[d]
						CD19	3	400		
5	63F	FCL, I[e]	4B	0	>2	CD37	3	500	2	PR[f]
						CD38	3	500		
						CD37	3	700	1	PR[f]
						CD38	3	700		
6	53M	CLL/SLL	4B	80	>2	CD37	3	900	2	MR[d]
						CD19	3	900		
7	51M	SLL	4A	18	>2	CD37	3	900	1	Stable[d]
						CD19	3	900		
8	38M	MCL	4B	0.8	>2[g]	CD37	3	800	1	Stable[d]
						CD19	3	800		
9	55F	DLBL	1E	0	0	CD37	3	500	0	CR[h]
						CD38	3	500		
10	28M	Mediast LBL	3B	0	>2	CD37	3	600	2	PR[i]
						CD38	2	400		

[a] According to Revised European American Lymphoma Classification. SLL: small lymphocytic lymphoma. FCL: follicle-centre lymphoma, grade I, II or III. CLL: chronic lymphocytic leukaemia. MCL: mantle-cell lymphoma. DLBL: diffuse large B-cell lymphoma. Mediast LBL: mediastinal subtype of diffuse large B-cell lymphoma.
[b] Ranked 1 (mild) to 4 (life-threatening) according to WHO criteria. Numbers refer to the manifestation of toxicity achieving the highest rank: this was fever in all patients except RH, where it was hypotension.
[c] Measured according to WHO criteria, with the reported degree of response sustained for one month or longer. CR: complete response. PR: partial response ($\geq$50% decrease in total tumour size). MR: minor response (25–50% decrease).
[d] The indicated response of the tumour masses was accompanied by an initial removal of >90% of neoplastic cells from the blood.
[e] A T-cell rich FCL.
[f] First remission lasted 18 months. Upon relapse a second course of antibody yielded a second partial remission.
[g] Previous treatment also included Campath-H antibody (humanized anti-CD25) and an autologous marrow transplant.
[h] A post-transplantation lymphoma. Complete remission remained intact 15 months after therapy.
[i] Therapy truncated by occurrence of subclavian vein thrombosis.

occurred in only three patients. The reductions occurred slowly, over a period of up to six weeks after ending treatment. They tended to be of useful duration: for example in patient 5 the remission lasted for 18 months, and was then reinstituted by a second course of antibody. The durable suppression of tumour which has not been entirely eradicated is probably related to the excellent metabolic half-life which can be achieved with chimeric antibody: for example in patient 5 the $t^1/_2$ of antibody remaining in the blood after completing the first course of antibody was >10 days. In patient 9 it is possible that the EBV-positive tumour was eradicated by a combination of therapeutic antibody and the host's anti-EBV response, but we do not have details of the expression of EBV antigens by the tumour. Overall we failed to observe any consistent difference between those tumours which responded therapeutically and those which did not.

Treatment with bispecific antibody/saporin [17] was offered to five patients with advanced lymphoma, all of whom had relapsed after multiple courses of chemotherapy. The infusions were of pre-formed immune complexes comprising saporin and two bispecific $F(ab'\gamma)_2$, anti-CD22/anti-saporin(1) and anti-CD22/anti-saporin(5). The antibodies were present in equal amounts, with a molar ratio of total antibody to saporin of 3.0. Infusions took place over periods of up two hours, with progressively increasing doses up to a maximum of 10 mg saporin weekly. The highest total given to a single patient was 34 mg saporin over a period of 140 days. Toxicity was minimal. Three patients experienced local inflammation over the vein used for infusion, and two complained of weakness and myalgia.

All five of these patients experienced some benefit. When present, tumour cells were cleared from the blood. Red cell, granulocyte and platelet counts improved, suggesting reduction of tumour in the marrow. Ascites and pleural effusions disappeared in the two patients exhibiting them. One patient showed a marked reduction in splenomegaly and two a reduction in the size of lymph nodes. Unfortunately none of these responses proved durable, and no patient could be said to be in partial remission by WHO criteria at one month post-therapy. Treatment ended in one patient because of an anti-antibody response, in three because the tumour was no longer responding, and in one because of non-compliance.

Assays of plasma concentrations revealed that the lymphoma cells could have experienced only a very brief exposures to saporin. The antibody underwent a fractional drop of about two thirds between one and 24 hours post-infusion, while the saporin level fell even more steeply and was undetectable (<4 ng/ml) at 24 hours.

Prospects

Our experience matches that of others in finding an irregular response of tumour to those antibodies dependent on recruitment of natural effectors.

Among the restricting factors which may operate here are a requirement for both antibody and effectors to permeate the tumour in sufficient amounts, the well known resistance of mammalian cells to lysis by homologous complement, and the possibility that MHC class I molcules on tumour cells can convey signals which impede ADCC by NK cells [18]. Once these poorly understood barriers are overcome the resulting remission can be prolonged, a feature probably due in part to prolonged survival of the therapeutic antibody.

In contrast, results achieved using immunotoxins resemble those described here with bispecific antibody/toxin: responses are more consistent but less durable. The toxin has only a brief metabolic half-life, whether given in immune complexes or as an immunotoxin (in which it is usually SS-bonded to the antibody moiety). Further exposures to toxin are limited by its toxicity (particularly towards vascular endothelium) and immunogenicity. There might however be a role for RIP-type toxins in initial attack on tumour, with an Fc-dependent antibody construct brought in later in the hope of improving and prolonging the initial remission. Such a stategy will require a good molecular knowledge of the tumour cell surfaces involved: one would be constrained not merely by variations in phenotype among different patients, or even among the cells of an individual tumour, but also by the suitability of a given antigen for the type of antibody attack which is envisaged. At present no tumours are understood better in this regard than the B-cell lymphomas. We feel also that the chemical engineering of antibody as outlined here offers great flexibility, both in predicting the usefulness of derivatives which one may proceed to synthesize by recombinant technology, and as manufacturing technology in its own right. Lymphomas arising in immunodeficient subjects, principally transplant recipients and AIDS patients, have proved ill suited to chemotherapy and so represent an opportunity and a challenge for immunological approaches such as we describe.

Acknowledgements

Our work is supported by Tenovus, the Cancer Research Campaign, the Leukaemia Research Fund, and the Wellcome Foundation.

References

1. Fischer A, Blanche S, Le Bedois J, Bordigoni P, Garnier J-L, Niaudet P, Morinet F, Le Deist F, Fischer AM, Griscelli C, et al. Anti-B-cell monoclonal antibodies in the treatment of severe B-cell lympoproliferative syndrome following bone marrow and organ transplantation. N Engl J Med 1991; 324: 1451–6.
2. Birkeland SA, Storm HH, Lamm LU, Barlow L, Blohme I, Forsberg B, Eklund B, Fjeldborg O, Friedberg M, Frodin L, et al. Cancer risk after renal transplantation in Nordic countries, 1964–1986. Int J Cancer 1995; 60: 183–9.

3. Leblond V, Sutton L, Dorent R, Davi F, Bitker M-O, Gabarre J, Charlotte F, Ghoussoub J-J, Fourcade C, Fischer A, et al. Lymphoproliferative disorders after organ transplantation: a report of 245 cases observed in a single center. J Clin Oncol 1995; 12: 961–8.
4. Bonardi MA, French RR, Amlot P, Gromo G, Modena D, Glennie MJ. Delivery of saporin to human B-cell lymphoma using bispecific antibody: targeting via CD22 but not CD19, CD37, or immunoglobulin results in efficient killing. Cancer Res 1993; 53: 3015–21.
5. Glennie MJ, Stevenson GT. Univalent antibody kills tumour cells in vitro and in vivo. Nature 1982; 295: 712–4.
6. Hamblin TJ, Cattan AR, Glennie MJ, MacKenzie MR, Stevenson FK, Watts HF, Stevenson, GT. Initial experience in treating human lymphoma with a chimeric univalent derivative of monoclonal anti-idiotype antibody. Blood 1987; 69: 790–7.
7. Stevenson GT, Pindar A, Slade CJ. A chimeric antibody with dual Fc regions (*bis*FabFc) prepared by manipulations at the IgG hinge. Anti-Cancer Drug Design 1989; 3: 219–30.
8. Stevenson GT, Glennie MJ, Kan KS. Chemically engineered chimaeric and multi-Fab antibodies. In: Clark M, (ed), Protein engineering of antibody molecules for prophylactic and therapeutic applications in man. Nottingham: Academic Titles 1993; 127–41.
9. Stirpe F, Gasperi-Campani G, Barbieri L, Falasca A, Abbondanza A, Stevens, WA. Ribosome-inactivating proteins from the seed of *Saponaria officinalis L.* (soapwort), of *Agrostemma gothago L.* (corn cockle) and of *Asparagus officinalis* (asparagus) and from the latex of *Hutex crepitans L.* (sandbox tree). Biochem J 1983; 216: 617–25.
10. Lane AC, Foroozan S, Glennie MJ, Kowalski-Saunders P, Stevenson GT. Enhanced modulation of antibodies coating guinea pig leukemic cells *in vitro* and *in vivo*. J Immunol 1991; 146: 2461–8.
11. Schroff RW, Farrell MM, Klein RA, Stevenson HC, Warner NL. Induction and enhancement by monocytes of antibody-induced modulation of a variety of human lymphoid cell surface antigens. Blood 1985; 66: 620–6.
12. French RR, Courtenay AE, Ingamells S, Stevenson GT, Glennie MJ. Cooperative mixtures of bispecific $F(ab')_2$ antibodies for delivering saporin to lymphoma in vitro and in vivo. Cancer Res 1991; 51: 2353–61.
13. Van Oosterhout YVJM, Van de Winkel JGJ, Preijers FWMB. Effect of isotype on internalization and cytotoxicity of CD19-ricin A immunotoxins. Cancer Res 1994; 54: 3527–32.
14. Thorpe PE, Wallace PM, Knowles PP, Relf MG, Brown ANF, Watson GJ, Knyba RE, Wawrzynczak EJ, Blakey DC. New coupling agents for the synthesis of immunotoxins containing a hindered disulfide bond with improved stability in vivo. Cancer Res 1987; 47: 5924–31.
15. Maloney DG, Liles TM, Czerwinski DK, Waldichuk C, Rosenberg J, Grillo-Lopez A, Levy R. Phase I clinical trial using escalating single-dose infusion of chimeric anti-CD20 monoclonal antibody (IDEC-C2B8) in patients with recurrent B-cell lymphoma. Blood 1994; 84: 2457–66.
16. Vitetta ES, Thorpe PE, Uhr JW. Immunotoxins: magic bullets or misguided missiles? Immunol Today 1993; 14: 252–8.
17. Bonardi MA, Bell A, French RR, Gromo G, Hamblin T, Modena D, Tutt AL, Glennie MJ. Initial experience in treating human lymphoma with a combination of bispecific antibody and saporin. Int J Cancer 1992; Suppl 7: 73–7.
18. Kärre K. Express yourself or die: peptides, MHC molecules, and NK cells. Science 1995; 267: 978–9.

33. Idiotypic vaccination against low grade follicular B cell lymphoma

JAN BRISSINCK, JIE ZHANG, MARGARET SHAW,
FREDA STEVENSON, ROBERT HAWKINS & STEPHEN RUSSELL

Introduction

B-cell non-Hodgkin's lymphomas are classified histologically into low-grade, intermediate grade and high-grade varieties. The low grade B-NHLs consist of small lymphocytic, follicular small cleaved and follicular mixed categories and comprise approximately 25 to 35% of newly diagnosed NHL. Low grade follicular lymphoma is usually disseminated (stage III-IV) at the time of diagnosis. The disease progresses very slowly without treatment, with a tendency to wax and wane with frequent spontaneous regressions and complete remissions [1]. The initial response to conventional therapies is good, however, after a period of time, relapse occurs and with each relapse the trend is for shorter remissions until the disease becomes refractory to therapy. Disease acceleration is often associated with a worsening prognosis. The median survival time is approximately 8 years regardless of the therapeutic modalities employed. A number of experimental therapies for the treatment of low grade follicular lymphomas including bone marrow transplantation, non-specific immune stimulants, cytokines, monoclonal antibodies, colony stimulating factors and idiotypic vaccines are currently under investigation.

Idiotypic vaccination

The clonally-derived population of transformed B cells in follicular NHL expresses abundant surface Ig which is not shed and whose idiotype represents a unique tumour specific antigen [2], distinguishing it from normal B cells. The surface immunoglobulin is composed of identical heavy chain-light chain heterodimers. Its antigen binding site is formed by pairing of two globular variable domains, one derived from each chain. The binding specificity of the surface immunoglobulin is mainly determined by the variability in the

J.L. Touraine et al. (eds.), Cancer in Transplantation. Prevention and Treatment, 299–304.

hypervariable loops of aminoacids embedded in the surface of the V domains of each chain. During B cell ontogeny, the V genes are derived by random assembly of smaller gene segments, such that each B cell expresses a unique combination of heavy and light chain V domains and hence a unique antigen binding site. Therefore, the antigen binding site is inherently antigenic and can itself be the target of an anti-idiotypic antibody response. There has thus been considerable interest in both active and passive immunotherapeutic strategies directed against the lymphoma idiotype on the assumption that anti-idiotypic antibodies and/or cytotoxic T lymphocytes will be capable of mediating tumour destruction.

Purified murine anti-idiotypic mAbs raised against idiotypic determinants of surface Ig expressed on follicular lymphomas have been used to treat patients in an advanced refractory stage of their disease. The antibodies were administered intravenously and several partial responses were observed, although only one patient achieved complete remission [3]. Further studies indicated that the targeted cells died by apoptosis [4]. Problems hampering the success of this approach included outgrowth of lymphoma cells expressing idiotypic variants due to somatic mutation [5], shedding of surface antigen, failure of the murine antibodies to recruit human effector functions and host response against the injected antibodies.

In light of these problems encountered with passive antibody administration, it was reasoned that active immunisation with the idiotypic immunoglobulin would be an attractive alternative. Active immunisation has the potential to induce a polyclonal anti-idiotypic antibody response against multiple idiotypic determinants on the lymphoma surface immunoglobulin thereby greatly reducing the likelihood of tumour escape by somatic mutation. Furthermore, anti-idiotypic antibodies of human origin should recruit human effector functions more efficiently and should reduce the risk of a HAMA response. Active immunisation also has the potential to stimulate cytotoxic and helper T cell responses against peptides derived from the idiotypic immunoglobulin. Studies in animal models have shown that idiotype specific immunity and protection against idiotype positive lymphoma cells can be induced by idiotype vaccination [6].

Clinical studies using this approach to treat B cell malignancies have been reported by Levy and co-workers [7]. Heterohybridomas were prepared from tumour biopsies by fusion, clones expressing Ig of the same immunophenotype of the tumour were expanded, idiotypic Ig was purified from culture supernatant and conjugated to keyhole limpet haemocyanin. Patients were treated with a series of immunisations comprising of the conjugated antibodies mixed with an immunological adjuvant. Prior to vaccination, the patients were treated with conventional chemotherapy until they had minimal residual disease or were in complete remission. Idiotype-specific humoral or cell mediated immune responses were seen in eight of eleven vaccinated patients with complete tumour regression and in eight of fifteen patients with measurable residual disease. There was indication of clinical benefit in the patients showing an immune response and the toxicity of the treatment was minimal. This study therefore confirms that idiotypic vaccination is a potentially beneficial approach to the treatment of follicular lymphoma. The major limitation is the time and labour involved in the generation of each patient-specific vaccine; typically it would take several months to identify and make the antibody for immunisation of a single patient.

A genetic approach to idiotypic vaccination

We have developed a more rapid method of identifying the immunoglobulin based on DNA sequencing which can be used to isolate the idiotypic antibody V genes from a lymphoma biopsy specimen in a matter of days. Using 'universal' primers which hybridise specifically to conserved 5′ and 3′ terminal sequences (framework one and the J-region) of human antibody V genes, the polymerase chain reaction (PCR) is used to amplify all rearranged V genes in the biopsy material [8, 9]. Heavy and light chain V gene sequences are amplified in separate reactions, and a random selection of the amplified DNA fragments are cloned into a T/A cloning vector (invitrogen) and introduced into electrocompetent bacteria. Plasmid DNA is extracted from the transformed bacterial colonies and the inserts are sequenced using flanking primers to prime the sequencing reaction. Since the lymphoma V genes are predominant in the starting material they are identifiable as recurring sequences. This has been confirmed in a series of B cell malignancies by comparing the recurring V gene sequences identified by PCR with the known lymphoma idiotype sequence identified by sequencing lymphoma-derived hybridomas [10]. Rapid isolation of the lymphoma-specific idiotypic V genes is therefore well demonstrated and avoids the need for production, screening and characterisation of multiple patient-specific hybridomas.

We chose to assemble the lymphoma V genes for expression as a single chain Fv in which the heavy and light chain V domains are connected by a short flexible peptide linker $(Gly_4Ser)_3$. Expressed in this form, free of the immunoglobulin constant domains, the idiotypic determinants of the lymphoma immunoglobulin are retained because forced pairing of the heavy and light chains ensures that the antigen combining site is reconstituted. Another advantage of the single chain Fv format for idiotypic vaccination is that it avoids the risk of potentially harmful immune responses against the immunoglobulin constant domains. The idiotypic VH and VL are assembled into the single chain Fv format by a two stage PCR reaction. The cloned VH and VL sequences are re-amplified using primers with specific extensions at their 5′ ends, introducing convenient restriction sites at the 5′ end of VH (Sfi I) and the 3′ site of the VL (Not I) and a part of the linker-coding sequence at the 3′ end of VH and the 5′ end of VL. The so created overlapping 3′

and 5′ ends of the amplified VH and VL sequences can now anneal to each other. In the second stage of the PCR assembly, both PCR products are mixed and extended from their central region of overlap to create an scFv template which is amplified using the Sfi I and Not I-tailed outer primers that were used in the first stage. The resulting PCR product can now be cloned into a bacterial or mammalian expression plasmid by use of the introduced Sfi I and Not I restriction sites.

Purification of the expressed single chain Fv protein is, however, time consuming and appears to be entirely unnecessary. Rather than introduce the expression plasmid into bacteria and purify the protein from the culture supernatant, the plasmid can be inoculated directly into the muscle whereupon is taken up and expressed by muscle cells near the injection site. It has been observed that DNA plasmid injected into the mouse muscle resulted in expression of the gene with greater efficiency than in other tissues [11]. The expression was found to be long lived and there is a linear relationship of expression with the dose of DNA injected. This process bypasses the need to purify protein or to use immunological adjuvants in the vaccination preparation. These observations have been extended to other species [12]. Animal studies showed that genetic vaccination is a more effective way of inducing an anti-idiotype response than vaccination with single chain Fv protein in Freund's adjuvant [13]. recently it has been demonstrated that plasmid vaccination induces T cell as well as anti-idiotypic B cell responses [14].

On the basis of these studies patient-specific idiotypic DNA vaccines for genetic immunisation against established low grade follicular lymphoma were generated. Apart from the speed and simplicity of the approach which avoids the need for immunological adjuvants, there are other potential advantages compared to previous protein-based vaccine strategies. The immunogen in the genetic vaccine is formatted as single chain Fv which will avoid potentially harmful responses against the immunoglobulin constant domains present in previously tested protein vaccines. Continued synthesis of the single chain Fv fragment in muscle cells following immunisation with DNA prolongs the supply of native antigen compared to challenge with preformed protein and there is an obvious analogy with live attenuated viral vaccines which stimulate superior immune responses compared to killed viral vaccines. Furthermore the single chain Fv should be expressed from inoculated cells in a folded form, helping to ensure that the humoral response is directed against native rather than denatured protein. By contrast, preformed protein inoculated with adjuvant may be significantly denatured and lead to production of antibodies against epitopes on denatured protein. Since the idiotypic immunoglobulin will be manufactured in muscle cells *in vivo*, it is possible that idiotype-derived peptides will be displayed at the surface of these cells in association with class I MHC molecules and will stimulate idiotype-specific CTL responses. Presentation to T cells might be further improved by expression of co-stimulatory molecules on the cells expressing the idiotypic antibody or by local production of interferon gamma to upregulate MHC expression.

The plasmid construct used in the mouse experiments has been redesigned for human use. The revised construct contains no retroviral sequences other than the RSV LTR which is known to drive gene expression efficiently in human cells. The expressed protein consists of a leader sequence which directs entry into the endoplasmatic reticulum, and the single chain Fv. The polyadenylation signals are derived from bovine growth hormone and the construct contains a colE1 origin of replication plus ampicillin resistance gene to allow its selection and amplification in E coli. There is also an F1 origin of replication to facilitate the preparation of single stranded DNA template for sequencing. We have started a phase I clinical trial to evaluate the safety of this construct for idiotypic vaccination as a treatment for follicular lymphoma and to determine the appropriate dose of plasmid to elicit an anti-idiotypic immune response. This study is conducted in patients with advanced disease, therefore, anti-idiotypic immune responses will probably be diminished due to immune paresis and anti-idiotype antibodies will be difficult to detect in the blood. We hope to conduct subsequent trials in patients with minimal residual disease following chemotherapy, provided the treatment proves not to be associated with toxic side effects.

References

1. Horning SJ, Rosenberg SA. The natural history of initially untreated low-grade non-Hodgkin's lymphomas. N Engl J Med 1984; 311: 1471–1475.
2. Stevenson GT, Stevenson FK. Antibody to a molecularly defined antigen confined to a tumour cell surface. Nature 1975; 254: 714–716.
3. Miller RA, Maloney DG, Warnke R, Levy R. Treatment of B-cell lymphoma with monoclonal anti-idiotype antibody. N Engl J Med 1982; 306: 517–522.
4. Vuist WMJ, Levy R, Maloney DG. Lymphoma regression induced by monoclonal anti-idiotype antibodies correlates with their ability to induce Ig signal transduction and is not prevented by tumour expression of high levels of Bcl-2 protein. Blood 1994; 83: 899–906.
5. Bahler DW, Levy R. Clonal evolution of a follicular lymphoma: evidence for antigen selection. Proc Natl Acad Sci USA 1992; 89: 6770–6774.
6. George AT, Stevenson FK. Prospects for the treatment of B cell tumours using idiotypic vaccination. Intern Rev Immunol 1989; 4: 271–310.
7. Hsu FJ, Kwak L, Campbell M, Liles T, Czerwinski D, Hart S, Syringelas A, Miller R, Levy R. Clinical trials of idiotype specific vaccine in B cell lymphomas. Ann NY Acad Sci 1993; 690: 385–387.
8. Ward ES, Gussow D, Griffiths AD, Jones PT, Winter G. Binding activities of single immunoglobulin variable domains secreted from *Escherichia Coli*. Nature 1989; 341: 544–546.
9. Marks JD, Hoogenboom HR, Bonnert TP, McCafferty J, Griffiths AD, Winter G. By-passing immunisation: human libraries from V-gene libraries displayed on phage. J Mol Biol 1991; 222: 581–597.
10. Hawkins RE, Zhu D, Ovecka M, Winter G, Hamblin TJ, Long A, Stevenson FK. Idiotypic vaccination against human B cell lymphoma. Rescue of variable region gene sequences

from biopsy material for assembly as single chain Fv personal vaccines. Blood 1994; 83: 3279–3288.

11. Wolff JA, Malone RW, Williams P, Chong W, Ascadi G, Jani A, Felgner PL. Direct gene transfer into mouse muscle *in vivo*. Science 1990; 247: 1465–1468.
12. Jiao S, Williams P, Berg RK, Hodgeman BA, Liu L, Pepetto G, Wolff JA. Direct injection in nonhuman primate myofibers *in vivo*. Hum Gene Therapy 1992; 3: 21–33.
13. Hawkins RE, Winter G, Hamblin TJ, Stevenson FK, Russell SJ. A genetic approach to anti-idiotype immunisation. J Immunother 1993; 14: 273–278.
14. Stevenson FK, Zhu D, King CA, Ashworth LJ, Kumar S, Hawkins RE. Idiotypic DNA vaccines against B cell lymphoma. Immunol Rev (1995) in press.

PART SEVEN

Conclusion

34. Immunosurveillance revisited

JEAN-LOUIS TOURAINE

More than 30 years ago, the immunosurveillance hypothesis was proposed by L. Thomas [1] and by F.M. Burnett [2–4]. The theory postulated that malignant diseases are initiated by spontaneous or induced mutations in individual cells. Such somatic-genetic alterations might be point-mutations and would occur randomly. The initial mutant cell multiplies clonally. Surveillance by the immune system, especially by T lymphocytes, recognizes the transformed cells as "almost foreign" or at least "not-self". Before the cell proliferation has reached a volume permitting tumor detection, the clone is eliminated by a mechanism comparable to that of delayed hypersensitivity or to allograft rejection. Each of us would develop several putative cancers that are rejected before being even suspected. Only when the efficiency of immunosurveillance would decrease, due to immunodeficiency or to aging for instance, the tumor would propagate and escape to this deficient immune system.

Arguments in favor of immunosurveillance

On first sight, the increased incidence of tumor occurrence in various immune defects seems to support the theory. Malignancies are indeed much more frequent in transplant patients treated with immunosuppressive drugs [5, 6], in children with congenital immunodeficiency diseases [7] and in young adults with AIDS [8] than in the general population.

The relatively recent identification of the precise role of oncogenes may also provide an explanation for the effect of a mutation that results in uncontrolled cell proliferation, and eventually tumor development.

Arguments against immunosurveillance

However, a number of phenomena do not appear to be in concordance with the initial concept of immunosurveillance:

- the theory fails to explain how surveillance is exerted in all tissues which are behind the blood-tissue barrier or in a so-called "immunologically privileged site";

J.L. Touraine et al. (eds.), Cancer in Transplantation. Prevention and Treatment, 307–310.

- many cancer cells do not exhibit specific antigens that can be recognized by T lymphocytes;
- many other factors contribute to the increased incidence of malignancies in aged people;
- many other specific and non-specific immune and genetic factors are involved in emergence of tumors;
- more importanly, the varieties of cancers which are found in immunosuppressed patients are somewhat different from those observed in the general population; some cancers, such as lung cancers, are extremely frequent in the general population and are no more frequent in immunosuppressed patients; by contrast, Kaposi's sarcomas are 500 fold more frequent, lymphomas are also extremely increased in incidence, as well as squamous cell carcinomas of the skin.

Theory of immunosurveillance revisited

Practically all malignancies which occur with a high incidence in immunosuppressed patients are virus-related cancers and a few other immunogenic cancers. Lymphomas are related to EBV, Kaposi's sarcoma to HHV-8, skin cancers to HPV, cervical cancers to HPV, hepatocellular cancers to HBV or HCV. Kidney carcinomas and melanomas are known to be immunogenic malignancies that can be treated by immunological methods and the metastases of which can regress after eradication of the large primary tumor. By contrast, in immunosuppressed patients, the chemically induced cancers do not appear to be increased in frequency. The other non-immunogenic cancers, the etiology of which is unknown, also are not more frequent in these patients. Such observations lead to the conclusion that the immune system does not exert a surveillance of all cells susceptible to undergo spontaneous mutation but may limit its activity to cells subjected to modification of surface antigens, especially as a result of a virus infection.

Immunodeficiency would merely mean that infection by oncogenic viruses are more frequent, as are the other virus infections, in patients with a deficiency of cell-mediated immunity. In addition, the immune defect is responsible for inefficiency of the mechanism in charge of rejection of virus-infected cells or of newly immunogenic cells.

Immunosurveillance revisited can propose a more limited function to the immune system in the prevention of tumors: fight against oncogenic viruses in the context of the general anti-virus immunity, fight against immunogenic cells such as kidney carcinoma or melanoma cells, and possible "surveillance" of T and B lymphocytes within the lymphoid system. Lymphocyte populations are exposed to a high risk of genetic "errors" due to virus infections and to frequent cell multiplications, and they have a sophisticated system for negative selection of "unwanted" lymphocytes. There is no evidence that, besides these particular cases, immunosurveillance exerts any role in the limitation of tumor development of any other kind.

To schematize the role of cell-mediated immunity against tumors and the possibility of escape from such an immunity, it can be said that:

- when tumor cells have no newly expressed antigens at the cell surface but have a decreased expression of HLA molecules, the host response mainly relies on NK cells;
- when tumor cells result from virus infection and transformation, some virus peptides are expressed in the groove of HLA molecules and the host can eradicate the tumor by a cytotoxic T lymphocyte response (which is generally an HLA-restricted phenomenon). The virus has the capability to mutate and the variant viruses that are then selected are those which do not induce the peptides more strongly recognized by the host cytotoxic T lymphocytes.

Perspectives for the transplant patients

From the finding that most tumors in transplant patients are virus-related and from the information on the immune system in such circumstances, it can be derived that there are hopes in the field of transplantation that eradication of an over-incidence of malignancies will be possible:

- vaccines can be envisionned against the very few viruses which are responsible for these very frequent cancers in transplant patients; the vaccination against HBV is already a step in that direction;
- infection with donor-related viruses can be limited more and more frequently by selecting donors or, in the future, by treating the transplants prior to transplantation itself;
- prevention of sexually transmitted viruses can be obtained by the use of condoms;
- avoidance of some co-factors, such as the sun responsible for an increased incidence of skin cancers, is possible;
- specific immunotherapy protocols will be developed and it is reasonable to assume that amplification of the patient's own cytotoxic T lymphocytes specific for the very tumor cells of the patient might be helpful;
- more importantly, reduction of prolonged and non-specific immunosuppression, as it is practiced usually today, will result in limitation of cancer incidence; the induction of immune tolerance will permit to avoid prolongation of immunosuppressive therapy, leaving the immune system intact with the only exception of a specific acceptance of donor antigens by the host; further virus infections or tumor development are not expected to occur frequently in such circumstances.

References

1. Thomas L. Discussion. In: Lawrence HS, editor. Cellular and humoral aspect of the hypersensitive states. Hoeber-Harfer, New York, 1959: 529–532.
2. Burnet FM. Somatic mutation and chronic disease. Br Med J 1965; 338–342.
3. Burnet FM. Self and not-self. Melbourne University Press, Australia, 1969: 3–310.
4. Burnet FM. Immunological surveillance. Oxford: Pergamon Press, 1970.
5. Kinlen LJ. Malignancies in man after organ transplantation. In: Schmähl D, Penn I, editors. Springer Verlag, Berlin Heidelberg, 1991: 18–26.
6. Penn I. Epidemiology of cancer in transplant patients. 1995. This issue.
7. Kersey JH, Spector BD, Good RA. Cancer in children with primary immunodeficiency diseases. J Pediat, 1974; 84: 263.
8. Gallo RC. AIDS and related malignancies. In: Science Challenging AIDS. Proceedings Based on the VIIth International Conference on AIDS; 1991 June 16–21; Florence. Karger, Basel, 1992.

PART EIGHT

Posters

LYMPHOPROLIFERATIVE SYNDROMES

CIRCULATING PLASMACYTOID CELLS : AN EARLY MARKER OF POST-TRANSPLANT LYMPHOPROLIFERATIVE DISORDERS

R. CAHEN[1], P. FELMAN[2], F. BERGER[3], P. TROLLIET[1], D. MOREL[2], J. PAGES[2], H.J. DELECLUZE[3], M. LABEEUW[1]

1 *Service de Néphrologie, Centre Hospitalier Lyon-Sud, 69310 Pierre Bénite*
2 *Laboratoire d'Hématologie, Centre Hospitalier Lyon-Sud, 69310 Pierre Bénite*
3 *Laboratoire d'Anatomie Pathologique, Hopital E. Herriot, Lyon*

Post-transplant lymphoproliferative disorders (PTLD) represent a dreaded complication in transplant patients. Early recognition and treatment is critical in reversing the disease. We report on 2 cases of PTLD in renal transplant recipients in whom plasmacytoid cells could be detected in peripheral blood several days before the clinical onset of the disease.

Both patients (case 1: male, 23 yrs; case 2: female, 35 yrs) received a sequential immunosuppressive regimen with ATG for 8 to 12 days, AZA, PRED and CsA started on day 7. Acute rejection crises occured in these 2 patients between days 11 and 55. Patient 1 presented 2 episodes of rejection, treated with 2 steroid pulses, a 12-day OKT3 course and 8 plasma exchanges; patient 2 presented 1 episode, treated with a steroid pulse and a 12-day OKT3 course. An infectious mononucleosis-like syndrome with fever, lymphadenomegaly, splenomegaly occured in both patients on post-transplant days 29 and 74. Lymph node and bone marrow specimens showed a proliferation made of lymphoplasmacytoid and plasma cells in case 1 and polymorphous lymphoid population with many large cells in case 2. The proliferation was shown to be polyclonal by immunophenotypic and immunogenotypic studies in each case. EBV serology showed a reactivation pattern. Expression of EBNA protein and the detection of EBV genome in tissue samples of both patients confirmed the diagnosis of EBV-associated PTLD. The 2 patients were given ganciclovir. The outcome was favorable for patient 1 after reduction of immunosuppressive treatment, but patient 2 died within a few days despite stopping immunosuppression.

Serum immunoelectrophoresis showed a polyclonal increase in immunoglobulins in 2 cases, with a restriction of heterogeneity in one. At the time of diagnosis, plasmacytoid cells were detected in the blood and represented 14 and 34% of the circulating cells in patients 1 and 2 respectively. Retrospective analysis of peripheral blood samples disclosed that plasmacytoid cells could be detected up to 14 days before the rise of serum immunoglobulins and the clinical onset of the disease.

Circulating plasmacytoid cells could be a useful warning sign of EBV-associated PTLD. A systematic search in transplant patients at risk for the development of PTLD may allow detection of the disease at an early stage, prior to clinical symptoms, when therapeutic intervention may be successful.

LYMPHOPROLIFERATIVE DISEASE IN HEART TRANSPLANT PATIENTS

Authors : C. Dufay, C. Besson, A. Pol, J.Saez De Ibarra, A. Prat, H. Warembourg.
Lille (France).

Since 1985, 239 heart transplantations have been done in Lille.

All the patients recieved a triple drug Immuno-Suppression (Cyclosporine, Azathiopine and Prednisone).

Five patients developed lymphoproliferative disease.

In three cases, the disease was limited to one localisation and in two cases it was disseminated.

The overall incidence of post-transplant lymphoproliferative disease was 2 %.

The peak occurrence after transplantation was 53,6 months (3 to 164 months).

The mortality was 40 % (two patients) : The first one developped limited disease at 66 months after transplantation and died 3 months later, the second one had a disseminated disease at 3 months and died 15 days later .

Three patients remain alive : Between them, two had a limited disease at 12 and 164 months (respectively),the follow up after diagnosis is 22 and 9 months. The third patient had a disseminated disease at 3 months and the follow up is 2 months.

All patients with a disseminated disease had an early onset (less that 1 year).

Due to acute rejection, the immunotherapy has been iscreased appropriately in four of the five patients who developed lymphoproliferative disease.

SUCCESSFUL MULTI-MODALITY THERAPY OF MONOCLONAL LYMPHOPROLIFERATIVE DISEASE IN A LUNG TRANSPLANT RECIPIENT

Adelheid End, Daniela Kandioler, Michael Grimm, Gerhard Dekan[1], Klaus Geissler[2], Mariette Vogl, Gerlinde Mitterbauer[3], Hendratti Pirc-Danoewinata[2], Walter Klepetko
Department of Surgery/Division of Cardiothoracic Surgery, Departments of [2]Medicine, [1]Pathology and [3]Laboratory Medicine, University of Vienna, Vienna, Austria

The incidence of posttransplant lymphoproliferative disease (PTLD) in lung transplant recipients is about 8 %. Prognosis of patients presenting with the monoclonal type is poor with a mortality rate up to 80 %. We report on a patient who was successfully treated by a combined therapy regimen. Double lung transplantation was performed in a 21-yr-old dwarf patient because of multiple lung cysts. Two months after operation mediastinal masses were diagnosed as monoclonal PTLD. Radiation therapy and reduction of immunosuppression failed; the PTLD showed rapid progression with appearance of additional multiple pulmonary tumors. Massive acute rejection (A4) was treated successfully by high-dose methylprednisolone for 4 days. On the 4th day, the first course of chemotherapy (CHOP) was started (Feb 28, 1992). High-dose aciclovir and ganciclovir were administered ex juvantibus and prophylactically at the same time although there were no signs of infection. As the tumor showed progression 14 days after the first chemotherapy and needle biopsy was not conclusive, the second course of chemotherapy was combined with iv infusions of monoclonal anti-CD24 antibodies. About two weeks later the tumor masses had disappeared except for a large residual node in the left upper lobe which remained constant despite continuing chemotherapy and administration of a second course of monoclonal antibodies. On Aug 24, 1992 this residual mass was resected surgically and turned out to be necrotic tissue. Up to now the patient is in a good clinical condition and free of recurrence. It is under discussion which part of the multiregimen, chemotherapy or monoclonal antibodies, contributed to the success of the therapy. As the prognosis of monoclonal PTLD is poor, however, an aggressive multi-modality approach is warranted. To our knowledge this is the first case treated successfully by both chemotherapy and monoclonal antibodies.

LYMPHOPROLIFERATIVE DISEASE LOCALIZED IN THE RENAL ALLOGRAFT. FRENCH MULTICENTRIC STUDY.

E. Renoult, M. Kessler
Centre Hospitalier et Universitaire de Nancy.

Lymphoproliferative disease (LPD) is a well-recognized complication of kidney transplantation. The B-cell proliferation may develop in a nodal site or in extranodal sites, including the transplant. In a previous retrospective analysis from a French multicentric analysis, 16 LPD localized in the renal allograft were recognized from 16 755 patients (0,095%) receiving a cadaveric renal transplant between 1952 and the beginning of 1993. All the cases were diagnosed from 1982.
Clinical and laboratory information was obtained for 15 of these patients. The mean age of the recipients was 44 years (range 19 - 67 years). Fourteen of the subjects received anti-lymphocyte globulin as induction therapy and most of the patients (13/15) received cyclosporine as their maintenance immunosuppressive treatment. Acute rejection was reported in 9 cases and was treated with methylprednisolone in 6 cases and with mono or polyclonal antibodies for 3 episodes. The mean interval from transplantation to diagnosis of LPD was 14 months (range, 1 - 44 months); 12 of the 15 patients (80%) developed LPD within 1 year of transplantation. Most of the recipients (12/15) showed symptoms. Fever (40%) and renal failure (46%) were the most common presenting signs. Renal ultrasound demonstrated hydronephrosis in 4 cases, a hilar mass in 5 cases, a mass lesion within the graft in 2 cases. Five patients had several organs (including the allograft) involved with LPD. Pathological examination showed a high grade malignant lymphoma with extensive necrosis and atypical large cells. Immunohistochemical study was consistent with B cell lymphoma in all of the 8 cases analyzed and monotypia was noted in 4 cases. The presence of Epstein-Barr virus genoma in the LPD was demonstrated in 5 of the 6 cases studied. Nine patients were managed with discontinuation of immunosuppression and transplant removal. To date, six patients (40%) died (five of them within two months after diagnosis). The remaining recipients are alive with no evidence of recurrence after 49 months (range 27 - 92 months).
In order to follow the incidence of this serious disease, the occurence of LPD (involving the graft) over the last two years was analyzed through a new collaborative study. Between January 1993 and January 1995, 2986 kidney transplants were done at 36 centres and 15 new cases of LPD were diagnosed (0.5%).
Taken as a whole, these results suggest LPD localized in the allograft are an increasingly problem that needs identification of contributing factors and new diagnostic and treatment protocols.

SKIN CANCERS

PREVENTION OF SKIN CANCER DURING ACITRETIN THERAPY IN RENAL-TRANSPLANT RECIPIENTS; A PLACEBO-CONTROLLED STUDY

J.N. Bouwes Bavinck[1] , L.M. Tieben[1], F.J. van der Woude[2], A.M. Tegzess[3], J. Hermans[4], B.J. Vermeer[1]
Departments of [1]Dermatology, [2]Nephrology and [4]Medical Statistics, University Hospital Leiden, and [3]department of Nephrology, University Hospital Groningen, the Netherlands.

Forty-four renal-transplant recipients were enrolled in a randomised, double-blind, placebo-controlled trial to test the possible skin-cancer-preventing effect of a six-month treatment with acitretin 30 mg daily. No deterioration in renal function occurred in any of the 38 evaluable patients treated. During the six-month treatment period 2 out of 19 patients (11%) in the acitretin group reported all together 2 new squamous cell carcinomas compared with 9 out of 19 patients (47%) in the placebo group who developed all together 18 new carcinomas: 15 squamous cell carcinomas, 1 Bowen's disease and 2 basal cell carcinomas (chi-square 6.27, $p = 0.01$). Interestingly, the effect of acitretin in preventing new skin cancers could largely be attributed to the group of 19 patients with a history of skin cancer. Most patients treated with acitretin had mild mucocutaneous side effects, but these were well manageable. Some patients experienced mild hair loss. With the exception of three patients no increase in serum cholesterol or triglyceride above pre-treatment levels was observed, and liver function remained unchanged in all patients. Acitretin 30 mg daily during six months had significantly more effect than placebo to prevent squamous cell carcinomas in a group of renal-transplant recipients who suffered severely from these lesions. This effect was most pronounced in patients with a history of skin cancer.

SKIN CANCER AFTER RENAL TRANSPLANTATION : EFFICACY OF IMMUNO-SUPPRESSIVE MONOTHERAPY ON RELAPSE RATE.

Branger B*, Dandurand M**, Abou S**, .

Nephrology department *, Dermatology department **, University Hospital, Nimes France.

Relapsing skin cancer is a well known complication of immunosuppression in renal transplant, mainly in sunny country. We report two demonstrative cases of frequent relapsing skin cancers with a benefit of immunosuppression reduction without compromising the kidney function.

Case reports: .Case 1. Mrs P.G.,white male of 61 years, was transplanted in 1982 with a cadaveric kidney. Primary renal desease was a polycystic kidney desease. The patient received six RBC pack transfusion.There were no anti-HLA antibody, the match was A1 X1, B8 B14 (donnor), A1 W31, B5 B8 (patient). No rejection episode was noted. Renal function was stable (creatininemia = 110±10 µmol/l) from the first week up to now. Immunosuppressive regimen associated prednisone (20 mg/d), azathioprine (150mg/d), and anti-lymphocyte globulins perfusion (daily during the first month). Complications were : hematuria (month 8, from the controlateral polycystic kidney), repeated legs vein thrombosis (2nd to 5th year). The first skin cancer appeared on the face in 1985, treated by surgery. Relapse appeared wthin one year, with multiple localisation on the neck and on the face. Despite local treatments including conventional surgery, cruosurgery, radiotherapy, skin cancers relaped every 3 to 6 months until 1991. Imuran was tapered from 100mg/d to 50 mg/d. In 1992 the immunosuppressive treatment resumed to prednisone 20 mg one another day. The skin cancer relapsing rate decreased to 6 to 12 months. One have to consider than the tissu typing of these cancers was basal cell carcinoma in all cases but one squamous cell carcinoma in 1991 .

Case 2. Mrs B.M., white male 59 years, was transplanted in january 1990 with a cadaveric kidney. Primary renal desease was a nephro-angiosclerosis. He developped 2 months before the transplantation a squamous cell carcinoma treated by surgery. The patient received three RBC pack transfusion.There were no anti-HLA antibody, the match was A1 A3, B8 B27 (donnor), A2 A9, B5 B18 , DR1 DR8 (patient). No rejection episode was noted. Renal function was stable (creatininemia = 80±10 µmol/l) from the first week up to now. Immunosuppressive regimen associated prednisone (20 mg/d, azathioprine (150mg/d), anti-lymphocyte globulins perfusion (daily during the first month) and ciclosporin A (400 mg to 200 mg/d). Complications were : arterial hypertension (month 3), diabetes mellitus secondary to corticotherapy (6 first months) and gum hyperplasia. The second skin cancer appeared on the right ear in 1991, treated by surgery. Relapse appeared wthin one year, with multiple localisation on the face: in all cases the tissu pathology showed squamous cell carcinoma. Cervical lymph nodes were invided in 1994 and surgery with radiotherapy permit to avoid any relapse until now. Imuran was tapered from 100mg/d to 0 in june 1990. Since 1992 the immunosuppressive treatment resumed to ciclosporine A 200/d.

Discussion: These observations illustrate the high rate of skin cancer in some transplant patients. Of a 64 transplant population followed from 1 to 18 years, only 4 patients presented skin cancers, but only two (reported cases) with a high relapse number. The immunosuppression reduction had a beneficial effect on cancers relapse rate.

Dermatological Lesions in Kidney Graft Recipients.

L. Coll, G. Pellerano, M. Brunet, M. Turin, L. Jost, F. Stengel.
CEMIC. Associated Hospital, Buenos Aires University. Argentine.

Between 1970 and 1993, 458 kidney transplants were performed at CEMIC, 230 of which, were in follow up at the moment of this prospective study. From May 1991 until July 1994, the same specialists, followed 100 kidney transplanted patients. The mean age was $\bar{X}$ 38.9 ± 13.2 years old (ys.); 70 % were men. The time in dialysis was $\bar{X}$ 31.5 ± 28.4 months (ms.) The mean immunosuppression (IMMS) time was $\bar{X}$ 46 ± 46.9 ms., 0 to 264 ms. The patients were under triple therapy, Methilprednisone, Azathioprine and Cyclosporine A, in 71 % of cases and double therapy, Methilprednisone and Azathioprine, in 29 %. Living related donors (LRD), were the source of kidney grafts in 71 % and cadaver donors (CD), in 29 %. In the group of study the mean age was X 52.6 ± 14.7 ys, the mean IMMS time was $\bar{X}$ 106.1 ± 81.7 ms., there was the same number of patients under triple and double therapy. The grafts were from CD in 75 %. Patients with more than 5 ys. of IMMS, presented 75 % of skin tumours, 63 % of pre tumoral lesions and 16 % of recidivants actinic queratosis. The 44 % of total population presented lesions associated to Human Papilloma Virus (HPV), in those with more than 8 ys. of IMMS, this percentage augmented to 100 %. Skin cancers appeared in 8 % of total population: Basocelular Epitheliomas (BE), 25 %; Epidermoide Carcinoma (EC), 25 %; and simultaneous BE y EC, 50 %. The ratio BE / EC, was 1:1, while the incidence of BE is higher in the immunocompetent population. The patients with EC had type II and III skin. The level of ultraviolet (UV) radiations is proportional to the south latitude: 34.4 S in Buenos Aires city. Sidney with the same incidence of skin tumours, is at 33.53 S. In the 87.5 % of cases the surgical treatment was successful. One patient died because of EC methastasis. Because of chronic rejection, 15 % of patients returned to dialysis. The HLA matching seems to be an important element, since most patients were cadaver graft recipients. As kidney transplanted patients survival increased, we have new problems to resolve, like prevention and treatment of tumoral lesions, being skin cancers the most frequent. This study showed that immunosuppressive state generated by drugs, aging, genetics, UV radiations, associated whith viral infección (HPV), are factors of skin cancers development. Education in sun exposition and protection must be done early in all potential graft recipients.

SKIN CANCERS AND PRECANCEROUS LESIONS IN RENAL GRAFTS.

Messina M, Segoloni GP, Damiani D,Angelini C,Giacchino F, Bertero M,Stratta P and Vercellone A. Nephrology and Transplant Unit,*Dermathological Clinic,-University of Turin ,Italy

It is well recognized that organ transplantation is associated with an increased number of tumors.Cutaneous malignancies are reported to be the most frequent in renal allograft recipients , in papers from Europe, USA and Australia.Their rate increases with duration of the graft, so that the cumulative risk rises to 40% or even 60% after 23 years.Some risk factors have been identified or hypotized:sunlight exposure, HPV infection,some precancerous lesions, azathioprine, cumulative immunosuppressive theraphy(IT), genetic factors(number of mismatches, absence of A11).

The Authors evaluate the population of 662 renal pts transplanted at their institution fom 11\81 to 4\94(minimun follow-up :1 yr)in respect of skin K.As a control group(C), pts with the same follow-up and without evidence of K were used.Analyzed factors were:ratio M\F, age, dialytic age, IT, % of surviving kidneys and pts, A,B,Dr mismatches,A11.IT consisted of Aza+ST or Cya(MonoT,DT,TT) with a regimen of ST in low doses,for maintenance and for rejection;ALG or OKT3 were sometimes employed.8 Kaposi'sarcoma (1,2%)and 23 Skin K(A) and precancerous lesions(B) (4,8%A+B)were found:11 BCC,5 SCC, 2 Keratoacanthomas,1 mixed K,2 Bowen'disease, 1 Merkeloma,1 tongue K,7 leukoplachias.Kaposi were analized apart.Statistical analysis (Student't and chi square test) were performed separately and altogether for A and B versus C .No significative difference was recorded in both analysis for all the examined parameters(excluding M\F ratio:8 vs 1.4). Respectively, for age, dialytic age,, follow-up, duration of the graft at the tumor,A+B versus C:47+-10 yrs,54+-40 mo,86+-33 mo,47+-25 mo vs.41+-9,49+-31,87+-39.As for IT (DT\TT\AZA\CyAMONO): 9\13\5\0 vs.7\15\8\1 (p=ns)Rejection\pts:0,59 vs 0,93 (p=ns).No correlation was found with mismatches or with A11(4\11 BCC and 1\5 SCC are A11+).% of surviving grafts and pts are superimposable(A+BvsC):70, 82 vs 74,93 %)In no case death or failure of the graft was somehow correlated with the K.In 1 pt skin K occurred after a precancerous lesion;in 2, we had recurrence.Theraphy always was surgical;in 9 IT was tapered.Kaposi's sarcoma had a different and more aggressive profile:earlier development(19+-16 mo, higher rejection rate(2,1),lower survival of kidneys(1\8) and pts(5\8).

In conclusion, in the Italian population of the Authors the prevalence of skin K and precancerous lesions is superimposable to data of the literature, or even lower.Skin K are not aggressive, excluding Kaposi'sarcomas.No association could be found with genetical factors nor IT.We are aware that the follow -up, not longer than 13 yrs,has to be considered a limiting factor for an in depth analysis.Nevertheless, we think that a not aggressive IT, together with a close survelliance of outpatients (nephrologists+dermathologist, with an early biopsy in suspicious lesions), in our geographical area, can be considered useful factors to restrain to an acceptable low rate the problem of skin cancers in transplanted patients.

OTHER MALIGNANCIES

DE NOVO MALIGNANCIES AFTER KIDNEY TRANSPLANTATION

F.Alföldy, A.Tóth, J.Járay, D.Görög, P.Borka, H.Podder, F.Perner

Semmelweis Medical University, Transplantation and Surgical Department Budapest

Purpose: We made a retrospective analysis on the incidence of the de novo malignancies in our kidney transplanted patients.

Material: 1009 kidney transplantation were performed in the period from 1973 to 1994 at our Department.

The mean age of the patients was 34,7 years. The average follow-up time was 5,8 years. Malignant tumour was found in 36 cases. In 2 cases tumours (1 kidney, 1 lung) occurred within 6 months after transplantation(it might have been a pre-existing, undetected tumour). In the other 34 cases the immunosuppressiv therapy had a great impact in the development of de novo malignancies. Tumour was not transferred with transplanted organs

Results: We found a higher tumour incidence (3,5%) in patients receiving immunosuppressiv therapy. The average time for diagnosing a tumour after kidney transplantation was 54 months. 32 patients had a single tumour, two patients had double tumour. According to the literature skin cancer was the most frequent tumour (11/36), Kaposi's sarcoma had the second highest incidence (7/36), although it is very rare in our population. The incidence of the oro-pharynegeal tumours (4/36) and kidney tumours (3/36) was also higher than in the non transplanted population.

The distribution of the other tumours was: 3 lung, 2 thyroid gland, 2 breast cancer , 1 liver, 1 larynx, 1 malignant thymoma and 1 NHL.

Conclusion: The incidence of the lymphoproliferative tumours was lower in our material than it is quoted in the literature. We found it only in patients who received Azathioprin-Prednisolon combination as immunosuppression.

The incidence of the Kaposi's sarcoma was higher than in the normal population, and it was found only in patients receiving Cyclosporin therapy.

Neoplastic diseases after liver transplantation

N. Bourgeois, V. Lefebvre, J. Van de Stadt, M. Gelin, M-O. Peny, C. Deprez, T. Velu, M. Adler
hopital Erasme, Université Libre de Bruxelles, Belgique

From January 1985 to January 1995, 125 adult patients underwent 135 liver transplantations (OLT). Hundred of them survived more than 3 months.
Six patients developped a malignant disease, 4 to 25 months after OLT.
None had treated rejection(s) before its onset.
Two men (43 and 47 years) transplanted for HBV-related cirrhosis developped a cutaneous Kaposi sarcoma of the ankles, 10 months after OLT. Both were treated with local cryotherapy ; their immunosuppressive therapy was lowered. They healed without rejection.
A 54 years male patient transplanted for HCV-related cirrhosis died 4 months after surgery from a fulminant EBV-related lymphoma.
In a 50 years man operated for cholangiocarcinoma, a 4 cms thoracic mass was resected 10 months after OLT, revealing also a EBV-related lymphoma. EBV genome was detected in the medulla. He was treated by 3 gr of acyclovir/day for 1 year. Immunosuppression was limited to low doses of cyclosporine. He is doing well 11 months after cessation of acyclovir.
A 44 years man, transplanted 22 months earlier for alcoholic cirrhosis, died in 4 months from a bronchial adenocarcinoma, despite chemotherapy and cessation of immunosuppression.
Finally, a 40 years woman died 4 months after transplantation (for an alcoholic cirrhosis) from a laryngeal carcinoma.
conclusion: Hundred patients, transplanted these last 10 years, survived more than 3 months afer OLT. Only a small proportion of them (3%) died from rapidly progresssive malignant disease favoured by immunosuppression. In some the neoplastic disease healed with appropriate therapy and reduction of immunosuppression.

«DE NOVO» CARCINOMA AFTER LIVER TRANSPLANT (L.T.)

Casanovas Taltavull, T., Baliellas, C., Sánchez Gili, M., Casanova, A., Benasco, C., Fabregat, J., Rafecas. A., Figueras, J., Gil-Vernet, S., Jaurrieta, E., Casais, L.A.
Liver Transplant Unit, Hospital of Bellvitge.

L'Hospitalet de Llobregat, Barcelona, SPAIN

Patients who have received a L.T. have a higher risk of developing «de novo» neoplasia than the general population.
The development of neoplasia is related to chronic Immunosuppression (IS) and latent viruses.
The mean frequency after L.T. is between 2-6%. There are a major incidence of lymphomas. The rate of lymphomas after L.T. is in Pittsburgh's experience 2,5% PTLPD (Post-transplant Lymphoproliferative disorder) is the most characteristic syndrome.
The aim of this study is the evaluation of factors which may be involved in our area.
Patients studied: In the series of 265 OLT in 234 patients in Hospital of Bellvitge (from Feb. 1984 to Feb. 1995). 142 males 38% antiVHC+ RIBA 3, and 92 females 27% antiVHC + RIBA 3. 10 cases CLKT (combined liver and kidney transplant).
We have observed 5 cases of «de novo» neoplasias (2,1% of patients transplanted). All were males, with ages from 41 to 60 years (50,4±6,8 years); 4/5 proven antiVHC (1/5 unknown not available); 5/5 had a past history of chronic alcoholism.
Diagnostic pre-OLT: Alcoholic liver cirrhosis (ALCI) 1 case; Posthepatitic C Cirrhosis (PHCC) 2 cases and PHCC and hepatocellular carcinoma 2 cases.
Initial IS= CyA+PD 2 cases; quadruple therapy 3 cases. Boluses of MP (Methylprednisolone) for acute rejection 3 cases. No patient received OKT3.
Current IS= CyA+Aza 3 cases; CyA+Aza+PD 2 cases.
Follow up until development of neoplasia was: 33, 88, 12, 13 and 9 months.
«De novo» neoplasias were: Hodgkin lymphoma (autopsy) squamous lung carcinoma and metastasis, undifferentiated lung carcinoma and metastasis, Kaposi's sarcoma (associated to hemophagocytosis) and liver lymphoma (of donor origin) which had syncronous artery hepatic thrombosis and required re-OLT.
Conclusions:
1) There is a partial discordance between the type of «de novo» neoplasia which we have observed and the experiences published. If the IS is similar, other predisponents should be investigated.
2) As a preliminary report we observed that from the availability to VHC serology all the cases were positive.
3) A very strict analysis of risk factors implicated should be carried out in each geographical area.

Primary Bronchogenic Carcinoma in Transplant Recipient

Delcambre F., Ramon P., Noel C., Pol A., Declerck N., Gosselin B., Wurtz A., Laffite JJ., Dracon M. and Pruvot FR. CHU-Lille France.

The risk of malignancy is a well-recognized event in long term transplant recipients. Incidence, average age of appearance, evolution, and response to treatment may differ from the general population and depend on varieties of neoplasms. Lung cancer has been reported as a specific risk of heart transplant recipients. We present 8 cases of lung cancer from 892 kidney, heart, and liver transplant recipients in which risk factors and management are discussed.

Patients and methods Among kidney (n = 564), heart (n = 240), and liver (n = 88) recipients transplanted from January, 1986 to December, 1994, eight cases of primary bronchogenic carcinoma were included in this study. All transplanted patients received cyclosporine. No correlation could be made between immunosuppression, rejection, CMV infection and appearance of cancer (table 1).

Table 1

	organ	age (1)	smoking risks (2)	ALG(3)	Immunosuppression (4)	Rejection crisis (n)	Rejection treatment	CMV disease
obs 1	kidney	64	20	+	CsA+ IM+ CS	0	-	-
obs 2	kidney	56	0	+	CsA+ CS	0	-	-
obs 3	liver	52	60	-	CsA+ IM+ CS	2	ALG	+
obs 4	liver (*)	50	50	-	CsA+ IM+ CS	2	OKT3+SAL	+
obs 5	heart	46	60	+	CsA+ IM+ CS	0	-	-
obs 6	heart	50	60	+	CsA+ IM+ CS	2	ALG	-
obs 7	heart	62	50	+	CsA+ IM+ CS	1	CS	-
obs 8	heart	54	60	+	CsA+ IM+ CS	0	-	-

(1): age at time of transplantation (years). (2): packs of cigarettes per day per years. (3): induction therapy. (4): CsA: cyclosporine ; IM: Imurel ; CS: Prednisone. (*) retransplantation for chronic rejection before cancer.

Results The delay between transplantation and diagnosis of lung cancer was either <1year (n=3) or > 4 years (n=5). A majority of patients (n=4, 3/4 heart recipients) had small cell lung cancers with high TNM stage of which three died from early (< 230j) dissemination. Four non small cell cancers could be resected with no post-operative death. Five patients survived more than 6 months (table 2).

Table 2

	Symptoms	Delay (1)	Histology	Stage (2)	Treatment	Survival
obs 1	chest X ray	6	epidermoid	pT2N2M0	lobectomy + RT (3)	alive 8 months
obs 2	chest X ray	48	small cell	T4N2M1	chemotherapy	alive 6 months
obs 3	fever	6	adenocarcinoma	pT2N0M0	bilobectomy	died 21 months (4)
obs 4	chest X ray	57	epidermoid	pT2N0M0	bilobectomy	alive 20 months (4)
obs 5	chest X ray	57	small cell	T1N2M0	chemotherapy	died 4 months
obs 6	dyspnea	69	epidermoid	pT2N1M0	pneumonectomy + RT	alive 10 months (4)
obs 7	chestX ray	11	small cell	T3N2M1	none	died 2 months (4)
obs 8	cough	82	small cell	T4N3M1	none	died 2 months

(1): months (2): at diagnosis (3): radiotherapy (4): with bone dissemination

Discussion **Incidence of bronchogenic cancer is high (0,9%) in transplanted patients and occurs at a younger age as compared to general population. Diagnosis is often made by chest X ray especially in small cell cancer. Pulmonary resection in non small cell cancer is a safe procedure in spite of immunosuppression, but prognosis is altered by secondary dissemination. Recipients with smoking history should be submitted to a special high frequency broncho-pulmonary investigation program.**

MISDIAGNOSED MALIGNANCY IN TRANSPLANTED ORGANS.

O.Detry, B.Detroz, M. D'Silva, J.O.Defraigne, M.Meurisse, P.Honoré, R.Limet, N.Jacquet
Department of Surgery and Transplantation, CHU Sart-Tilman, Liège, Belgium

Organ transplantation has become the treatment of choice for a growing number of terminally ill patients. The increase number of procedures increase the number of complications related to transplantation and to the immunosuppression. We report our experience in the transferral of malignancy by grafting cancerous organs into recipients, which is a rare but desastrous complication of transplantation.

CASE REPORTS

Donor 1 was a 30-year-old female died from nontraumatic cerebral hemorrhage. A multiorgan harvest was performed, and the liver and the left kidney were explanted and transplanted to recipient 1 and 2, respectively. The right kidney was rejected for vascular and urological abnormalities. Necropsy revealed a nodule in the right kidney, and three hemorrhagic nodules in the right lung. Histopathological analysis of these nodules demonstrated the presence of a choriocarcinoma. Later serum analyses revealed very high levels of ß-HCG.

Recipient 1 was a-20-year-old female who received the left kidney from donor 1. Graft CT-scan demonstrated a 2-cm nodule, and the immunosuppression was interrupted. Transplantectomy was performed on postoperative day 12 but ß-HCG levels rose. A chemotherapy was undergone, which succeeded in normalizing the ß-HCG level. Two years later, the patient was retransplanted and since then shows no evidence of recurrence.

Recipient 2 received the liver from donor 1. His ß-HCG levels rose dispite normal graft CT scan. The patient died on day 39 from pulmonary complications, and autopsy showed 3 choriocarcinoma metastasis in the hepatic graft.

Donor 2 was a-35-years-old female died from a nontraumatic cerebral hemorrhage. Paraaortic adenopathy was noticed during multiorgan harvesting. The liver, the heart and the kidneys were transplanted in 4 different centers. The results of the histopathological examination conducted that the paraaortic and pulmonary nodes were positive for a disseminated epidermoid epithelioma, originating from the cervix uteri.

Recipient 3 was a 25-year-old man who received the liver from donor 2 in our department. The patient was retransplanted on postoperative day 7 and no evidence of malignancy was detected on histopathological analysis examination on the graft.

Donor 3 was a 55-year-old female who died from cerebral hemorrhage in another country. We received one kidney, and we found a 4-cm nodule in this organ. Frozen section of this lesion showed a renal adenocarcinoma and transplantation was aborted in our center and in the centers which received the other kidney and the heart from the same donor.

DISCUSSION

As these cases demonstrate, the transferral of malignancy with organ transplantation may rarely but dramatically complicate the postoperative outcome of recipients. Its medical management is difficult, and its psychological impacts on the recipients may be desastrous. The transplant centers, both small and large, must be prepared for such an eventuality. Due to the organ shortage, the transplant teams enlarge the indications of harvesting, accepting older donors for instance, but the "malignant" donors must be avoided. The use of donors with previously successfully treated cancer should be totally excluted, excepted the primary supratentorial cerebral tumors. However, as in our cases, the donor's cancer is often non diagnosed. Careful examination of the abdomen and the thorax must be performed during the harvesting, and histopathological analysis of suspected nodules must be available before the transplantation. Peroperative echography and postharvesting autopsy may be helpful. If a recipient was transplanted with a kidney harvested from a cancerous patient, the immunosuppression must be discontinued and the graft must be explanted. Specific chemotherapy must be initiated if primary tumor is proven sensitive to treatment. Hepatic allografts are not immediately expandable, and they must remain in situ until another graft is available.

NEPHROGENIC ADENOMA (NA) OF THE BLADDER IN RENAL TRANSPLANTED PATIENTS

Guermani P, Pigato M, Manzo M- Division of Urology ,Molinette Hospital Turin - Italy
Segoloni GP, Messina M, Angelini M- Clinic of Nephrology and Transplantation Unit, University of Turin

NA is a rare abnormality, not a neoplasm but an immature urothelial metaplasia, first described by Davis in 1949 in a 40 -yrs- old man with a history of urinary tract infections. It is an adenomatous form of metaplasia associated with chronic urinary tract infections, trauma, urinary tract surgery, calculi, tubercolosis, schistosomiasis. The lesion is generally isolated but may be multiple in almost 20% of cases; its size ranges from microscope to the entire bladder involvement.Some cases have been reported in association with renal transplantation, where predisposing factors can be defined: bladder implantation of the ureter, recurrent urinary tract infections, vescicoureteral reflux, immunosuppressive therapy.The AA. describe the occurrence of 3 cases in a population of 796 patients transplanted at their institution from 11/81 to 4/95.

Case 1: a 38- yrs - old female pt was transplanted on 11-05-82. Immunosuppressive therapy consisted of Aza and steroids at the beginnig; after of Aza and Cya in low doses. No rejection treatment was ever performed. Serum creatinine was normal in spite of frequent urinary tract infections. A cystoendoscopy was prescribed subsequently to episodes of painless hematuria (2/93). It demonstrated some bladder diverticuli and some papillary lesions which were excised; urethral underlying pathology was treated by urethrotomy according Turner-Warwick. Histological examination showed NA. In 2 cystoendoscopies after 6 and 12 months a recurrence was noted and excised. No other recurrence was found in subsequent routine cystoendoscopies. Serum creatinine is still 1 mg%.

Case 2: a 49 -yrs- old man - HBV positive - was transplanted on 21/11/81; Immunosuppressive therapy consisted of Aza and steroids till 02/05/88, then of Cya and steroids. The patient was treated for rejection 3 times with steroids. His medical history was uneventful as for infections or genitourinary pathologies for ten years. In 1992 a bladder outlet obstruction caused by benign prostatic hyperplasia was diagnosed and treated endoscopically. NA was histologically detected in the lesions excided (trigone zone). After 2 years no recurrence was demonstrated.
Serum creatinine is unchanged (1,6 mg %).

Case 3: a 44 -yrs - old man was transplanted on 06-04-82. In his medical history 2 treatments for rejection (respectively with ALG and Steroids) were recorded. A renal biopsy performed in 05-94 for proteinuria and worsening renal function (Crs 4,2 mg%), demonstrated a picture of transplant glomerulopathy. Some months after, two episodes of sudden hematuria occurred. US was normal, no urinary infection was noted. A cystoendoscopy was prescribed; NA was diagnosed on the excided lesion (3/95). Serum creatinine is unchanged; presently, a follow up is not yet available.

In conclusion, the AA think that the frequence of NA is underevaluated in transplanted pts, a population where risk factors for NA are known. Even if NA is not to be considered a neoplasm in the general population, the development of atypical cells in immunosuppressed pts cannot be excluded. Besides, recurrences are reported and the natural history of NA and of its recurrences is not well known.

In transplanted pts with frequent and/or hematuria, if US and routine blood and urine tests are not helpful to clearify the diagnosis, we think that a more aggressive approach is advisable (cystography and cystoendoscopy). A part from the unfortunate discover of a malignancy, the presence of "minor" lesions, as NA, must not be underestimated. Its early excision is mostly successfull, not highly riskful and preemptive towards more drastic and disturbing therapies -as cystectomy- which may be unavoidable when the lesions are too large and numerous.

TRANSMISSION OF RENAL CARCINOMAS WITH CADAVERIC DONOR KIDNEYS: A FIVE YEARS FOLLOW UP

Guermani P, Alladio F, Manzo M- Division of Urology, Molinette Hospital Turin - Italy
Segoloni GP, Messina M, Damiani D- Clinic of Nephrology and Transplantation Unit, University of Turin

Despite careful pretransplant investigations and rigorous selection of donors, it is not possible always to avoid any transfer of infraclinical malignancy. It must be stressed that most transmitted cancers were in the pioneering era of transplantation, while today the situation occurs very rarely.
Data from Cincinnati Register in 1991 report on 164 pts who received organs from donors with cancers versus more than 130.000 grafts perfomed. When dealing with the field of renal tumour, routine blood and urine analysis and ultrasonography (US) may fail in detecting small intraparenchimal lesions; so cancer may be noted only intraoperatively or at a variable time after surgery. The clinical management of the recipient is yet to be defined.
Many factors either clinical or ethical must be weighed when taking the decision about transplantectomy-the most attractive option-or excision of the noduli, also successfully reported even if more rarely. The AA. report their experience about inadvertent transplantation of malignancy in 2 out of 788 transplants performed at our institution from November 1981 to March 1995.
Case 1: a 54 -yrs- old man was transplanted on 3/1990 from a donor 58 - yrs - old. Disease on his native kidney was chronic GN. Surgery was uneventful. A few days after, US routine examination and a CT scan demonstrated a tumor (2 cm.in diameter); serum creatinine was normal. One month later a local excision was performed, with intraoperative US detection of the mass.
Pathological examination showed a renal adenocarcinoma clear cell type 1 pT1 G1.
Case 2: a 52 - yrs- old female was transplanted on 3/1992 from a donor 44 - yrs- old. Disease on his native kidney was APKD. During surgery a mass of the hilus was detected and resected with some surrounding renal tissue free of tumour. Histological examination in the operativing room revealed an adenoma and definitively a renal adenocarcinoma clear cell type 1 pT1 G1.
Respectively after 5 and 3 yrs s.Cr. were 1,9 and 1 mg%, tumour markers were normal as well as CT scan, Xray, and US routinely performed.
Immunosuppressive therapy was Cya monotherapy now (DT was adopted for 4 yrs) in case 1 and DT in case 2 . In both cases an informed consent was obtained from the patients; in case 2 the patient spontaneusly choosed not to undergo a transplactectomy after the local excision we decided to perform during surgery of the graft. Recipients of other organs (2 kidney, 1 liver, 1 heart) are alive and well or dead (the cardiac patient), all of them without any evidence of metastatic tumor.
In conclusion, the AA report about their long term (3 and 5 yrs) favourable experience with a conservative surgery of renal carcinomas inadvertently transplanted. We think that this treatment option, somehow more riskful than the classical transplactectomy, may be nowadays proposed in selected case always having obtained a precisely informed consent from patients.

TUMORS AFTER RENAL TRANSPLANTATION

M. Haberal, H. Karakayalı, E. Velidedeoğlu, G. Arslan, H. Akkoç, N. Büyükpamukçu, N. Bilgin

Başkent University Hospital, Ankara, Turkey

Immunosuppressive therapy in organ transplant recipients is complicated by an increased incidence of malign diseases, particularly with certain tumors. From November 1975 to December 1994, 1034 kidney transplantations were performed on 997 patients in our centers. Among these kidney recipients, 23 malignant diseases were observed in 22 patients (2.2%) in the post-transplant period. Thirteen (59.9%) of these patients were male and 9 (40.1%) were female; their mean age was 37.6 years (range 10-59). Eighteen (81.8%) of these transplants were from living-related donors and 4 (18.2%) were from cadaver donors. The immunosuppressive therapy consisted of Prednisolone + Azathiopurine + Cyclosporin A in 12 (54.5%) patients, Prednisolone + Cyclosporine A in 4 (18.2%) patients and Prednisolone + Azathiopurine in 6 (27.3%) patients. We observed basal cell carcinoma in 3 (0.3%) patients, squamous cell carcinoma in 3 (0.3%) patients, Kaposi's sarcoma in 5 (0.5%) patients, lymphoma in 5 (0.5%) patients, bladder carcinoma in 2 (0.2%) patients, colon carcinoma in 1 (0.1%) patient, cervix carcinoma in 1 (0.1%), breast carcinoma in 1 (0.1%), acute myelositic leukemia in 1 (0.1%) and thyroid carcinoma in 1 (0.1%) patient. In one of the patients, 9 months after the diagnosis of bladder carcinoma, an adenocarcinoma of the caecum was observed. All patients were treated with the appropriate surgical and/or medical treatment modalities. Eleven patients died 9 to 129 months (mean 61.5 months) after transplantation, and the other 11 patients are still alive. Seven of the patients have good renal functions, and the mean follow-up period after the diagnosis of malign diseases in this group was 36.5 months (range 2-103 months). In conclusion, due to the increased incidence of certain malignancies in transplant recipients, these patients must be followed closely.

THE INCIDENCE OF MALIGNANCY IN THE POPULATION OF 1 . 2 8 0 KIDNEY TRANSPLANTATIONS - A COMPLETE SINGLE CENTER ANALYSIS

Authors: Igna, D.; Keller, H.; Kirste, G.

University Hospital Freiburg im Breisgau
Department of Surgery, Section of Transplantation Surgery,
D-79106 Freiburg i. Br., Hugstetter Strasse 55

Malignancies in patients after transplantation procedure are still a major obstacle of immunosuppressive therapy. Up to now it is unclear whether certain type or frequency of malignancy can be observed depending on quantity and quality of immunosuppresive therapy.

In this report the incidence of malignancy depending on sex, age, localisation, immunosuppression is compared with the incidence of malignancy for skin, colon and uro-genital system in general population of Baden-Württemberg.

The immunosuppressive protocol was 2 x 3 mg/kg/body weight Ciclosporin adjusted to a trough level of 150 - 250 ng/ml; 3 mg/kg/body weight Azathioprin tapered to 0.5 mg at day five; 100 mg Cortison tapered to 10 mg at day 28.

A population of 1.280 patients after kidney transplantation in the University Hospital Freiburg between 1976 and 1995 was retrospectively and descriptively analysed for "de novo" cancers post transplantation. There are 62 cases (4,2 %) in the age between 28 and 70 years reported.

Clinical presentation of the neoplasms was similar to those decribed in the general population. All of them underwent standard treatment for tumors. Among 62 cases we observed only 6 recidives and 2 inoperable cancers, one with a high malignant cerebral non-hodgkin-lymphoma.

Most of the tumors were detected at an early stage due to regular consulting in the transplant outpatient ward. There are 18 patients presented with skin tumors, 15 with gastrointestinal tumors, 7 with urogenital tract tumors and 22 with other localisations.

There is no difference in the immunosuppressive therapy among patients with tumors or without nor any special protocols for antirejection therapy. Only one case with a tumor of lymphoprolifertative tissue could be observed.

Evidently malignancies of the lymphoproliferative tissue can be avoided by low dose immunsosuppressive therapy. The incidence of other types of tumors is depending on the underlying kidney disease and may be of the management on dialysis.

THE MALIGNANCIES AFTER KIDNEY TRANSPLANTATION IN THAILAND

Sopon Jirasiritham, M.D.

Department of Surgery, Faculty of Medicine, Ramathibodi Hospital, Mahidol University, Bangkok, Thailand

It is well recognized that the incidence of malignancy increased quite significantly in kidney transplant recipients. The most common malignancies, reported from the western atmosphere, are the squamous cell carcinoma of skin and lymphoproliferative tumors. In Asian country, the predominant malignancy after transplantation is gastrointestinal tract i.e., gastric cancer and hepatocellular carcinoma.

We studied our experience in kidney transplant patients who developed malignancy. In our series, we performed 257 consecutive cases of kidney transplantations from 1986 to 1994. The donor types were 67 living related donors and 190 cadaveric donors. All patients were all followed up in a special transplantation clinic. The duration of post-transplantation periods ranged from 3 months to 9 years with the average of 3.8 years. The immunosuppressive regimen composed of cyclosporine and low dose steroid in most patients except for a fews who received triple immunosuppressant due to chronic rejection. The 1-year and 3-year graft survival were 87%, 75% for cadaveric donor group and 96.5%, 96.5% for living related donor group respectively.

We experienced 4 cases of malignancies. These were 2 hepatocellular carcinomas, 1 squamous cell carcinoma of the lung and 1 squamous cell carcinoma of skin. The malignancies were diagnosed 40-62 months after transplantation. Both cases of hepatocellular carcinoma were carriers of hepatitis B surface antigenemia (HBsAg+). Both expired from liver failure 1, 3 months after diagnosis. The squamous cell carcinoma of the lung was treated by lobectomy and still alive with close follow-up. The squamous cell carcinoma of skin was widely excised and no recurrence was detected so far.

In Thailand, the incidence of hepatocellular carcinoma is about 0.01%, so the incidence of hepatocellular carcinoma in the kidney transplantation patient (0.78%) is obviously higher. We believed that the presence of HBsAg played a significant role. We noticed that no lymphoma in our series inspite of the fact that non-Hodgkin lymphoma was the most common hematologic malignancy in Thailand. We need further study to explain this fact.

In conclusion, only 4 cases (1.5%) of malignancies were experienced in kidney transplant patients. These composed of 2 hepatocellular carcinoma, and 2 squamous cell carcinoma. No lymphoma was observed. Multiple factors might contribute to this low figure of malignancy comparing to other institutes.

KAPOSI'S SARCOMA IN KIDNEY TRANSPLANT RECIPIENTS

A.Tóth, F.Alföldy, J.Járay, D.Görög, P.Borka, I.Fehérvári, F. Perner

Semmelweis Medical University, Transplantation and Surgical Department Budapest

Purpose: We analysed the manifestation and clinical course of Kaposi's sarcoma cases in kidney transplant recipients
Material/Method:. We performed 1009 kidney transplantation from 1973 to 1994.
During the follow-up of patients 36 malignant tumours were detected, they occurred in 34 patients.
Skin cancers were the most frequently found tumours (11/36), Kaposi's sarcoma showed the second highest incidence (7/36). Three of them had cutaneous and 4 visceral manifestations.
All our cases were HIV, EBV, hepatits B surface antigen negative.
Three patients had serological proved CMV infection.
We could not find those HLA antigens (HLA-A2, B15 and DR5), which are regarded as risk factors in the development of Kaposi's sarcoma.
Result: The main features of Kaposi's sarcoma in our material were:
1. Rapid development after transplantation (mean time 10 months), in comparison with the other tumours, where this period was 58 months after transplantation.
2. All our Kaposi's sarcoma patients were male.
The male/female ratio in the transplanted population is 1,5:1. This rate increases in the de novo tumours following transplantation to 2,6:1.
3. All patients received Cyclosporin immunosuppressiv therapy.
4. In these cases the frequency of rejection episodes was high (5/7). They were treated with high dose steroids (4 cases) or/and with anti lymphocyte globulin (1 case).
5. There is a great difference in the clinical course of the cutaneous and visceral manifestations.
a. The skin lesions on the lower extremities, the "classical form" developed slower (13 months) . They reacted well to irradiation.
b. The visceral form of Kaposi's sarcoma developed very rapidly after transplantation. (mean time 7 months)
In two cases Kaposi's sarcoma was diagnosed only at autopsy.
In the other two cases which were diagnosed in vivo, we were not able to prevent the fatal outcome neither by discontinuation of immunsuppression nor by Interferon treatment.
Conclusion: Awareness of development of certain malignancies is essential especially in male patient following kidney transplantation.

Malignancy in Kidney Transplant Patients

V. Třeška, J. Valenta, E. Veselá
Department of Surgery, University Hospital
Pilsen, Czech Republic

Out of 241 kidney transplant patients in four patients (1.6%) five de novo malignancies (2.0%) developed (lymphoma, thyreoid cancer, basalioma, renal pelvis cancer and laryngeal cancer). Three patients (1.2%) were transplanted with a history of previous malignancy (Wilms´ tumor, seminoma and Grawitz´s tumor).

The 32-year patient with a history of Wilms´ tumor in whom a thyreoid cancer developed 5 months after Tx and a basalioma 42 months after Tx is living 5 years later with a good graft function. The 54-year man in whom a laryngeal cancer developed one year after Tx is living with a functioning graft 3 months after laryngectomy. A 58-year woman died of an advanced lyphoma 51 months after Tx and a 44-year woman in whom a large renal cancer was diagnosed 48 months after Tx died after a complicated nephrectomy.

Out of the three patients with a previous malignancy the man with the Wilms´ tumor in whom two more malignancies developed following kidney transplantation is living, a 54 years old man with a bilateral Grawitz´s tumor died of generalization 3 years after Tx, and the 30-year man who was in a very poor condition after chemotherapy for seminoma died after transplantation of sepsis.

Renal transplantation can be carried out successfully even in pateints with previous malignancy and also in de novo malignancies the graft may be saved. The morbidity and mortality rates, however, are high.

DE NOVO MALIGNANCY FOLLOWING ORTHOTOPIC LIVER TRANSPLANTATION (OLT) FOR ALCOHOLIC CIRRHOSIS (AC).

VANLEMMENS C[1], MONNET E[2], BRESSON-HADNI S[1], BECKER MC[1], MINELLO A[1], HEYD B[1], MANTION G[1], KANTELIP B[1], HILLON P[1], MIGUET JP[1]. Unité de Transplantation Hépatique[1], Département de Santé Publique[2], CHRU Jean Minjoz - Faculté de Médecine - 2 Place Saint Jacques - 25030 BESANÇON CEDEX.

AC is the most common cause of end-stage liver failure in Europe and the United States. Since at present OLT is the best treatment for end-stage liver diseases, AC has recently become an increasing indication of OLT and its results are comparable with those of subjects transplanted for non alcoholic liver diseases (non ALD). However, the long-term results of OLT for patients with AC are still unknown, and information concerning the incidence of new malignancies following OLT is lacking. The aim of our study was to establish the prevalence and characteristics of the new cancers among patients transplanted for AC (group A) at our liver transplant unit and to compare these results with those of the other patients transplanted for non AC (group B). Patients and methods : between March 1986 and December 1994, a total of 163 adult patients underwent OLT. 27 patients who died before the first month post-OLT were excluded from the study. Thus, 61 patients (52 men) in group A and 75 (40 men) in group B were studied. The mean age at the time of OLT was comparable between the 2 groups of patients (group A = 50.7 years ± 8.1 SD ; group B = 49.3 ± 12.4 SD) ($p = 0.9$). The mean duration of follow-up since OLT was also comparable in the 2 groups of patients (group A = 37.9 months ± 25.8 SD ; group B = 42.2 months ± 36.3 SD) ($p = 0.3$). Standard immunosuppresive treatment was the same in the 2 groups and consisted of steroids, ciclosporine and azathioprine. A total of 5 patients from the group A and 10 patients from the group B received OKT 3. Results : 10 (9 men) out of the 61 group A patients (16.4 %) developped new tumors, whereas only 2 (1 man) out of the 75 group B patients (2.7 %) acquired de novo cancers (breast carcinoma and squamous cell carcinoma) ($p = 0.0001$). The incidence rate of de novo malignancy after OLT among the group A patients (= 49.6 for 1000 person-years) was significantly higher than that of group B patients (7 for 1000 person-years) ($p = 0.0001$, relative risk = 7.1, $CI_{95\%}$ [1.5 - 32.5]). The incidence of lymphoma was higher in patients from group A [4 patients out of the 61 (6.4 %)] than that of group B patients (0 %) ($p = 0.087$). Among the 6 other patients from group A with de novo tumors : 3 men consecutively developped two tumor types (throat carcinoma and oesophagus carcinoma in 2 cases, prostate carcinoma and squamous cell carcinoma in 1 case), 2 men and 1 woman developped lung, throat and breast carcinoma respectively. The average length of time from OLT to the onset of cancer was shorter for lymphoma (2.5 months) than for the other tumors (36 months in group A and 48 months in group B). The 4 patients with lymphoma died whereas among the 6 other patients who acquired de novo malignancy in group A, 2 died but from other causes than de novo cancers. Conclusion : OLT for AC is associated with a higher risk of de novo malignancies as compared with the other indications. The precocity and rapidity of lymphoma in these alcoholic patients is striking and raises the question of the responsability of alcoholism in the evolution of these lymphoma. The occurrence of oesophagus and throat cancers in such patients is less surprising, since they are usually heavy smokers.

MISCELLANEOUS

SEQUENTIAL ASSESSMENT OF PERIPHERAL B-CELLS AND DETECTION OF VIRAL INFECTIONS IN KIDNEY RECIPIENTS. M.C.BENE[1], E.RENOULT[2], M.N.KOLOPP-SARDA[1], S.MATTEI[3], J.P. VILLEMOT[3], M.KESSLER[2], G.C.FAURE[1]. Immunology Laboratory[1], Kidney[2] and Heart[3] Transplantation. Centre Hospitalier Universitaire de Nancy.

B-lymphocytes are the preferential target of the Epstein-Barr virus which is able to immortalize them and lead to the development of lymphoproliferative disorders. Other viruses can induce transient variations in immunoglobulin levels suggesting B-cell activation. We investigated whether changes in peripheral B-cell proportions could be associated with infectious episodes in transplanted patients.

We isolated, in a retrospective study of patients transplanted during the past two years, records properly documented for concomitant clinical, serological and immunological follow-up. The latter included sequential assessment of peripheral lymphocyte subsets (CD3, CD4, CD8, CD57). Special interest was given to B-cell levels, measured by immunofluorescence labelling of surface immunoglobulins (BCR) with an FITC-goat Fab'2 to human immunoglobulins Fab and flow cytometry (EPICS Profile I or XL, Coultronics, Hialeah, FL).

In a first group of 12 patients, an Epstein Barr virus (EBV) infection was recognized as a primary infection (n=8) or a reactivation (n=4). Two of the patients, a kidney transplant recipent and a heart and kidney transplant recipient, had developed a documented lymphoproliferative disease. The first patient died, and the other one has survived after removal of the kidney tranplant which appeared to be the single involved site. One patient presented with an infectious mononucleosis-like illness. The 9 other patients developed transient serum anti-EBV viral capsid antigens (VCA) IgM antibodies after a clinically mild viral syndrome. In this series of EBV-infected patients, a significant increase in peripheral B-cell levels was noted, resulting in persistently elevated B-cells in 7 cases. This immunological characteristic appeared 2 weeks to 5 days (mean: 11 days) before seroconversion or clinical diagnosis in 7 patients, and was concomitant to clinical or serological signs in the other 5. Peripheral lymphocytes were tested for spontaneous *in vitro* transformation in 6 cases, and proliferation was evidenced in 4.

In another group of 17 kidney transplant recipients (including 3 heart and kidney transplant recipients) with cytomegalovirus (CMV) primary infection (n=6) or reactivation (n=11), a similar variation from the patient's baseline level of peripheral B-cells was noted in all but one case. Sequential assessment of B-cell levels however showed that this variation was transient, and normal levels were resumed within a few days. This peak of peripheral B-cells was detected between 1 to 4 weeks prior to seroconversion (mean: 4,5 weeks) in 14 cases, and/or concomitantly in 6 cases.

These data suggest that the simple sequential assessment of peripheral B-cell levels can provide information regarding virus-mediated B-cell activation. Significant variations from a patient's baseline should prompt serological investigations for EBV or CMV infection or reactivation. Patients with persistently high B-cell levels, suggestive of EBV infection, could perhaps benefit from appropriate therapeutic anti-viral regimen.

HCV CHRONIC INFECTION IN HD (HEMODIALYSED) CANDIDATES TO KT (KIDNEY TRANSPLANT). INFLUENCE OF VIRUS C GENOTYPES ON RESPONSE TO IFN TREATMENT.

Casanovas Taltavull, T., Baliellas, C., Perelló, A., Cervantes, X., Benasco, C., Andrés, E., González, M.T., Gil-Vernet, S., Pérez, J.L., Niubó, J. Casanova, A., Casais, L.A.
Liver Transplant Unit, Hospital of Bellvitge
L'Hospitalet de Llobregat, Barcelona, SPAIN

IFN is the most accepted treatment for HCV chronic infection in immunocompetent patients. But IFN is not without risk in transplanted patients, because possible deleterious effects on the graft.
Patients infected with HCV genotype II (Okamoto) have more severe liver disease and a poorer response to IFN than patients with other viral strains.
We did a pilot study of treatment with IFN in 10 end stage renal disease (ESRD) patients candidates to KT who were on HD.
The aim of this study was to evaluate the following:
1) HCV genotypes, clinical and therapeutical implications in ESRD patients.
2) Clinical tolerance and specific side effects of treatment in uremic patients
3) Beneficial effects of treatment on CLD (Chronic Liver Disease).
4) The outcome of the KT

Characteristics of the patients and treatment

10 patients (7 males, 3 females) age 44,4±11,7 years (range 20-59). Causes of nephropathy: 3 Proliferative Chronic Glomerulonephritis; 2 IgA Nephropathy; 1 Hemolytic-Uremic Syndrome; 1 Focal and Segmental Glomerulosclerosis; 2 Chronic Pyelonephritis; 2 Nephrosclerosis. ALT≥3N for more than 12 months, AntiHCV by RIBA 3, RNA-HCV+, by PCR, genotyped by Okamoto technique. Liver biopsy proven chronic hepatitis. Histologic diagnostics: 1 Chronic Persistent Hepatitis, 1 Chronic Lobulillar Hepatitis, 8 Chronic Active Hepatitis.
Treatment recombinant or lymphoblastoid IFN alpha. 3 MU three times weekly after HD sessions during 6 months, tapering to 1,5 MU three weekly, completing one year.

Results (in relation with the objectives):

1) Pre treatment:	10 cases PCR +;	Genotypes:	6 GII
			1 GII+I
			3 not typable
Immediately after treatment:	9 cases PCR + (genotype not done)		
	1 case PCR -		
6-26 months after treatment:	2 cases PCR + (GII remained)		
	8 cases PCR -		

2) 7/10 patients completed 1 year. 3 completed 4 months (1 patient of those did not respond). IFN had to be discontinued in 3 patients, because hematologic side effects and depression, alitiasic colecystitis with peritonitis and fever related to chronic rejection.
3) 9 patients had complete and maintained response, of these, 2 patients had only a 4 months treatment because side effects.
4) 6 patients received KT (28 m., 18 m., 17 m., 15 m., 10 m., 1 month evolution). All remain with ALT N and PCR -. One suffered acute vascular rejection and had to go back to HD, 2 remain with creatinine x 2 N, and 3 N creatinine.

Conclusions:

- In HD patients candidates to KT, with chronic HCV infection, we propose liver biopsy in the PCR + cases to establish a prognosis. IFN treatment is only indicated in cases with severe disease.
- HCV genotypes should not be used to determine which patients receive therapy. In our experience response to IFN has been good in GII genotype.
- Some patients had adverse effects related to IFN or to uremic state. These require strict clinical surveillance.
- After KT no recurrence ofhepatitis was observed. PCR remained -. The response to IFN in this group is better than the general population.
- The evolution of the graft was not altered by IFN.
- This result: justify further studies with a larger number of patients.

ESSENTIAL FATTY ACID DEFICIENCY IN CHILDREN WITH EXTRAHEPATIC BILIARY ATRESIA : INFLUENCE OF ORTHOTOPIC LIVER TRANSPLANTATION.

M Chambon[1], A Lachaux[1], A Lapillonne[2], V Chirouze[3], O Boillot[4], V Fournier[1], M Lièvre[5], D Gille[4], M Hermier[1].
1 Hépatogastroentérologie et Nutrition Pédiatriques, 2 Néonatologie, Hôp. E. Herriot, Lyon. 3 IMEDEX, Chaponost. 4 Transplantologie Hépatique, Pavillon D, Hôpital E. Herriot, 4 Pharmacologie Clinique, Av. Lacassagne, Lyon.

<u>OBJECTIVE</u> :

Cholestatic children with EBA have an impaired ability to absorb dietary fat and exhibit LCPUFA deficiency. The aim of this study was to assess their LCPUFA status before and after OLT, and the effect of infusion of essential fatty acid (EFA) before OLT.

<u>METHODS</u> :

Six children with EBA waiting for OLT were included in this study. All of them failed to recover from biliary obstruction 3 months after hepatic portoenterostomy and now have total bilirubin levels > 250 mmol/l. LCPUFA values in red-blood cell were prospectively studied before (every 3 months) and after (every six months) OLT. Mean age was 9.2 ± 1.4 months at the time of OLT, and four of six children received on parenteral nutrition (PN) with EFA supplementation for 14 to 60 days before OLT.

<u>RESULTS</u> :

Table I - Laboratory datas (% of total fatty acids, mean ± SD)

Age (months)	Linoleic Ac	Arachidonic Ac	Docosahexaenoic Ac (DHA)
1.5-4	9.01±1.68	16.67±0.39	5.89±1.18
8-11	6.16±2.19	14.26±0.58*	2.36±0.28*
After PN	10.43±3.24	15.06±0.80	3.43±1.10
6 months post-OLT	9.32±0.66	20.22±1.07*	3.90±0.59**

* $p<0.01$: 1.5-4 vs 8-11 et 8-11 vs 6 months post OLT ;
** $p<0.05$: 8-11 vs 6 months post OLT.

<u>CONCLUSION</u> :

LCPUFA deficiency was rapidly noticed in EBA, increased when portoenterostomy had failed and disappeared in less than six months after OLT.

GAMMAPATHIES IN TRANSPLANTED CHILDREN: 18 MONTH FOLLOW-UP OF 39 PATIENTS BY QUARTERLY IMMUNOFIXATION.

(PH.DESPREZ*, A.LAHLOU*, M.L.WIESEL, M.FISCHBACH*, U.SIMEONI*, J.GEISERT*)**

***Service de Pédiatrie I, CHU Hautepierre, 1 avenue Molière 67200 Strasbourg**

****Centre Régional de Transfusion Sanguine, 10 rue Spielmann 67000 Strasbourg**

Between November 1992 and March 1994, 39 transplanted children were assessed quarterly for gammapathies. Mean age at transplantation was 10,1 years. We assessed 11 liver-transplant recipients, 25 kidney-transplant recipients and 3 lung-transplant recipients .
The follow-up included Immunofixation (IF) carried out with the help of monospecific antibodies allowing identification of monoclonal bands detected during electrophoresis (Hydragel IF°, Sebia, France).
20 children did not have abnormal IF. 19 patients (49 %) had transient anomalies (6 patients) or regular anomalies (13 patients), ranging from oligoclonal pattern (15 patients) to mono or bi-clonal pattern (4 patients).
Oligoclonal patterns were found in all transient abnormal IF and disappeared after adjustment of immunosuppression. All 7 patients treated with OKT3 demonstrated abnormal IF. One of them died of lymphoproliferative syndrome induced by EBV primo-infection. Another patient with oligoclonal pattern experimented a regressive lymphoid hyperplasia after the study.
No statistically significant difference was noted between abnormal IF in liver-transplant population (64%) and abnormal IF in kidney-transplant population (48%). Mean age for each population were respectively 5,9 years and 11,3 years.

IF seems to be a useful tool for assessing and adjusting immunosuppression in transplanted children. Anomalies are frequent and cannot constitute a reliable cancer screening.
Slight differences noticed between liver-transplant population and kidney-transplant population need further investigations to assess importance of age at transplantation, viral status, immunosuppression protocol and relative weight of graft.

Unusual infections after pulmonary transplantation

ETIENNE B, LEVREY H, BERTOCCHI M, RABODONIRINA M, CELARD M, ETIENNE J, VANDENESH F, PIENS MA, PAULUS S, BASTIEN O, MORNEX JF.

Hôpital Louis Pradel & Université Claude Bernard, Lyon, France.

Infections occur frequently after pulmonary transplantation. They account for at least 1/3 of the deaths. Many bacterial, fungal and viral agents can cause those infections. Rare agents are more difficult to identify and may, in some instances, raise issues regarding the management of transplanted patients. Among 100 pulmonary transplants performed between july 1988 and december 1994 (31 heart lung, 52 single lung and 17 double lung), 3 developed such rare infections.

A 52 years old man, presenting with end stage idiopathic pulmonary fibrosis, underwent heart-lung transplantation in january 1991. The clinical course was uneventful for the first 2.5 years. In october 1993, a marked decline in the Forced Expiratory Volume in 1 Second led to the diagnosis of a bronchiolitis obliterans syndrome (i.e. a chronic rejection) and the immunosuppression regimen was increased. In july 1994, he was admitted for asthenia, weight loss and diarrhea. *Enterocytozoon bieneusi* was found in the stools. A two-weeks treatment with parenteral nutrition and iv metronidazole allowed a weight gain and a mild improvement in the diarrhea. Three months later, symptoms relapsed, *E. bieneusi* was recovered from the stools and duodenal biopsy samples. Treatment including nutrition and albendazol (1200 mg/day) was unable to control the symptoms. Infections observed in highly immunosuppressed individuals raise the question of the benefit of increasing the immunosuppressive treatment when patients develop a form of chronic rejection.

A 61 years old man, presenting with α1-antitrypsin deficiency asssociated pulmonary emphysema, underwent a double lung transplantation in february 1992. Few months later, he developed a bronchiolitis obliterans syndrome leading to end stage obstructive lung disease. In december 1994 he was admitted for a sudden and severe fever. Blood and cerebrospinal fluid cultures disclosed *Listeria monocytogenes*. Despite treatment with high doses of amoxicilline he died 5 days after diagnosis. *Listeria* spp infections are known to be associated with a poor prognosis in immunosuppressed patients. In this context raw milk drinking and crusted cheese eating must be discussed.

A 54 years old man, presenting with primary pulmonary hypertension, underwent a heart-lung transplantation in march 1990. The clinical course was uneventful untill october 1994 when he was admitted for axillary lymphadenopathy. Pathologic diagnosis was cat scratch disease and serum anti *Rochalimaea hensleae* antibodies were present. A 2 months treatment with trimethoprim-sulfamethoxazole was succesful. Such an infection raise the problem of patients habits such as pet handling.

These examples emphasize difficulties in establishing the diagnosis of rare infections and suggest that care should be taken in the management of the immunosuppressive treatment and advices regarding hygiene and way of life should be given to patients.

TRANSIENT HYPERPHOSPHATASEMIA AFTER LIVER TRANSPLANTATION IN INFANCY.

A Lachaux[1], M Chambon[1], O Boillot[2], C Le Gall[1], I Loras[1], I Canterino[3], JM Pouillaude[3], D Gille[2], L David[1], M Hermier[1].
1 Hépatogastroentérologie et Nutriton Pédiatriques, 2 Transplantologie Hépatique, 3 Radiologie Pédiatrique, Hôpital Edouard Herriot, Lyon.

Marked increase of alkaline phosphatase (AP) value in an infant after liver transplantation (LT) can suggest liver or bone disease. Lake of recognition of transient hyperphosphatasemia in infancy (THI) can be followed by intensive and unnecessary investigation.

PATIENTS AND METHODS

A boy aged 9 months born with biliary tract atresia had a LT. Two years and three months after LT, during routine examination, a spectacular increase of the serum AP value was observed (Table I). Maintenance immunosuppression was based on cyclosporine (5 mg/kg/day) and prednisolone (0.30 mg/kg/every two days).

RESULTS :

Delay post LT	25 m	27m+1w	27m+2w	27m+3w	28 m	29 m
AP UI/L	238	2450	4600	3510	674	246
GGT UI/L	28	17	18	13	13	26
ALT UI/L	36	34	22	30	24	46
AST UI/L	58	56	38	53	45	43
TB µmol/L	11	16	12	11	12	13

During the two months following the discovery of marked increased of serum AP value, liver function tests (including aminotransferase, γglutamyltransferase, bilirubin, prothrombin time) and measurements of calcium, phosphate, parathyroid hormone, osteocalcin and vitamin D were normal. Liver sonography and doppler were normal. Isoenzyme fractionation gave a bone skeletal phosphatase value of 50 %, a liver phosphatase value of 37 % and a gut phosphatase value of 12 %.

DISCUSSION

The cause of THI remains obscure and in the previously reported cases this affection was found both in sick and healthy infants. Thus THI have been described in infants with digestive (eg Crohn) or infections (eg viral or bacterial) diseases and also in patients with congenital immune deficiency.

This case is the first of THI reported in infancy after LT. THI must be worth known in order to avoid unuseful investigation.

GILBERT 'S SYNDROME. A POSSIBLE CAUSE OF HYPERBILIRUBINEMIA AFTER ORTHOTOPIC LIVER TRANSPLANTATION.

A Lachaux[1], A Aboufadel[1], M Chambon[1], O Boillot[2], C Le Gall[1], D Gille[2], M Hermier[1].
1 Hépatogastroentérologie et Nutrition Pédiatriques, 2 Transplantologie Hépatique, Hôpital Edouard Herriot, Lyon.

Unconjugated hyperbilirubinemia is a common feature after liver transplantation. Possible causes are : hemolysis, episodes of rejection or cholangitis. Gilbert's syndrome transferred by the donor liver should be considered an additional potential cause, and screening for this disorder might be useful.

PATIENTS AND METHODS :

Over a period of 3 years (March 91 - March 94), liver transplantation was performed in 26 infants. The age ranges from 8 months to 16 years. These patients were followed up in our out patient unit on a regular basis. The presumptive diagnosis of Gilbert's syndrome was made in those patients having an unconjugated serum bilirubin level > 17 µmol/l and a direct serum bilirubin level ≤ 8 µmol/l while their serum levels of aminotransferase alkaline phosphatase and γ glutamyl transpeptidase were normal. There was no evidence of biliary obstruction by ultrasonography. Hemolysis was excluded on the basis of normal serum levels of hemoglobin, haptoglobin, reticulocyte count, erythrocyte autoantibody levels and in the absence of immunoallergic erythrocyte autoantibody directed against RBC sensitized by cyclosporine.

RESULTS

Patients in this study had 1 year or more of follow up. Two of the 26 patients presented an intermittent pattern of unconjugated hyperbilirubinemia with levels > 17 µmol/l.

Delay post LT	PATIENT 1		PATIENT 2	
	TB (mini/maxi) (µmol/l)	CB (mini/maxi) (µmol/l)	TB (mini/maxi) (µmol/l)	CB (mini/maxi) (µmol/l)
1st year	9/67	0/8	13/84	0/8
2nd year	19/77	0/11	38/63	0/8
3rd year	6/51	0/7	38/64	2/5

CONCLUSION

Gilbert's syndrome is the most common cause of non hemolytic unconjugated hyperbilirubinemia with a prevalence of 3-7 % in the general population. Transplant patients may receive liver grafts from affected donors. The awarness of this syndrome may avoid a costly and invasive evaluation in the liver transplant recipient, however recognizing this disorder can be delayed by the reduction of unconjugated bilirubin concentrations when high doses of steroids are administered in the early post transplant period. In the case of a post transplant patient with a serum bilirubin profile that suggests Gilbert's, the simplest test is to obtain a fasting and a post prandial serum bilirubin levels.

DISSEMINATED TUBERCULOSIS WITH PULMONARY MILIARY AND PHARYNGEAL LOCALISATION IN 2 KIDNEY TRANSPLANTED PATIENTS.

Marrast AC.[1], Daoud S.[1], Garnier JL.[1], Lefrançois N.[1], Müller P.[2], Philit F.[3], Dubernard JM.[1], Touraine JL.[1]
1 Service de Transplantation, Hôpital Edouard Herriot, Lyon, FRANCE.
2 Service d'ORL, Hôpital Edouard Herriot, Lyon, FRANCE.
3 Service de Pneumologie, Hôpital Louis Pradel, Lyon, FRANCE

We observed 2 cases of disseminated tuberculosis with pulmonary miliary.
The first patient was 22 years old. He underwent a living related kidney transplantation Tx in 1988, at the age of 16, for a congenital uropathy, which required an ileoplasty. He was vaccinated for BCG and his tuberculin test was positive before Tx. Creatininemia stabilized at 180 micromol/l. No rejection episode was noticed. Immunosuppressive regimen associated Ciclosporine 5 mg/kg/day, Prednisolone 0,15 mg/kg/day and Azathioprine 1,5 mg/kg/day. He suffered in January 1994 from an acute Mycoplasma Pneumoniae pneumonia with a favorable outcome after administration of Ofloxacine 400 mg/day for 2 months. He was admitted in February 1995 for hectic fever associated with tonsilitis, pharyngitis and interstitial pneumonitis evolving for 2 weeks despite Amoxicillin therapy. The tonsil biopsy culture was positive for acid-fast bacilli on Ziehl-Neelsen Stain. Microscopic anatomy showed granulomata with huge epithelial cells. The thoracic CT scan showed miliary infiltration. Cultures of sputum, bronchial aspiration, urine and tonsil tissue were positive for Mycobacterium Tuberculosis.
The second patient was a 60 year old Algerian. She had been treated with hemodialysis over 20 years, for an unknown chronic nephropaty. She had no known history of tuberculosis. She underwent cadaveric kidney transplantation in 1994. Initial immunosuppressive regimen associated Ciclosporine 5 mg/kg/day, Prednisolone 1 mg/kg/day and Azathioprine 2mg/kg/day and anti lymphocyt globulins 2 mg/kg/day for 10 days. Creatininemia stabilized at 90 micromol/l, 10 days after transplantation. No rejection episode was noticed. She was treated for Herpes and Cytomegalovirus infection 1 month after transplantation. She was admitted 3 months later for hectic fever. Thoracic X-Ray showed interstitial pneumonia. Sputum culture was positive for acid-fast bacilli on Ziehl-Neelsen Stain. Thoracic CT scan showed miliary infiltration. Culture of sputum, bronchial aspiration were positive for Mycobacterium Tuberculosis. Clinical out come were favorable for both patients under quadritherapy : Rifampicin 10 mg/kg/day, Isoniazid 5 mg/kg/day, Pyrazinamid 30 mg/kg/day, Ethambutol 20/kg/day. Ciclosporine and corticoid posology adjustements were required.
These observations remind that in cases of long term fever , tuberculosis should be suspected even if there has been no previous history of tuberculosis in the patient, in the context of the current epidemy.

SUCCESSFUL FIBRINOLYSIS FOLLOWING THROMBOSIS IN A GRAFTED KIDNEY ARTERY.

Marrast AC.[1], Rouvière O.[2], Lefrançois N.[1], Dawhara M.[1], Garnier JL.[1], Daoud S.[1], Ramackers JM.[3], Lyonnet D.[2], Martin X.[1], Touraine JL.[1]

1 Service de Transplantation, Hôpital Edouard Herriot, Lyon, France.
2 Service de Radiologie, Hôpital Edouard Herriot, Lyon, France.
3 Service de Médecine nucléaire, Hôpital Edouard Herriot, Lyon, France.

A 25 year old man was admitted to the transplant unit for an acute kidney graft pain which occured 20 hours before associated with oliguria. The chronic renal failure was due to reflux nephropathy. He underwent a kidney graft in November 1988. 2 kidney rejection episodes occured 10 days and 1 month after transplantation with a favorable out come. Baseline creatinemia stabilized around 150 micromol/l. Vascular graft thrill was noticed in January 1990. Systolodiastolic hypertension occured in February 1992, worsening progressively, with an impairement of the graft function. Angiography confirmed a slightly tight and stretched anastomotic and post anastomotic stenosis of the transplant artery. Transluminal angioplasty was performed with good inital results on hypertension and renal function. The thrill and hypertension reapered 10 months later. A new endoluminal dilatation was performed. Hypertension persisted but stenosis was non significant. Hypertension required Nifedipin 40 mg/day and Atenolol 50 mg/day. Creatininemia stabilized around 120 micromol/l. He was admitted in March 1995 for an acute graft pain and anuria. Angiography revealed complete thrombosis of the transplant artery. In situ fibrinolysis was performed with Recombinant Human Tissue-type Plasminogen Activator (Actilyse*). An in situ bolus of 10 mg was performed followed by an infusion of 40 mg for 45 mn. Total infusion was 1mg/kg. Continuous infusion of Heparin was started 12 hours after. An angiography performed 12 hours later confirmed the total desobstruction of the artery. Renal scintigraphy using Tc Mag 3 as tracer showed a good perfusion of the upper pole. He recovered diuresis after 3 days and satisfactory renal function after 3 weeks.

The creatininemia stabilized around 360 micromol/l 1 month after the accident.

This case illustrates a successful fibrinolysis following thrombosis in a grafted kidney artery, 7 years after Tx. Recovery of the graft's function was possible altough fibrinolysis was performed 20 hours after the onset of the symptoms.

ATYPICAL URINARY CITOLOGY IN KIDNEY TRANSPLANT RECIPIENTS.

Massara C, Basolo B, Funaro L, *F. Bayle, **De Marchi A., Formica M, ***Guermani P, Rollino C, Segoloni GP, **Coverlizza S, Piccoli G.
Nephro-Urology Institute (Dir. Prof. A. Vercellone). University of Turin. Italy.
* Service de Nephrologie. CHU Grenoble. France.
**Morbid Anatomy. Giovanni Bosco Hospital. Turin. Italy.
*** Urology Department. S. Giovanni Battista Hospital. Turin. Italy.

Several reports have demonstated that organ transplant recipients receiving life-long immunosuppression develop a disproportional higher incidence of malignancies when compared with expected cancer rates in age-matched control population. In the long term survival following transplantation, cancers represent a major cause of morbidity and late failure in patients (pts) otherwise living with a well functioning graft. In some reports carcinomas represent 37.6% of all malignancies and recently uroepithelial abnormalities seem to be increased in transplant recipients.

At this pourpose urinary citology was investigated in 57 kidney transplant recipients (21 females, 36 males) (mean age 48.8 yrs , range 24 - 73 yrs) with a mean follow-up post transplantation of 80.5 months (range 11-241 months). We selected patients (pts) without diuresis from native kidney, urinary calculi, recurrent cystitis, polycystic kidney disease, clinical cyclosporine nephrotoxicity, history of analgesic nephropathy. Urinary samples were treated by membrane filtration technique and the cells obtained were stained with Papanicolau . According to the "Tutorial of Citology" Chicago 1988, abnormalities in uroepithelial cells were classified as Positive, Atypical or Negative.

118 urinary samples of 57 pts were collected: Positive cells were presents in 5.6% (3/57) pts, Atypical cells in 12.3 % (7/57) pts. All of these are males. There is no difference between pts with negative citology and those with uroepithelial abnormalities as regard to : 1) patients age [48.8 yrs (range 24-73 yrs) vs 47.8 yrs (range 33-64 yrs); p=n.s.], 2) time of transplantation follow-up [80.5 months (range 11-241 months) vs. 61.4 months (11-162 months); p= n.s.], 3) immunosuppression schedule.

Serial studies performed in 5 pts did not show evolution of the abnormalities, and in one case they disappeared.

Positive cells persisted in 2 pts: intravenous pielography and histological bladder "mapping" were negative.

In conclusion uroepithelial abnormalities were present in high percentage in our selected pts (17.9%), sometimes withouth time regression. Follow-up may be short in persistently positive cases, but at the moment carcinoma degeneration was presumably excluded. Our preliminary data obtained in this particular population seem to indicate that other significances of these cellular abnormalities may be supposed: pharmacological effects ?, hormonal interferences?, urothelial kynetic alterations?, subclinical infections?. Further investigations occurs to clarify the etiology and the evolution of this phenomena.

INTEREST OF RADIONUCLIDE IMAGING IN DIAGNOSIS OF A CASE OF NON EVIDENT URINARY FISTULA AFTER RENAL TRANSPLANTATION.

JM Ramackers[1], C N'Guyen[1], N Lefrançois[2], M Dawhara[3], AC Marrast[2], X Martin[3], JL Touraine[2], JM Dubernard[3], JO Peyrin[1].
Service de Médecine Nucléaire[1], Service de Transplantation rénale et Immunologie Clinique[2], Service d'Urologie et Chirurgie de Transplantation [3], Hopital E. Herriot, LYON.

Urinary fistula is a serious complication which usually occur early after renal transplantation and whose timely diagnosis is important before irreversible impairment of the graft. Ultrasonography, radiologic urography and cystography, computed tomography (CT), but also scintigraphy may lead to diagnosis of urinary leaks.
We report a case of a 28 Yr-old man who recently underwent renal transplantation. Initial evolution was uneventful, with recovery of good renal function, until the seventh postoperative day when the patient developped a minor deterioration of renal function and violents abdominal pains. According to CT results, echography showed a little intraperitoneal effusion and suspected a muscular parietal hematoma. Renal scintigraphy using 99mTc-MAG-3 was performed periodically to evaluate renal function in the transplanted kidney. It displayed, at fisrt day of complication, an additional image at the upper pole of the bladder, which was not seen on previous scintigraphy, growing during exploration time, and considered most likely to be due to urinary leakage. In order to confirm this etiology, retrograde cystography was indicated, but showed no contrast leakage through the bladder and ureter. Nevertheless, a new scintigraphy was performed because symptoms remained, and confirmed the previous suspected urinary fistula with a more typical aspect, especially on later images. So, surgical exploration was undertaken at the eleventh postoperative day, and revealed a little fistula located at the urinary anastomosis. Follow-up was marked by rapid clinical and biological improvement, and urinary leakage was disappeared on scintigraphic contol.
Radionuclide study is a non invasive imaging technique which can be willingly iterated, and is very useful in monitoring renal function of transplanted kidney, as well as identifying surgical complications as urinary leakage with high sensitivity.

DISCONTINUATION OF IMMUNOSUPPRESSIVE TREATMENT AFTER KIDNEY TRANSPLANTATION

S. Daoud, J.L. Garnier, N. Lefrançois, A.C. Marrast & J-L. Touraine
Transplantation and Clinical Immunology Unit, Pav. P, Hôpital E. Herriot, 69437 Lyon cedex 03, France

Data were collected over a period of 24 years (since the early 70s). During this period, 12 definite case-reports of treatment discontinuation were recorded.
As compared to the number of kidney transplants in our department during this period (> 2300),the number of our cases is surprisingly low [1].
There are several reasons explaining a likely underestimation of the incidence of treatment discontinuation by the patients :
- In this retrospective study, only patients hospitalized for significant impairment of renal function were accounted for. Patients who temporarily suspended treatment without renal function impairment were not taken into account.
- Among the numerous hospitalizations for impairment of renal function, only patients who acknowledged partial or total discontinuation of immunosuppressive treatment.

Among the patients studied, a number of predisposing factors appeared frequently :
- The most important factor was an intercurrent event :
  happy event (wedding...)
  unsuccessful event (depression, alcohol abuse ...)
  life condition responsible for difficulty in obtaining medications (travel...)
- Men stopped treatment more often than women did (9 men / 3 women)
- A certain psychosocial context was often involved (weakness, loneliness, denial of disease to friends).

Other factors were extremely variable :
- The age when the treatment was stopped (16 to 54 of age)
- The period of time between treatment discontinuation and hospitalization varied from 15 days to 18 months in case of total discontinuation but it could be 2 years or longer when only Azathioprine was stopped.
- The type and duration of dialysis (EER) prior ot the transplant did not appear to significantly induce a different therapeutical compliance.
- The interval of time between the transplant and the treatment discontinuation (from 1 month to 6 years).

Consequences of therapy discontinuation in our patients :
The treatment discontinuation resulted in a documented acute rejection of the transplant from 8 patients. All patients were treated with corticosteroids and 3 of them additionally received OKT3, one additionally received ALG
The results of this treatment of advanced and frequently late rejection were poor :
- In 3 cases, hemodialysis was immediately and definitely required.
- In the 9 other patients a chronic rejection later developed.

Reference :

1- S. De Geest, L. Borgermans, H. Gemoets, I. Abraham, H. Vlaminck, G. Evers & Y. Vanrenterghem. Incidence, determinants, and consequences of subclinical noncompliance with immunosuppressive therapy in renal transplant recipeints. Transplantation, 1995, 59 : 340-347.

Name Index

MIX
Papier aus verantwortungsvollen Quellen
Paper from responsible sources
FSC® C105338

If you have any concerns about our products,
you can contact us on
ProductSafety@springernature.com

In case Publisher is established outside the EU,
the EU authorized representative is:
Springer Nature Customer Service Center GmbH
Europaplatz 3, 69115 Heidelberg, Germany

Printed by Libri Plureos GmbH
in Hamburg, Germany